Pharmacology Handbook

Pharmacology Handbook

Edited by **Sean Boyd**

New Jersey

Published by Foster Academics,
61 Van Reypen Street,
Jersey City, NJ 07306, USA
www.fosteracademics.com

Pharmacology Handbook
Edited by Sean Boyd

International Standard Book Number: 978-1-63242-321-4 (Hardback)

The publisher's policy is to use permanent paper from mills that operate a sustainable forestry policy. Furthermore, the publisher ensures that the text paper and cover boards used have met acceptable environmental accreditation standards.

Trademark Notice: Registered trademark of products or corporate names are used only for explanation and identification without intent to infringe.

Printed in the United States of America.

Contents

Preface

The researches compiled throughout the book are authentic and of high quality, combining several disciplines and from very diverse regions from around the world. Drawing on the contributions of many researchers from diverse countries, the book's objective is to provide the readers with the latest achievements in the area of research. This book will surely be a source of knowledge to all interested and researching the field.

The history of pharmacology travels along with that of scientific methodologies and the novel frontiers of pharmacology give way to a novel world in search of drugs and advanced technologies. Constant growth in this field has also altered significantly the way of designing a fresh drug. Modern drug discovery is actually based on profound knowledge regarding the disease and both molecular as well as cellular mechanisms involved in its development. The aim of this book is to provide valuable information regarding the field of clinical pharmacology and diagnosis.

In the end, I would like to express my deep sense of gratitude to all the authors for meeting the set deadlines in completing and submitting their research chapters. I would also like to thank the publisher for the support offered to us throughout the course of the book. Finally, I extend my sincere thanks to my family for being a constant source of inspiration and encouragement.

Editor

Part 1

Clinical Pharmacology

Pharmacological Approaches to Improve Ageing

Pedro J. Camello, Cristina Camello-Almaraz and Maria J. Pozo
Department of Physiology, University of Extremadura, Cáceres,
Spain

1. Introduction

Aging is generally considered as a progressive and irreversible set of structural and functional changes, due both to the genetic background of the individual and the oxidative damage and modifications of intracellular signaling mechanisms. Although the anatomical and physiological alterations associated to aging (e.g. sarcopenia, cognitive and sensorial decline, functional loss in cardiovascular system...) are not a disease, they reduce the functional reserve of the organism, ultimately leading to pathological alterations and death.

Improvements of nutrition, hygiene and public health, and medical diagnosis and treatments have dramatically extended life expectancy in the last decades. However, the rate of human aging is to the moment an elusive target in biomedical interventions. The achievement of a slowing of human age is not necessarily linked to an increase of morbid, unhealthy population, but is likely to postpone the onset of age-related pathologies (Blagosklonny, 2010). Pharmacological intervention to decelerate aging and age-related diseases is highly attractive because it would target all the population during many years. If successful, antiaging therapy will be more efficient in reducing mortality than to fight separately each age-related disease (Olshansky *et al.*, 2007). Research on anti-aging interventions has evolved along the main theories of aging. We describe here the available explanations for aging before presenting the updated status of each approach.

2. Oxidative stress, aging and antioxidant treatments

2.1 Mitochondrial free radicals theory of aging

After formulation of the "rate of living" hypothesis at the beginning of the last century, proposing that longevity is determined by the metabolic rate (Pearl, 1928), the main explanation for aging has been oxidative damage due to free radicals, especially when comparative studies made clear that metabolic rate alone could not explain longevity (see Speakman & Selman, 2011). The oxidative theory of aging (Harman, 1956) proposes that aging is driven by the damage inflicted to cellular components by reactive oxygen species (ROS) produced by mitochondria in the course of respiration, and has evolved into the mitochondrial free radicals theory of aging pointing to this organelle as a key factor in aging (Harman, 1972;Miquel *et al.*, 1980), including some refinement (de Grey, 2004). Briefly, endogenous ROS (and some nitrogen reactive species derived from them) modify lipids, DNA and proteins, leading to functional and structural alterations of the cell, both directly and by modifications of the nuclear and mitochondrial genomic material (Pak *et al.*, 2003), the later especially exposed to ROS due to proximity and to the lack of histones (Yakes & Van, 1997).

ROS are formed in the inner mitochondrial membrane by transfer of electrons to molecular oxygen from complex I and III of the electron transport system (ETS) during the flow of electrons from reduced NADH and FADH generated by metabolism. At resting, about 0.1% of consumed oxygen (in spite of the erroneous figure of about 2%) (Fridovich, 2004) produces the highly reactive superoxide anion, enzymatically mutated to H_2O_2 and then to H_2O. It is important to note that the rate of ROS formation is not determined by the level of O_2 consumption, but by electrochemical potential of the inner membrane (generated by the H^+ gradient created by the ETS) and by the amount, efficiency and reduction level of complex I and III (Skulachev, 2004). This led to the "uncoupling to survive" theory of aging: H^+-permeating proteins at the inner mitochondrial membrane inhibit ROS production and are correspondingly enhanced in more long-lived species and in some life-extending manipulations (Brand, 2000).

To limit oxidative damage cells have developed enzymatic (superoxide dismutase, catalase,...) and non-enzymatic (glutathione) antioxidants to scavenge and metabolize radicals and have reduced the most ROS-sensitive components of proteins and lipids, i.e. methionine and cysteine contents of mitochondrial proteins and the number of double bonds of unsaturated fatty acids (lipid oxidation forms long lasting reactive carbonyl species which attack lipids, proteins and DNA) (Pamplona & Barja, 2011).

Although a causal link for mitochondrial radical production in aging has been generally accepted in the last three decades, the actual status is rather controversial. This view was supported by correlative studies between longevity and mitochondrial ROS production (Ku *et al.*, 1993;Sohal *et al.*, 1990). These reports did not controlled for phylogeny, body mass and metabolic rate level (Speakman, 2005), but posterior controlled studies confirmed the correlation and extended it to mitochondrial DNA oxidation (see Pamplona & Barja, 2011). On the other hand, initial studies with transgenic mice showed that inhibition or enhancement of endogenous antioxidant enzymes respectively shortens (Yamamoto *et al.*, 2005) or extends (Hu *et al.*, 2007;Schriner *et al.*, 2005) lifespan, but more recent studies did not reproduce this (Lapointe & Hekimi, 2010;Page *et al.*, 2010) or were ambiguous (Perez *et al.*, 2009). In addition, although mice with defective mitochondrial DNA repair enzymes show normal ROS production they age faster (Trifunovic *et al.*, 2005), supporting the idea that mitochondria alterations drive senescence even with normal oxidative damage.

The conflicting results of genetic experiments and the poor effects of antioxidants therapy in longevity (see 2.2) have been used to refute the free radical theory of aging (e.g., Lapointe & Hekimi, 2010;Perez *et al.*, 2009). However, it is likely that ROS production and not antioxidant defenses is the main factor determining longevity, as indicated by comparative and phylogenic studies on the correlation between longevity and antioxidants (Pamplona & Barja, 2011). This is supported by the finding that caloric restriction (CR) (the most successful life-extending manipulation) decreases mitochondrial ROS output and DNA oxidation (Migliaccio *et al.*, 1999), and by life extension in mice with genetic ablation of the protein p66shc (which produces mitochondrial ROS in response to insulin/IGF-1 signaling and stress factors) (e.g. Vendelbo & Nair, 2011).

It is clear that even if mitochondrial ROS were not the only cause of aging, is unlikely that oxidative stress and mitochondria do not participate in the aging process. Several modifications of the theory have focused on the mitochondrial DNA alterations induced by radicals (de Grey, 2004;Pamplona, 2011). Other authors have proposed that although high ROS concentration are detrimental, physiological levels protect from aging by increasing stress defense systems, so that non physiological increases of antioxidant activity can paradoxically accelerate aging (mitochondrial hormesis or mitohormesis, Tapia, 2006).

2.2 Antioxidative therapies

Given the large evidence linking oxidative stress with aging, the use of antioxidants has been a repeated approach in anti-aging research for decades. Even if aging itself is not due to oxidative damage, this approach could extend average life by reducing the mortality of a number of pathological conditions associated to oxidation.

The most frequently assayed antioxidants are present in vegetables and fruits, not only vitamins E (tocopherols), A (carotenes) and C, but also flavonoids (from tea and *Ginkgo biloba)*, phenolic compounds (e.g. resveratrol in grapes), catechins and others. A number of artificial antioxidants have also been assayed (deprenyl, NDGA, PBN, thioproline,...). It must be noted that efficiency not only depends on their oxidant scavenging activity, but also in humans bioavailability factors (absorption, lifetime,...) so that animal studies are a requisite even for initial evaluation of the potential utility of an antioxidant.

Part of the initial studies in rodent models showed that some antioxidants could extend average and/or maximum lifespan (see Meydani *et al.*, 1998;Spindler, 2011). Unfortunately no measurements of the oxidative stress were performed in the initial reports, a requisite to confirm that a treatment lowers oxidative stress (Knasmuller *et al.*, 2008). Also, the effects could be due to a decrease in caloric intake of the animals and not by direct antioxidant effects, but when other authors controlled this variable still found an increase in mice lifespan (Bezlepkin *et al.*, 1996;Miquel & Economos, 1979). Recently, an extensive meta-analysis of the rodent lifespan studies reveals that a range of antioxidants (from chemicals such as deprenyl to naturally occurring compounds such as polyphenols) extend lifespan independently of the CR effect observed in other studies (Spindler, 2011).

In human, the available information is epidemiological or observational, including transversal studies about alimentary habits. Vitamins C, E and A operate synergistically against lipid peroxidation (see a review in Fusco *et al.*, 2007), and vitamin C can also regenerate vitamin E levels (Niki *et al.*, 1995). There is a negative correlation between plasmatic levels of antioxidants, mainly vitamin E, and incidence of cardiovascular diseases and some types of cancer (see Fusco *et al.*, 2007 and Hercberg *et al.*, 2009). This correlation is also present for fruits and vegetables intake (Genkinger *et al.*, 2004) and flavonoids and polyphenols (Manach *et al.*, 2005) and for other age-related diseases such as Alzheimer disease (Viña *et al.*, 2004) or diabetes (Czernichow *et al.*, 2006).

The life-extending effects of antioxidants in humans must be inferred from trials assessing the mortality of age-related pathologies. Contrary to the observational studies, randomized trials have not confirmed the expected decrease of mortality after long-term antioxidant treatment. In the trial SUVIMAX, with low doses of antioxidants, a reduction in mortality after 7.5 years of treatment was observed only in men (Hercberg *et al.*, 2004), which could be explained by a possible lower level of endogenous antioxidants compared to women, similar to a trial in a Chinese population with poor nutritive status (Blot *et al.*, 1993). Other large scale trials have not found beneficial effects of vitamin E supplementation (alone or with other antioxidants) on the incidence of cardiovascular and cancer mortality (Jacobs *et al.*, 2003;Lee *et al.*, 2005;Lonn *et al.*, 2005). It has been suggested that only individuals with low levels of antioxidant would benefice from these treatments, as found in lung cancer rates and selenium supplement (Reid *et al.*, 2002).

A concerning outcome of the controlled trials is the finding that supplementation can have detrimental effects in some groups (Hercberg *et al.*, 2009;Pham & Plakogiannis, 2005). Therefore, the official recommendation is an adequate intake of antioxidant-enriched aliments until more evidence makes clear if supplementation is safe (Fusco et al., 2007).

The discrepancy between the epidemiological and interventional studies could be due to limitations in the design of the studies. As pointed above, the "shotgun" approach of "flooding" the tissues with an antioxidant is likely inefficient or even detrimental *per se* (see 2.1) and it depends critically on the dosage (supplementation does not guarantee redox normalization (Knasmuller et al., 2008)) and the moment of application (in rodent models lifespan effects require initiation at late (PBN) or early age (vitamins mixture, NDGA) (Bezlepkin *et al.*, 1996;Spindler, 2011)). Also, it is likely that only certain combinations of antioxidants can block the redox network of multiple endogenous radicals (as shown in experimental models, (Rebrin *et al.*, 2005)). Last, the plasma measurements commonly used in human studies are not an unequivocal account of systemic redox (Knasmuller et al., 2008). On the other hand, the epidemiological results could be due to differences in lifestyles and genetic and environmental influences, all of them factors cancelled in randomized controlled trials.

A great interest has been raised by resveratrol, a polyphenol found in grapes and red wine. Resveratrol extends longevity in mice fed a high calorie diet (Baur *et al.*, 2006), but not under normal diet (Pearson *et al.*, 2008) and, relevant for human studies, improves in rodent models several markers for senescence and oxidative stress, mimicking caloric restriction (see Minor *et al.*, 2010a). Moreover, resveratrol also improves endothelial function in human patients with coronary heart disease (Lekakis *et al.*, 2005) (see also section 4).

The mechanism of action of resveratrol is however different to other antioxidants. Its main targets seem to be activation of sirtuins, deacetylases that activate transcription of antioxidant enzymes and promote mitogenesis (Vendelbo & Nair, 2011), although recent data indicate that its action on Sirt1 is indirect. It is noteworthy that Sirt1 and Sirt3 interact with metabolic pathways related to aging (see 4), working as sensors of energy availability (Guarente, 2000): upon low energy levels, increased NAD+ concentration activates Sirt1, which in turn operates on FOXO3, a transcription factor correlated with longevity in humans (Willcox *et al.*, 2008) that increases transcription of antioxidants in response to caloric restriction. Sirt3 is genetically linked to longevity in humans (Rose *et al.*, 2003), declines with age (Lanza *et al.*, 2008) and also activates FOXO3 (Sundaresan *et al.*, 2009).

A special mention is deserved by melatonin, the hormone released during the night by the pineal gland (see section 3). In addition to its chronobiological function it is one of the most potent antioxidants known. Melatonin not only acts as a direct antioxidant and inductor of the antioxidant enzymes, but it also generates, after oxidative cleavage, a series of derivatives with potent antioxidant activity (see Hardeland *et al.*, 2009). Melatonin accumulates in nuclei and mitochondria, protecting against oxidation of genetic material and it has been repeatedly shown to be an excellent antioxidant in conditions of oxidative stress, both in animals and humans (for recent reviews see Anisimov *et al.*, 2006 or Pozo *et al.*, 2010). Melatonin has also been shown in animal models to slow functional changes associated to aging in a number of systems (Camello-Almaraz *et al.*, 2008;Gomez-Pinilla *et al.*, 2008;Pascua *et al.*, 2011). More important, melatonin extends lifespan in more than 50% of rodent studies and has well established anticarcinogenic properties for mammary and colon cancer in animal models (Anisimov et al., 2006). Although to date there are no human mortality data in healthy individuals treated with melatonin, the results from clinical assays are promising. For example, a meta-analysis shows in human patients of solid tumors a decrease in risk of death at 1 year (Mills *et al.*, 2005), and numerous animal and human (clinical) studies support the potential of this hormone to limit cancer development (see a review in Karasek, 2004). Additionally, controlled trials in humans have shown the absence of toxicity and significant side effects (Singer *et al.*, 2003).

3. Hormonal replacement as antiaging therapy

The observation that several endocrine secretions decay with aging (sexual hormones, growth hormone (GH), melatonin and others (Pandi-Perumal *et al.*, 2008), laid the basis for attempts for hormonal replacement as antiaging therapy.

3.1 Melatonin

Melatonin, discovered 50 years ago, is a hormone synthesized by the pineal gland, retina, gastrointestinal tract and immune cells. Melatonin plasma levels follow a circadian rhythm: it is secreted by the pineal gland during the dark phase of the day, because light input into retinal cells activates nerve impulses to the suprachiasmatic nuclei of hypothalamus (SCN), which in turn suppresses the excitatory sympathetic input to the pineal gland and the release of melatonin. Thus, melatonin monitors the onset and duration of the dark phase, synchronizing the central circadian oscillator (SCN) and the peripheral organs with the environmental light-dark cycle, but is also involved in vasomotor control, sleep initiation,... (Pandi-Perumal et al., 2008). In humans the rhythmic secretion starts around the 6th month of age, peak levels are achieved at 4 - 7th years, melatonin concentration drops at puberty and diminishes gradually in old people (Karasek, 1999). Melatonin acts through plasma membrane and nuclear receptors and by interaction with intracellular signalling proteins and it has potent antioxidant properties (this aspect has been treated above).

The decline in melatonin secretion with age is accompanied by a progressive deterioration of the central circadian oscillator (Hofman & Swaab, 1994) and by sleep disruption, a feature of aging in humans (Neubauer, 1999). Although a meta-analysis did not find conclusive evidence that melatonin was effective to improve sleep parameters in patients with insomnia due to great discrepancies in pharmacological preparation, dose and time of treatment and measurements of melatonin and circadian parameters (Buscemi *et al.*, 2005), a more recent meta-analysis supports the effectiveness of exogenous melatonin in patients with delayed sleep phase disorder (van Geijlswijk *et al.*, 2010). The study found three requisites for optimal melatonin therapy: adequate dose (too low is inefficient, too high is hypnotic), administration 3-6 hours before the so-called dim light melatonin onset and choice of appropriate patients (with a delayed biological timing).

A recent improvement is a formulation that releases melatonin slowly in the gut after oral administration and increases its plasma concentration over the following 8-10 h (Circadin®, Neurim Pharmaceuticals, Israel), which has been approved by the European Medicines Evaluation Agency in June 2007 for the short-term treatment of primary insomnia. Several studies have shown its efficiency and safety for short-term treatment (3 weeks) of adults and old people (Luthringer *et al.*, 2009), including a double-blind, placebo-controlled randomized trial evaluating the short and long-term effects of Circadin (Wade *et al.*, 2010). Circadin also seems to improve blood pressure rhythms (Grossman *et al.*, 2006).

The effects of melatonin on sleep rhythm are due to its plasma membrane receptors (MT1 and MT2) in the suprachiasmatic nucleus. MT1 receptors inhibit firing of suprachiasmatic neurons and MT2 receptors entrain circadian rhythms and have phase-shifting effects (Hunt *et al.*, 2001). This finding lead to the design of specific agonists ramelteon (Rozerem®, Takeda Pharmaceuticals, Japan) and agomelatine (Valdoxan®, Servier and Novartis). Ramelteon, approved by the FDA (July 2005) for the treatment of insomnia, has been assayed for the treatment of primary insomnia in humans (Erman *et al.*, 2006). Although these studies found it effective and safe, the European Medicines Evaluation Agentcy found the efficacy of ramelteon insufficient for marketing authorization. Agomelatine binds to melatonin receptors but is also an antagonist of serotonin 5-HT2C receptors used to decrease anxiety and promote sleep (Lemoine *et al.*, 2007). Its efficacy, tolerability and safety have been assessed by several randomized, placebo and active-controlled studies (Kennedy & Emsley, 2006) and improves the disrupted sleep of depressed patients (Lemoine et al., 2007).

3.2 GH

The growth hormone (GH) and its key mediator insulin-like growth factor-I (IGF-I) regulate somatic growth and development, metabolism and body composition, but seems to be also related to aging. The pulsatile GH secretion shows an age-related decay after the high amplitude pulses of the postnatal and puberty stages (Finkelstein *et al.*, 1972), and correlates to aging-related changes in body composition (sarcopenia, osteopenia, increase in fat content,...) (Veldhuis *et al.*, 1995). This correlation, together with the fact that replacement therapy in GH deficient adults and elderly improves body composition, lipoprotein profile, exercise capacity and bone density (Rudman, 1985), elicited interest in the possible use of GH as antiaging therapy. However, a higher mortality has been found in patients critically ill treated with GH (Takala *et al.*, 1999) and in rodents and humans suffering high levels of GH (acromegaly) (Sheppard, 2005). This is in keeping with the increased lifespan of mutant mice with defects in GH/IGF-1 secretion/pathways (Bartke, 2003) and by some data on human lifespan (Suh *et al.*, 2008). Therefore, the clinical use of GH is only approved in US for treatment of GH deficiency, idiopathic short stature and HIV/AIDS.

3.3 Vitamin D

In addition to its key role in calcium homeostasis, there are evidences that vitamin D can influence longevity by decreasing the morbidity of age-related diseases, such as cancer or cardiovascular diseases, in addition to osteoporosis (not treated in this review). The active form of vitamin D3 (1,25(OH)2-cholecalciferol or calcitriol) binds to nuclear receptors (VDRs) to modulate the transcription of genes involved in systemic and intracellular Ca^{2+}

homeostasis and in cellular proliferation. The later are also due to fast, non genomic effects mediated by plasma membrane VDRs (Dusso *et al.*, 2005).

The main actions of vitamin D of interest as antiaging therapy are its anti-inflammatory and anti-cytokine effects in humans (shown in controlled trials (Schleithoff *et al.*, 2006)), and its ability to promote neuronal survival in different experimental models (Regulska *et al.*, 2006). In fact, human observational studies show a negative correlation of levels of vitamin D3 with cardiovascular disease (Zittermann *et al.*, 2005) (an inflammatory process), and with cognitive performance in elderly (Llewellyn *et al.*, 2009;Oudshoorn *et al.*, 2008). Additional support for vitamin D3 as antiaging treatment comes up from evidences that serum concentration of vitamin D decreases with age (Utiger, 1998) and its role in the control of cell cycle and apoptosis, which are altered in aging: calcitriol reduces proliferation of normal and cancer cells (Ylikomi *et al.*, 2002) and up-regulates apoptosis of cells damaged by redox stress and DNA alteration (Higami & Shimokawa, 2000).

The beneficial effects of vitamin D in age-associated diseases is expected to result in a prolongation of average lifespan. A study showed that vitamin D deprivation decreased the lifespan of male, but not female, rats (Thomas *et al.*, 1984). In humans, a recent meta-analysis of randomized trial showed a clear reduction in all-cause mortality in old individuals under vitamin D supplementation (Autier & Gandini, 2007). However, some reports have raised concerns with the safety of calcitriol supplementation (Stolzenberg-Solomon, 2009), although limitations in the design of the studies avoid definitive conclusions.

4. Caloric restriction

CR is the most robust non-genetic nutritional experimental intervention for slowing aging, and maintaining health and vitality in organisms ranging from budding yeast (*Sacharomyces cerevisiae*) to humans (Fontana *et al.*, 2010b). It is defined as a reduction of total macronutrient intake without causing malnutrition, with food intake reduced by 30-40% compared to *ad libitum* levels. Experiments involving CR in rodents in 1935 provided the first promise for modulation of lifespan (McCay *et al.*, 1935). Since then CR has been repeatedly proved to be effective in extending average and maximum lifespan and delaying the onset of age-associated pathologies in diverse species (for review see (Minor *et al.*, 2010a;Omodei & Fontana, 2011)). It was not until the 1990s that CR became widely viewed as a scientific model that could provide insights into the underlying mechanisms of aging and lifespan extension. The fact that CR significantly increased the average and maximum lifespan in many simpler eukaryotes, including the common model organisms used in aging research, *Drosophila melanogaster*, *Caenorhabditis elegans* and *Saccharomyces cerevisiae* pointed out that CR represents an evolutionarily conserved mechanism for modulating longevity and opened the possibility of using genetic tools in these models that helped to unveil intracellular pathways related to pro-longevity.

Alternative approaches to CR are a controlled reduction of a particular macronutrient of the diet (dietary restriction, DR) or temporal variations of food intake (intermittent fasting, IF). Particularly, protein restriction, PR, where a percentage of calories derived from protein is replaced by fat or carbohydrate, has been investigated in rodents and decreases in mitochondrial reactive oxygen species production and DNA and protein oxidative modifications have been reported (Ayala *et al.*, 2007), which could explain the increase in lifespan previously reported for PR (Leto *et al.*, 1976). Similar effects were obtained with reduction of the amino acid methionine (Naudi *et al.*, 2007), but they could not be replicated by restricting lipid intake alone (Sanz *et al.*, 2006a) or carbohydrate intake alone (Sanz *et al.*, 2006b). IF, a regimen of either alternate day fasting or fasting for a day after 2 days of feeding, both increases lifespan and delays or prevents some age-related diseases (reviewed in Mattson & Wan, 2005). However, CR is by now the most powerful nutritional intervention to prolong life.

4.1 Effects of caloric restriction

It is totally accepted that the effects of CR on lifespan and mortality in rodents increase linearly with the extent of the restriction until reaching approximately a 50-60% of restriction at which lifespan is negatively affected. In addition, the effect of CR on lifespan is stronger when initiated at weaning and weaker later in life (reviewed in (Fontana, 2009b;Speakman & Hambly, 2007;Speakman & Mitchell, 2011)). In fact, CR increases rather than decreases mortality if initiated in advanced age (Forster *et al.*, 2003). CR inhibits growth and body size after maturation and reduces body weight, as consequence of changes in the endocrine profile as discussed below. CR also inhibits fertility, especially in females, but there is an increase in their reproductive performance when they are subsequently returned to *ad libitum* feeding (Selesniemi *et al.*, 2008)

CR induces transcriptional alterations that are indicative of metabolic reprogramming, a change in how energy is generated and how fuel is utilized. A key metabolic change during CR is a shift from fat storage to fat utilization impacting stress signaling pathways and ROS production (Anderson & Weindruch, 2010). Immediately following food intake there was a period of endogenous fatty acid synthesis that was then followed by a period of prolonged fatty acid oxidation, which induces large changes in the respiratory quotient (RQ) (Speakman & Mitchell, 2011). In addition, during CR there is an increase in the AMP/ATP ratio which leads to the activation of the AMP-activated protein kinase (AMPK) that promotes fat oxidation increasing the transport of fatty acids into the mitochondrion. In fact, marked phosphorylation of AMPK has been found after long term CR (Edwards *et al.*, 2010). Because fatty acid substrates enter the electron transport chain predominantly via complex II rather than complex I, the main ROS generator is bypassed when the metabolism is switched predominantly to fatty acid oxidation. This might represent a mechanism minimizing oxidative stress under CR.

The hormonal profile of long-term CR is characterized by a suppression of the gonadal, thyroid and GH-insulin-like growth factor I (GH-IGF-I) axes, an increase in the insulin sensitivity and an increase in the daily peak levels of plasma corticosterone that takes part in successfully coping with stressors (Xiang & He, 2011). CR also results in decreased levels of leptin and increased blood concentration of ghrelin and adiponectin, a modulator of a number of metabolic processes appearing to have anti-inflammatory, anti-diabetic, and anti-atherogenic properties that seem to play an important role in life extension effect of CR (Chiba *et al.*, 2002;Lago *et al.*, 2007).

The reductions in IGF-I and insulin signaling that occur under CR have been suggested to be causally linked to the lifespan enhancing effects of CR. This is in part based on the observation that several rodent models that present mutations that modified insulin/GH/IGF-I signals, live longer than controls and there is considerable phenotypic overlap between long-lived mutant mice and normal mice on chronic CR. These models include, amongst others, *Prop-1* (Ames mice) and *pit-1* (Snell mice) mutant dwarf mice, GH receptor/binding protein homozygous knockout mice (*GHR/BP-/-* or GHRKO), insulin receptor substrate 1 knockout mice (*Irs1-/-*)... Most of these mice have a body weight smaller than their normal siblings and present decreased levels of IGF-I , and increased sensibility to insulin (Chiba *et al.*, 2007), except *Irs1-/-* mice whose IGF-I levels are unchanged and show a mild but lifelong insulin resistance having increased lifespan and reduced markers of aging (Selman *et al.*, 2008). In GHRKO mice CR increased lifespan only in females and failed to further enhance the remarkable insulin sensitivity and the insulin signaling cascade in GHRKO mutants (Bonkowski *et al.*, 2006;Bonkowski *et al.*, 2009). These data imply that somatotropic signaling is critically important in mediating the effects of CR on lifespan and also support the notion that enhanced sensitivity to insulin plays a prominent role in the actions of CR and GH resistance on longevity. It was originally reported that long-term severe CR did not reduce serum IGF-I concentration or the IGF-I/IGF binding protein ratio in humans but total and free IGF-I concentrations were significantly lower in moderately protein-restricted individuals (Fontana *et al.*, 2008). In addition, it has been recently shown that CR for 4 years leads to reduced IGF-I serum levels in formerly obese women relative to normal-weight women eating *ad libitum* (Mitterberger *et al.*, 2011), which suggests that growth hormone/IGF-I axis is also important in the effects of CR in humans.

4.2 Caloric restriction in non-human primates

Most CR research on longevity in mammals has been performed in rodents, mainly in mice. However, studies designed to evaluate the effects of CR on species closer to humans are of great interest in order to translate the knowledge to humans. Two prospective investigations of the effects of CR on long-lived nonhuman primate species began nearly 25 years ago and are still under way. These studies (randomized controlled trials) revealed beneficial effects of CR on physiological functions and the retardation of disease. In the study conducted in the Wisconsin National Primate Research Center a recent report showed that animals on 30% of CR appeared subjectively younger than controls, the body weight was reduced and the age-related sarcopenia attenuated. Improvements in metabolic function (improved insulin sensitivity and glucose tolerance) and preservation of grey matter volume in subcortical regions were reported. In addition, there was a lower incidence of neoplasia, cardiovascular disease and type 2 diabetes mellitus. Survival analysis considering only age-related deaths revealed a significant effect of CR in increasing survival, but when assessing "all-cause" mortality CR did not provide a statistically significant lifespan increase (Colman *et al.*, 2009). In any case, the reduction of age-related diseases and the potential increase in longevity are promising. Data regarding CR-induced longevity from the National Institute of Aging's are not yet available, although a decrease in age-related diseases and beneficial effects on other physiological parameters have been provided (Mattison *et al.*, 2007).

4.3 Caloric restriction in humans

The studies about human responses to CR have some limitations that should be taken into account when interpreting the results. An important amount of data come from members of the CR Society International (www.calorierestriction.org) which has the mission to promote the use of CR in humans. In agreement with the research results from animal studies, voluntary CR in humans results in sustained beneficial effects on the major atherosclerosis risk factors, and has protective effect against obesity and insulin resistance. In addition, the CR society members have reduced circulating levels of insulin, PDGF, TGF-β and pro-inflammatory cytokines (reviewed in Fontana, 2009a). Nonetheless, despite high serum adiponectin and low inflammation, approximately 40% of CR individuals exhibited an exaggerated hyperglycemic response to a glucose load. This impaired glucose tolerance is associated with lower circulating levels of IGF-1, total testosterone, and triiodothyronine, which are typical adaptations to life-extending CR in rodents (Fontana *et al.*, 2010a). Assuming the importance of these findings, it should be noted that these volunteers are clearly a self selected population and this is not a randomized controlled trial.

There is a randomized controlled trial for the effects of CR on humans, and that is the CALERIE (Comprehensive Assessment of the Long term Effects of Reducing Intake of Energy) trial sponsored by the NIA in the USA. In the phase 1 of the trial all the studies have been performed in non-obese healthy but overweight subjects, therefore it is difficult to separate beneficial effects due to the weight loss or to CR. The most relevant findings of phase 1 trials were the reduced body weight and total fat mass, the reduced fasting levels of insulin, leptin and T3 and the increased insulin sensitivity. Activity energy expenditure and core body temperature were decreased in response to the CR. In addition, CR decreased cardiovascular risk, increased some antioxidant defenses and reduced markers of inflammation (reviewed in (Speakman & Hambly, 2007)). Interestingly, "in vitro" studies utilizing CR human serum to examine effects on markers of health and longevity in cultured cells resulted in increased stress resistance and an up-regulation of genes (sirt1 and PGC1α) proposed to be indicators of increased longevity (Allard *et al.*, 2008). In the phase 2 trial of the study, a two-year CR period was selected to attempt to provide for a sustained period of weight stability following weight loss that would more accurately unveil the effects of CR in humans (Rickman *et al.*, 2011). Whether CR extends life in humans and the magnitude of this potential effect also remain unclear and far for been resolved

4.4 Intracellular pathways mediating CR effects

For many individuals, the hardships of maintaining a CR lifestyle are too great to justify the improved health profile and potential life-extension benefits. Nevertheless, identifying the genetic and physiological mediators of CR could aid in the discovery of compounds/treatments that would act on those pathways, thereby mimicking the positive aspects of CR without imposed food restriction.

TOR, a serine/threonine protein kinase that belongs to the family of phosphoinositide-3-kinase (PI3K)-related kinases (PIKK), is the primary candidate involved in the regulation of lifespan in animals under CR. Its name, Target Of Rapamycin, indicates that it mediates the effects of rapamycin, an antifungal and immunosuppressant agent that inhibits TOR. In mammalian cells, TOR participates in the mammalian complex 1 (mTORC1) that is sensitive to rapamycin and controls cell size, proliferation and lifespan via a variety of downstream pathways. mTORC1 is a homodimer that has four components in addition to the Serine/Threonine kinase mTOR: Raptor, mLST8, PRAS40 and Deptor. Raptor binds mTOR and recruits the downstream kinase substrates (S6K and 4E-BP) in a manner that enables their phosphorylation by the mTOR catalytic domain. Other proteins that participate in TORC1 regulation are Tuberous Sclerosis Complex proteins TSC1 and TSC2, with a GTPase-activating (GAP) domain, and the Ras-like small GTPase RHEb, the preferred substrate of the TSC2 GAP activity. TSC complex inhibits TOR signaling as the result of its ability to deactivate Rheb (reduced GTP/GDP) (reviewed in Kapahi et al., 2010).

TORC1 integrates responses to growth factor stimulation, changes in energy status, nutrients, oxygen levels and various types of stress. Thus growth factors like IGF and insulin, via Akt, directly phosphorylate several sites on TSC2, which decrease the inhibitory activity of TSC and the increase TORC1 activity. A drop in the cell energy content, as that induced by glucose deprivation, is reflected in the rise of the AMP/ATP ratio that triggers AMP-dependent activation of AMPK. In turn, AMPK reduces the activity of TORC1 by direct phosphorylation and stimulation of Tsc2 activity and inhibition of Raptor. Amino-acid regulation is exerted predominantly through Rag GTPases (RagA, RagB, RagC, and RagD) that sense amino acid levels. In the presence of amino acids the complex interacts with raptor and promotes TORC1 through relocalization to RHEB rich cellular compartments. Conversely, deprivation of amino acid inhibits mTORC1 with leucine or arginine withdrawal mimicking total amino acid deprivation. Amongst the environmental stresses to which cells are exposed, TORC1 also senses hypoxia. Low levels of oxygen, through stabilization of HIF1α induce the transcription of hypoxic response genes, mostly REDD1 that inhibits TORC1 activity by a TSC2-dependent mechanism. In addition, hypoxia reduces ATP levels, and then it controls TORC1 through AMPK. Genotoxic stress represses TORC1 activity through p53-mediated increased expression of PTEN, TSC2 and REDD1 (reviewed in Kapahi et al., 2010;Ma & Blenis, 2009;Speakman & Mitchell, 2011).

TORC1 controls cell growth maintaining the adequate balance between anabolic processes such as protein synthesis and catabolic processes like autophagy. As commented before, S6K and 4E-BP1 are the best-known substrates of TORC1 and through them TORC1 regulates protein synthesis by regulating the activity of the translational machinery and also specifically controlling the translation of subset of mRNAs that are thought to promote cell growth and proliferation (Ma & Blenis, 2009). The limiting step of protein synthesis is translation initiation. The recruitment of the small ribosomal subunit to mRNA requires the participation of the translation initiation factor 4F (eIF4F) complex. 4E-BP binds eIF4E, a component of this complex, and prevents translation initiation. When hyperphosphorylated by mTORC1, 4E-BP1 dissociates from eIF4E, allowing the initiation of translation. Evidence suggests that S6Ks modulate the functions of translation initiation factors during protein synthesis and also coordinate the regulation of ribosome biogenesis, which in turn drives efficient translation (see for review (Ma & Blenis, 2009)). S6K1 interacts back with the insulin signaling pathway by phosphorylating the insulin receptor substrates IRS1 and IRS2, which seems related to insulin resistance. Consistent with the important role of S6K on mediating mTOR induced lifespan extension, S6K1$^{-/-}$ mice have gene expression profiles similar to those of CR mice, and females have extended longevity with evidence of fewer age-related diseases (Selman et al., 2009).

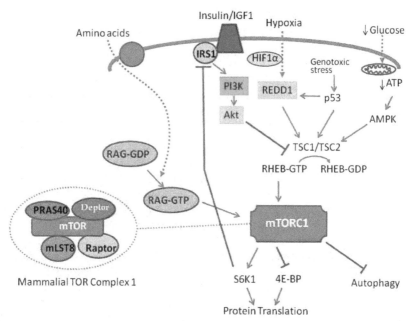

Fig. 1. mTORC1 and insulin/IGF1 signalling and lifespan.

In mammalial cells mTORC1 receives positive inputs from RHEB-GTP, but it is inhibited when RHEB is bound mainly to GDP. TSC1/TSC2 complex, through its GTPase-activating domain favors GDP-bound RHEB and then it mediates mTORC1 inhibition. Several extracellular and intracellular pathways activate (by phosphorylation) TSC complex, such as the ATP sensor AMPK that is stimulated when cellular energy decreases, the hypoxic response gene REDD1 that senses hypoxia, and p53 that senses genotoxic stress. TSC complex is inhibited by Akt-mediated phosphorylation, which results in mTORC1 activation. An important pathway for Akt activation is the insulin/IGF signaling. The amino acid level in the cell controls the state of Rag GTPases. The presence of amino acids enhances Rag-GTP and activates mTORC1 through relocalization to RHEB rich cellular compartments. Activation of mTORC1 increases mRNA translation and protein synthesis through phosphorylation of S6K1 and 4E-BP and inhibits autophagy, which results in cell growth and also in senescence. Inhibition of mTORC1 increases autophagy, reduces protein synthesis and cell grothw/differentiation decreasing senescence and extending lifespan.

Accumulating evidence demonstrates that longevity pathways, including mTOR, interact with the macroautophagic process. Autophagy is a lysosome-mediated degradative process of eukaryotic cells to digest their own constituents during development or starvation. Macroautophagy (hereafter referred as autophagy) is a type of autophagy that involves the formation of subcellular double membrane-bound structures called autophagosomes to sequester cytoplasmatic materials and deliver them into lysosomes for breakdown by acid hydrolases. According to the current knowledge, the first signalling component downstream of mTOR in the autophagy pathway in mammals is ULK1, a serine/threonine kinase. ULK1 plays a key role at the nucleation (the early event when membrane structures are initiated) and formation of the preautophagosome structures. mTOR-induced ULK1 phosphorylation avoids the recruitment of proteins to the autophagosome membranes inhibiting downstream events essential for autophagy (reviewed in (Jung *et al.*, 2010)).

Sirtuins are a family of NAD+-dependent protein deacetylases that exert multiple cellular functions by interacting with, and deacetylating a wide range of signaling molecules, transcription factors, histones and enzymes (Yamamoto *et al.*, 2007). In mammals, the family is represented by seven members (SIRT1-7) with different cellular locations. Several studies have demonstrated that CR regulates sirtuin system and that a functional sirtuin system is required for lifespan extension to occur (Bamps *et al.*, 2009;Cohen *et al.*, 2004). Thus, CR does not have any effects of lifespan extension in SIRT1 deficient mice (Boily *et al.*, 2008). By contrast, elevation of SIRT1 expression results in a phenotype resembling that of caloric restriction (Bordone *et al.*, 2007). In humans SIRT1 gene expression also appears to be responsive to caloric restriction (reviewed in (Kelly, 2010)). SIRT1 elicits anti-senescence activity by targeting a wide range of protein substrates that are critically involved in regulating key cellular processes, such as oxidative stress, DNA damage, mitochondrial biogenesis and autophagy. Targets for SIRT1-mediated deacetylation include p53, NFkB, PGC-1a (peroxisome proliferator-activated receptor-c coactivator 1a], eNOS, mTOR and FoxOs. It is also of great importance the interaction of SIRT1 with LKB/AMPK. While acute activation of the LKB1/AMPK pathway confers adaption to stress, sustained stimulation of this pathway leads to irreversible senescence. SIRT1-mediated deacetilation of LKB, and consequent ubiquintination and degradation serves to prevent persistent AMPK signaling, reinforcing the anti-age effects of SIRT1 (reviewed in (Wang *et al.*, 2011)).

4.5 Therapies based on caloric restriction

The knowledge of the intracellular pathways related to aging led to the development of drugs, named generically caloric restriction mimetics (CRM) that replicate the effects of CR. These drugs targets the main pathways affected by CR: insulin/IGF1, mTOR, and sirtuins.

4.5.1 Insulin/IGF1 pathway

The firts CRM used was 2-deoxy-D-glucose (2DG), a compound that inhibits glycolisis. In keeping with the effects of CR, 2DG in rodents reduced body temperature, body weight and circulating glucose and insulin and increased glucocorticoids and heat-shock proteins. In addition, reduced tumors and increased stress resistance to neurotoxins and cold shock (Le Couteur *et al.*, 2011;Minor *et al.*, 2010a). Despite of these findings, long-term administration of 0.4% 2DG did not enhanced lifespan but increased mortality due to cardiac toxicity and adrenal tumors (Minor *et al.*, 2010b), which indicates that this drug could have therapeutic value for short-term treatment but it would not be indicated for aging interventions.

The biguanide antidiabetic drug metformin has been shown to molecularly recapitulate most of the pro-longevity effects occurring upon CR (Dhahbi *et al.*, 2005) and to suppress S6K1 activity in cultured proliferating epithelial cells (Vazquez-Martin *et al.*, 2009). In keeping with these effects, it has been reported that chronic metformin treatment of mice from different strains predisposed to high incidence of mammary tumors decreased body temperature, increased mean and maximal lifespan and postponed tumors and age-related switch-off of estrous function. These effects were dependent on the gender and the strain of mice (reviewed in (Anisimov, 2010)). In humans a retrospective study has reported an impressive 56% decrease in breast cancer risk among diabetic receiving metformin (Bodmer *et al.*, 2010), which together with the animal studies suggest that metformin could increase lifespan in humans. Metformin treatment phenocopies the effects of amino acid-deprivation on mTORC1, suggesting that this drug may inhibit mTORC1 via modulation of Rag signaling (Kalender et al., 2010). The effects of metformin on mTOR and its effector S6K1 can also be due to the well recognized activation of AMPK by the drug (Hardie, 2011), which as described above, inhibits mTORC1. Other bioguanides such as buformin and phenformin have shown promising results in rodent tumor suppression, but they have to be withdrawn from the clinical practice due to association with lactic acidosis (Minor et al., 2010a).

4.5.2 mTOR pathway

Rapamycin, a macrolide antibiotic with antitumor and immunosuppressant actions, selectively and effectively inhibits mTORC1 as CR does, as discussed above. The inhibitory action of rapamycin on TOR signaling requires the formation of the rapamycin/FKBP12 complex, which interferes with the proper interaction between raptor and mTOR, rather than or in addition to a more direct inhibition of mTOR catalytic activity. Many roles of mTORC1 on cell growth and survival have been unveiled by the use of rapamycin. Rapamycin is, by now, the pharmacological treatment that more resembles CR-induced lifespan extension. One of the most important contributions to this field has been the report of the National Institute on Aging Intervention Testing Program (ITP) showing that rapamycin supplementation late in life (20 months of age) induced a significant mean lifespan extension in both male and female mice fed a standard diet. This study was conducted in three different sites in the USA and used genetically heterogenous mice to avoid genotype-specific effects on disease susceptibility. According to this study, rapamycin may extend lifespan by postponing death from cancer, by retarding mechanisms of ageing, or both (Harrison et al., 2009). Rapamycin treatment increases autophagy, reduces cell senescence and have anti-inflammatory as well as antitumor effects. In addition rapamycin and rapamycin analogs (rapalogs) ameliorate age-related diseases such as cancer, metabolic syndrome, neurodegenerative and cardiovascular diseases (reviewed in (Sharp & Richardson, 2011)).

4.5.3 Sirtuin pathway

Resveratrol, in addition to its antioxidant properties, has been reported to mediate yeast lifespan extension through the activation of the sirtuin family of deacetylases (Howitz et al., 2003). This led to the idea that resveratrol might act as a CRM, and was supported by results on rodents showing impressive protection against age-related diseases including neurodegeneration, cancer, cardiovascular diseases and obesity (Markus & Morris, 2008). Regarding the targets of resveratrol, biochemical studies indicate that resveratrol may not activate sirtuins directly but thorugh activation of AMPK (Hwang et al., 2009). Although in mice fed with a high fat diet resveratrol induces lifespan extension and its commonly associated features (increased insulin sensitivity and AMPK activity, reduced IGF-I levels, …) (Baur et al., 2006), there are no reports of increased lifespan in healthy mammals. This may indicate that resveratrol induces effects by targeting intracellular pathways activated by CR without slowing aging. The effects of resveratrol have led to development of more potent SIRT1 activators. These newly synthesized compounds (by a pharmaceutical biotechnology company called Sirtris Pharmaceuticals) are potent small-molecule activators of SIRT1 that are structurally unrelated to natural polyphenols. There are promising data regarding the effects of these compounds in mouse models and some of them are in phase II clinical trials for type 2 diabetes, opening an approach for other age-related diseases (reviewed in Camins et al., 2010).

5. Conclusion

The evolution of our understanding of the biological basis of aging has focused antiaging research on antioxidant, metabolic and hormonal replacement therapies. Although beneficial effects of antioxidant therapies are not in doubt, controlled trials have revealed poor efficiency for hormonal and antioxidant treatments. Thus, more controlled and properly designed trials are needed to determine the potential of these approaches. The recent advances in knowledge about metabolic signalling pathways involved in the aging process especially in mTOR/Insulin/IGF-1 pathway that mediate the beneficial effects of CR, have opened new venues for the development of effective antiaging or CRM treatments. The results reported for rapamycin treatment starting later in life are of great interest in terms of the potential use of this inhibitor of mTORC1 for slowing aging and probably its combination with resveratrol, an stimulator of Sirt1 that improves age-related diseases without increasing lifespan in mammals, will render a more potent and efficient treatment. In addition, future research in how the different pathways integrate and interact to mediate CR effects will provide us with new pharmacological interventions that can slow the process of aging. An important issue in the prescription of these drugs to healthy humans is that aging is not recognized as a condition to be treated. Thus, the anti-aging drugs should be introduced in human if they affect disease, and later on, when showed effective the day will come when they become anti-aging drugs.

6. Acknowledgments

Financial support from BFU2011-24365, RETICEF (RD06/0013/1012), Junta de Extremadura (GR10009) and FEDER.

7. References

Allard, J.S., Heilbronn, L.K., Smith, C., Hunt, N.D., Ingram, D.K., Ravussin, E. & de, C.R. (2008). In vitro cellular adaptations of indicators of longevity in response to treatment with serum collected from humans on calorie restricted diets. PLoS One Vol.3, No.9, (2008), pp. e3211

Anderson, R.M. & Weindruch, R. (2010). Metabolic reprogramming, caloric restriction and aging. Trends Endocrinol Metab Vol.21, No.3, (March 2010), pp. 134-141

Anisimov, V.N. (2010). Metformin for aging and cancer prevention. Aging (Albany NY) Vol.2, No.11, (November 2010), pp. 760-774

Anisimov, V.N., Popovich, I.G., Zabezhinski, M.A., Anisimov, S.V., Vesnushkin, G.M. & Vinogradova, I.A. (May 2006). Melatonin as antioxidant, geroprotector and anticarcinogen. Biochim Biophys Acta Vol.1757, No.5-6, (May 2006), pp. 573-589

Autier, P. & Gandini, S. (2007). Vitamin D supplementation and total mortality: a meta-analysis of randomized controlled trials. Arch Intern Med Vol.167, No.16, (September 2007), pp. 1730-1737

Ayala, V., Naudi, A., Sanz, A., Caro, P., Portero-Otin, M., Barja, G. & Pamplona, R. (2007). Dietary protein restriction decreases oxidative protein damage, peroxidizability index, and mitochondrial complex I content in rat liver. *J Gerontol A Biol Sci Med Sci* Vol.62, No.4, (April 2007), pp. 352-360

Bamps, S., Wirtz, J., Savory, F.R., Lake, D. & Hope, I.A. (2009). The Caenorhabditis elegans sirtuin gene, sir-2.1, is widely expressed and induced upon caloric restriction. *Mech Ageing Dev* Vol.130, No.11-12, (November 2009), pp. 762-770

Bartke, A. (2003). Can growth hormone (GH) accelerate aging? Evidence from GH-transgenic mice. *Neuroendocrinology* Vol.78, No.4, (October 2003), pp. 210-216

Baur, J.A., Pearson, K.J., Price, N.L., Jamieson, H.A., Lerin, C., Kalra, A., Prabhu, V.V., Allard, J.S., Lopez-Lluch, G., Lewis, K., Pistell, P.J., Poosala, S., Becker, K.G., Boss, O., Gwinn, D., Wang, M., Ramaswamy, S., Fishbein, K.W., Spencer, R.G., Lakatta, E.G., Le, C.D., Shaw, R.J., Navas, P., Puigserver, P., Ingram, D.K., de, C.R. & Sinclair, D.A. (2006). Resveratrol improves health and survival of mice on a high-calorie diet. *Nature* Vol.444, No.7117, (November 2006), pp. 337-342

Bezlepkin, V.G., Sirota, N.P. & Gaziev, A.I. (1996). The prolongation of survival in mice by dietary antioxidants depends on their age by the start of feeding this diet. *Mech Ageing Dev* Vol.92, No.2-3, (December 1996), pp. 227-234

Blagosklonny, M.V. (2010). Why human lifespan is rapidly increasing: solving "longevity riddle" with "revealed-slow-aging" hypothesis. *Aging (Albany NY)* Vol.2, No.4, (April 2010), pp. 177-182

Blot, W.J., Li, J.Y., Taylor, P.R., Guo, W., Dawsey, S., Wang, G.Q., Yang, C.S., Zheng, S.F., Gail, M., Li, G.Y. & . (1993). Nutrition intervention trials in Linxian, China: supplementation with specific vitamin/mineral combinations, cancer incidence, and disease-specific mortality in the general population. *J Natl Cancer Inst* Vol.85, No.18, (September 1993), pp. 1483-1492

Bodmer, M., Meier, C., Krahenbuhl, S., Jick, S.S. & Meier, C.R. (2010). Long-term metformin use is associated with decreased risk of breast cancer. *Diabetes Care* Vol.33, No.6, (June 2010), pp. 1304-1308

Boily, G., Seifert, E.L., Bevilacqua, L., He, X.H., Sabourin, G., Estey, C., Moffat, C., Crawford, S., Saliba, S., Jardine, K., Xuan, J., Evans, M., Harper, M.E. & McBurney, M.W. (2008). SirT1 regulates energy metabolism and response to caloric restriction in mice. *PLoS One* Vol.3, No.3, (2008), pp. e1759

Bonkowski, M.S., Dominici, F.P., Arum, O., Rocha, J.S., Al Regaiey, K.A., Westbrook, R., Spong, A., Panici, J., Masternak, M.M., Kopchick, J.J. & Bartke, A. (2009). Disruption of growth hormone receptor prevents calorie restriction from improving insulin action and longevity. *PLoS One* Vol.4, No.2, (2009), pp. e4567

Bonkowski, M.S., Rocha, J.S., Masternak, M.M., Al Regaiey, K.A. & Bartke, A. (2006). Targeted disruption of growth hormone receptor interferes with the beneficial actions of calorie restriction. *Proc Natl Acad Sci U S A* Vol.103, No.20, (May 2006), pp. 7901-7905

Bordone, L., Cohen, D., Robinson, A., Motta, M.C., van, V.E., Czopik, A., Steele, A.D., Crowe, H., Marmor, S., Luo, J., Gu, W. & Guarente, L. (2007). SIRT1 transgenic mice show phenotypes resembling calorie restriction. *Aging Cell* Vol.6, No.6, (Dec. 2007), pp. 759-767

Brand, M.D. (2000). Uncoupling to survive? The role of mitochondrial inefficiency in ageing. *Exp Gerontol* Vol.35, No.6-7, (September 2000), pp. 811-820

Buscemi, N., Vandermeer, B., Hooton, N., Pandya, R., Tjosvold, L., Hartling, L., Baker, G., Klassen, T.P. & Vohra, S. (2005). The efficacy and safety of exogenous melatonin for primary sleep disorders. A meta-analysis. *J Gen Intern Med* Vol.20, No.12, (December 2005), pp. 1151-1158

Camello-Almaraz, C., Gomez-Pinilla, P.J., Pozo, M.J. & Camello, P.J. (2008). Age-related alterations in Ca2+ signals and mitochondrial membrane potential in exocrine cells are prevented by melatonin. *J Pineal Res* Vol.45, No.2, (September 2008), pp. 191-198

Camins, A., Sureda, F.X., Junyent, F., Verdaguer, E., Folch, J., Pelegri, C., Vilaplana, J., Beas-Zarate, C. & Pallas, M. (2010). Sirtuin activators: designing molecules to extend life span. *Biochim Biophys Acta* Vol.1799, No.10-12, (October 2010), pp. 740-749

Chiba, T., Yamaza, H., Higami, Y. & Shimokawa, I. (2002). Anti-aging effects of caloric restriction: Involvement of neuroendocrine adaptation by peripheral signaling. *Microsc Res Tech* Vol.59, No.4, (November 2002), pp. 317-324

Chiba, T., Yamaza, H. & Shimokawa, I. (2007). Role of insulin and growth hormone/insulin-like growth factor-I signaling in lifespan extension: rodent longevity models for studying aging and calorie restriction. *Curr Genomics* Vol.8, No.7, (Nov. 2007), pp. 423-428

Cohen, H.Y., Miller, C., Bitterman, K.J., Wall, N.R., Hekking, B., Kessler, B., Howitz, K.T., Gorospe, M., de, C.R. & Sinclair, D.A. (2004). Calorie restriction promotes mammalian cell survival by inducing the SIRT1 deacetylase. *Science* Vol.305, No.5682, (July 2004), pp. 390-392

Colman, R.J., Anderson, R.M., Johnson, S.C., Kastman, E.K., Kosmatka, K.J., Beasley, T.M., Allison, D.B., Cruzen, C., Simmons, H.A., Kemnitz, J.W. & Weindruch, R. (2009). Caloric restriction delays disease onset and mortality in rhesus monkeys. *Science* Vol.325, No.5937, (July 2009), pp. 201-204

Czernichow, S., Couthouis, A., Bertrais, S., Vergnaud, A.C., Dauchet, L., Galan, P. & Hercberg, S. (2006). Antioxidant supplementation does not affect fasting plasma glucose in the Supplementation with Antioxidant Vitamins and Minerals (SU.VI.MAX) study in France: association with dietary intake and plasma concentrations. *Am J Clin Nutr* Vol.84, No.2, (August 2006), pp. 395-399

de Grey, A.D. (2004). Mitochondria in homeotherm aging: will detailed mechanisms consistent with the evidence now receive attention? *Aging Cell* Vol.3, No.2, (April 2004), pp. 77

Dhahbi, J.M., Mote, P.L., Fahy, G.M. & Spindler, S.R. (2005). Identification of potential caloric restriction mimetics by microarray profiling. *Physiol Genomics* Vol.23, No.3, (November 2005), pp. 343-350

Dusso, A.S., Brown, A.J. & Slatopolsky, E. (2005). Vitamin D. *Am J Physiol Renal Physiol* Vol.289, No.1, (July 2005), pp. F8-28

Edwards, A.G., Donato, A.J., Lesniewski, L.A., Gioscia, R.A., Seals, D.R. & Moore, R.L. (2010). Life-long caloric restriction elicits pronounced protection of the aged myocardium: a role for AMPK. *Mech Ageing Dev* Vol.131, No.11-12, (Nov. 2010), pp. 739-742

Erman, M., Seiden, D., Zammit, G., Sainati, S. & Zhang, J. (2006). An efficacy, safety, and dose-response study of Ramelteon in patients with chronic primary insomnia. *Sleep Med* Vol.7, No.1, (January 2006), pp. 17-24

Finkelstein, J.W., Roffwarg, H.P., Boyar, R.M., Kream, J. & Hellman, L. (1972). Age-related change in the twenty-four-hour spontaneous secretion of growth hormone. *J Clin Endocrinol Metab* Vol.35, No.5, (November 1972), pp. 665-670

Fontana, L. (2009b). The scientific basis of caloric restriction leading to longer life. *Curr Opin Gastroenterol* Vol.25, No.2, (March 2009b), pp. 144-150

Fontana, L. (2009a). The scientific basis of caloric restriction leading to longer life. *Curr Opin Gastroenterol* Vol.25, No.2, (March 2009a), pp. 144-150

Fontana, L., Klein, S. & Holloszy, J.O. (2010a). Effects of long-term calorie restriction and endurance exercise on glucose tolerance, insulin action, and adipokine production. *Age (Dordr)* Vol.32, No.1, (March 2010a), pp. 97-108

Fontana, L., Partridge, L. & Longo, V.D. (2010b). Extending healthy life span--from yeast to humans. *Science* Vol.328, No.5976, (April 2010b), pp. 321-326

Fontana, L., Weiss, E.P., Villareal, D.T., Klein, S. & Holloszy, J.O. (2008). Long-term effects of calorie or protein restriction on serum IGF-1 and IGFBP-3 concentration in humans. *Aging Cell* Vol.7, No.5, (October 2008), pp. 681-687

Forster, M.J., Morris, P. & Sohal, R.S. (2003). Genotype and age influence the effect of caloric intake on mortality in mice. *FASEB J* Vol.17, No.6, (April 2003), pp. 690-692

Fridovich, I. (2004). Mitochondria: are they the seat of senescence? *Aging Cell* Vol.3, No.1, (February 2004), pp. 13-16

Fusco, D., Colloca, G., Lo Monaco, M.R. & Cesari, M. (2007). Effects of antioxidant supplementation on the aging process. *Clin Interv Aging* Vol.2, No.3, (2007),377-387

Genkinger, J.M., Platz, E.A., Hoffman, S.C., Comstock, G.W. & Helzlsouer, K.J. (2004). Fruit, vegetable, and antioxidant intake and all-cause, cancer, and cardiovascular disease mortality in a community-dwelling population in Washington County, Maryland. *Am J Epidemiol* Vol.160, No.12, (December 2004), pp. 1223-1233

Gomez-Pinilla, P.J., Gomez, M.F., Sward, K., Hedlund, P., Hellstrand, P., Camello, P.J., Andersson, K.E. & Pozo, M.J. (2008). Melatonin restores impaired contractility in aged guinea pig urinary bladder. *J Pineal Res* Vol.44, No.4, (May 2008), pp. 416-425

Grossman, E., Laudon, M., Yalcin, R., Zengil, H., Peleg, E., Sharabi, Y., Kamari, Y., Shen-Orr, Z. & Zisapel, N. (2006). Melatonin reduces night blood pressure in patients with nocturnal hypertension. *Am J Med* Vol.119, No.10, (October 2006), pp. 898-902

Guarente, L. (2000). Sir2 links chromatin silencing, metabolism, and aging. *Genes Dev* Vol.14, No.9, (May 2000), pp. 1021-1026

Hardeland, R., Tan, D.X. & Reiter, R.J. (2009). Kynuramines, metabolites of melatonin and other indoles: the resurrection of an almost forgotten class of biogenic amines. *J Pineal Res* Vol.47, No.2, (September 2009), pp. 109-126

Hardie, D.G. (2011). Sensing of energy and nutrients by AMP-activated protein kinase. *Am J Clin Nutr* Vol.93, No.4, (April 2011), pp. 891S-6

Harman, D. (1956). Aging: a theory based on free radical and radiation chemistry. *J Gerontol* Vol.11, No.3, (July 1956), pp. 298-300

Harman, D. (1972). The biologic clock: the mitochondria? *J Am Geriatr Soc* Vol.20, No.4, (April 1972), pp. 145-147

Harrison, D.E., Strong, R., Sharp, Z.D., Nelson, J.F., Astle, C.M., Flurkey, K., Nadon, N.L., Wilkinson, J.E., Frenkel, K., Carter, C.S., Pahor, M., Javors, M.A., Fernandez, E. & Miller, R.A. (2009). Rapamycin fed late in life extends lifespan in genetically heterogeneous mice. *Nature* Vol.460, No.7253, (July 2009), pp. 392-395

Hercberg, S., Czernichow, S. & Galan, P. (2009). Tell me what your blood beta-carotene level is, I will tell you what your health risk is! The viewpoint of the SUVIMAX researchers. *Ann Nutr Metab* Vol.54, No.4, (2009), pp. 310-312

Hercberg, S., Galan, P., Preziosi, P., Bertrais, S., Mennen, L., Malvy, D., Roussel, A.M., Favier, A. & Briancon, S. (2004). The SU.VI.MAX Study: a randomized, placebo-controlled trial of the health effects of antioxidant vitamins and minerals. *Arch Intern Med* Vol.164, No.21, (November 2004), pp. 2335-2342

Higami, Y. & Shimokawa, I. (2000). Apoptosis in the aging process. *Cell Tissue Res* Vol.301, No.1, (July 2000), pp. 125-132

Hofman, M.A. & Swaab, D.F. (1994). Alterations in circadian rhythmicity of the vasopressin-producing neurons of the human suprachiasmatic nucleus (SCN) with aging. *Brain Res* Vol.651, No.1-2, (July 1994), pp. 134-142

Howitz, K.T., Bitterman, K.J., Cohen, H.Y., Lamming, D.W., Lavu, S., Wood, J.G., Zipkin, R.E., Chung, P., Kisielewski, A., Zhang, L.L., Scherer, B. & Sinclair, D.A. (2003). Small molecule activators of sirtuins extend Saccharomyces cerevisiae lifespan. *Nature* Vol.425, No.6954, (September 2003), pp. 191-196

Hu, D., Cao, P., Thiels, E., Chu, C.T., Wu, G.Y., Oury, T.D. & Klann, E. (2007). Hippocampal long-term potentiation, memory, and longevity in mice that overexpress mitochondrial superoxide dismutase. *Neurobiol Learn Mem* Vol.87, No.3, (March 2007), pp. 372-384

Hunt, A.E., Al-Ghoul, W.M., Gillette, M.U. & Dubocovich, M.L. (2001). Activation of MT(2) melatonin receptors in rat suprachiasmatic nucleus phase advances the circadian clock. *Am J Physiol Cell Physiol* Vol.280, No.1, (January 2001), pp. C110-C118

Hwang, J.T., Kwon, D.Y. & Yoon, S.H. (2009). AMP-activated protein kinase: a potential target for the diseases prevention by natural occurring polyphenols. *N Biotechnol* Vol.26, No.1-2, (October 2009), pp. 17-22

Jacobs, E.J., Connell, C.J., Chao, A., McCullough, M.L., Rodriguez, C., Thun, M.J. & Calle, E.E. (2003). Multivitamin use and colorectal cancer incidence in a US cohort: does timing matter? *Am J Epidemiol* Vol.158, No.7, (October 2003), pp. 621-628

Jung, C.H., Ro, S.H., Cao, J., Otto, N.M. & Kim, D.H. (2010). mTOR regulation of autophagy. *FEBS Lett* Vol.584, No.7, (April 2010), pp. 1287-1295

Kalender, A., Selvaraj, A., Kim, S.Y., Gulati, P., Brule, S., Viollet, B., Kemp, B.E., Bardeesy, N., Dennis, P., Schlager, J.J., Marette, A., Kozma, S.C. & Thomas, G. (2010). Metformin, independent of AMPK, inhibits mTORC1 in a rag GTPase-dependent manner. *Cell Metab* Vol.11, No.5, (May 2010), pp. 390-401

Kapahi, P., Chen, D., Rogers, A.N., Katewa, S.D., Li, P.W., Thomas, E.L. & Kockel, L. (2010). With TOR, less is more: a key role for the conserved nutrient-sensing TOR pathway in aging. *Cell Metab* Vol.11, No.6, (June 2010), pp. 453-465

Karasek, M. (1999). Melatonin in humans-where we are 40 years after its discovery. *Neuro Endocrinol Lett* Vol.20, No.3-4, (1999), pp. 179-188

Karasek, M. (2004). Melatonin, human aging, and age-related diseases. *Exp Gerontol* Vol.39, No.11-12, (November 2004), pp. 1723-1729

Kelly, G. (2010). A review of the sirtuin system, its clinical implications, and the potential role of dietary activators like resveratrol: part 1. *Altern Med Rev* Vol.15, No.3, (September 2010), pp. 245-263

Kennedy, S.H. & Emsley, R. (2006). Placebo-controlled trial of agomelatine in the treatment of major depressive disorder. *Eur Neuropsychopharmacol* Vol.16, No.2, (Feb.2006), pp. 93-100

Knasmuller, S., Nersesyan, A., Misik, M., Gerner, C., Mikulits, W., Ehrlich, V., Hoelzl, C., Szakmary, A. & Wagner, K.H. (2008). Use of conventional and -omics based methods for health claims of dietary antioxidants: a critical overview. *Br J Nutr* Vol.99 E Suppl 1, (May 2008), pp. ES3-52

Ku, H.H., Brunk, U.T. & Sohal, R.S. (1993). Relationship between mitochondrial superoxide and hydrogen peroxide production and longevity of mammalian species. *Free Radic Biol Med* Vol.15, No.6, (December 1993), pp. 621-627

Lago, F., Dieguez, C., Gomez-Reino, J. & Gualillo, O. (2007). The emerging role of adipokines as mediators of inflammation and immune responses. *Cytokine Growth Factor Rev* Vol.18, No.3-4, (June 2007), pp. 313-325

Lanza, I.R., Short, D.K., Short, K.R., Raghavakaimal, S., Basu, R., Joyner, M.J., McConnell, J.P. & Nair, K.S. (2008). Endurance exercise as a countermeasure for aging. *Diabetes* Vol.57, No.11, (November 2008), pp. 2933-2942

Lapointe, J. & Hekimi, S. (2010). When a theory of aging ages badly. *Cell Mol Life Sci* Vol.67, No.1, (January 2010), pp. 1-8

Le Couteur, D.G., McLachlan, A.J., Quinn, R.J., Simpson, S.J. & de, C.R. (2011). Aging Biology and Novel Targets for Drug Discovery. *J Gerontol A Biol Sci Med Sci* (August 2011)

Lee, I.M., Cook, N.R., Gaziano, J.M., Gordon, D., Ridker, P.M., Manson, J.E., Hennekens, C.H. & Buring, J.E. (2005). Vitamin E in the primary prevention of cardiovascular disease and cancer: the Women's Health Study: a randomized controlled trial. *JAMA* Vol.294, No.1, (July 2005), pp. 56-65

Lekakis, J., Rallidis, L.S., Andreadou, I., Vamvakou, G., Kazantzoglou, G., Magiatis, P., Skaltsounis, A.L. & Kremastinos, D.T. (2005). Polyphenolic compounds from red grapes acutely improve endothelial function in patients with coronary heart disease. *Eur J Cardiovasc Prev Rehabil* Vol.12, No.6, (December 2005), pp. 596-600

Lemoine, P., Guilleminault, C. & Alvarez, E. (2007). Improvement in subjective sleep in major depressive disorder with a novel antidepressant, agomelatine: randomized, double-blind comparison with venlafaxine. *J Clin Psychiatry* Vol.68, No.11, (November 2007), pp. 1723-1732

Leto, S., Kokkonen, G.C. & Barrows, C.H. (1976). Dietary protein life-span, and physiological variables in female mice. *J Gerontol* Vol.31, No.2, (March 1976), pp. 149-154

Llewellyn, D.J., Langa, K.M. & Lang, I.A. (2009). Serum 25-hydroxyvitamin D concentration and cognitive impairment. *J Geriatr Psychiatry Neurol* Vol.22, No.3, (September 2009), pp. 188-195

Lonn, E., Bosch, J., Yusuf, S., Sheridan, P., Pogue, J., Arnold, J.M., Ross, C., Arnold, A., Sleight, P., Probstfield, J. & Dagenais, G.R. (2005). Effects of long-term vitamin E supplementation on cardiovascular events and cancer: a randomized controlled trial. *JAMA* Vol.293, No.11, (March 2005), pp. 1338-1347

Luthringer, R., Muzet, M., Zisapel, N. & Staner, L. (2009). The effect of prolonged-release melatonin on sleep measures and psychomotor performance in elderly patients with insomnia. *Int Clin Psychopharmacol* Vol.24, No.5, (September 2009), pp. 239-249

Ma, X.M. & Blenis, J. (May 2009). Molecular mechanisms of mTOR-mediated translational control. *Nat Rev Mol Cell Biol* Vol.10, No.5, (May 2009), pp. 307-318

Manach, C., Mazur, A. & Scalbert, A. (2005). Polyphenols and prevention of cardiovascular diseases. *Curr Opin Lipidol* Vol.16, No.1, (February 2005), pp. 77-84

Markus, M.A. & Morris, B.J. (2008). Resveratrol in prevention and treatment of common clinical conditions of aging. *Clin Interv Aging* Vol.3, No.2, (2008), pp. 331-339

Mattison, J.A., Roth, G.S., Lane, M.A. & Ingram, D.K. (2007). Dietary restriction in aging nonhuman primates. *Interdiscip Top Gerontol* Vol.35, (2007), pp. 137-158

Mattson, M.P. & Wan, R. (2005). Beneficial effects of intermittent fasting and caloric restriction on the cardiovascular and cerebrovascular systems. *J Nutr Biochem* Vol.16, No.3, (March 2005), pp. 129-137

McCay, C.M., Crowell, M.F. & Maynard, L.A. (1935). The effect of retarded growth upon the length of life span and upon the ultimate body size. *J Nutr* Vol.10, (May 1935), pp. 63-79

Meydani, M., Lipman, R.D., Han, S.N., Wu, D., Beharka, A., Martin, K.R., Bronson, R., Cao, G., Smith, D. & Meydani, S.N. (1998). The effect of long-term dietary supplementation with antioxidants. *Ann N Y Acad Sci* Vol.854, (Nov. 1998), pp. 352-360

Migliaccio, E., Giorgio, M., Mele, S., Pelicci, G., Reboldi, P., Pandolfi, P.P., Lanfrancone, L. & Pelicci, P.G. (1999). The p66shc adaptor protein controls oxidative stress response and life span in mammals. *Nature* Vol.402, No.6759, (November 1999), pp. 309-313

Mills, E., Wu, P., Seely, D. & Guyatt, G. (2005). Melatonin in the treatment of cancer: a systematic review of randomized controlled trials and meta-analysis. *J Pineal Res* Vol.39, No.4, (November 2005), pp. 360-366

Minor, R.K., Allard, J.S., Younts, C.M., Ward, T.M. & de, C.R. (2010a). Dietary interventions to extend life span and health span based on calorie restriction. *J Gerontol A Biol Sci Med Sci* Vol.65, No.7, (July 2010a), pp. 695-703

Minor, R.K., Smith, D.L., Jr., Sossong, A.M., Kaushik, S., Poosala, S., Spangler, E.L., Roth, G.S., Lane, M., Allison, D.B., de, C.R., Ingram, D.K. & Mattison, J.A. (2010b). Chronic ingestion of 2-deoxy-D-glucose induces cardiac vacuolization and increases mortality in rats. *Toxicol Appl Pharmacol* Vol.243, No.3, (March 2010b), pp. 332-339

Miquel, J. & Economos, A.C. (1979). Favorable effects of the antioxidants sodium and magnesium thiazolidine carboxylate on the vitality and life span of Drosophila and mice. *Exp Gerontol* Vol.14, No.5, (1979), pp. 279-285

Miquel, J., Economos, A.C., Fleming, J. & Johnson, J.E., Jr. (1980). Mitochondrial role in cell aging. *Exp Gerontol* Vol.15, No.6, (1980), pp. 575-591

Mitterberger, M.C., Mattesich, M., Klaver, E., Piza-Katzer, H. & Zwerschke, W. (2011). Reduced Insulin-Like Growth Factor-I Serum Levels in Formerly Obese Women Subjected to Laparoscopic-Adjustable Gastric Banding or Diet-Induced Long-term Caloric Restriction. *J Gerontol A Biol Sci Med Sci* (August 2011)

Naudi, A., Caro, P., Jove, M., Gomez, J., Boada, J., Ayala, V., Portero-Otin, M., Barja, G. & Pamplona, R. (2007). Methionine restriction decreases endogenous oxidative molecular damage and increases mitochondrial biogenesis and uncoupling protein 4 in rat brain. *Rejuvenation Res* Vol.10, No.4, (December 2007), pp. 473-484

Neubauer, D.N. (1999). Sleep problems in the elderly. *Am Fam Physician* Vol.59, No.9, (May 1999), pp. 2551-2560

Niki, E., Noguchi, N., Tsuchihashi, H. & Gotoh, N. (1995). Interaction among vitamin C, vitamin E, and beta-carotene. *Am J Clin Nutr* Vol.62, No.6 Suppl, (December 1995), pp. 1322S-1326S

Olshansky, S.J., Perry, D., Miller, R.A. & Butler, R.N. (2007). Pursuing the longevity dividend: scientific goals for an aging world. *Ann N Y Acad Sci* Vol.1114, (October 2007), pp. 11-13

Omodei, D. & Fontana, L. (2011). Calorie restriction and prevention of age-associated chronic disease. *FEBS Lett* Vol.585, No.11, (June 2011), pp. 1537-1542

Oudshoorn, C., Mattace-Raso, F.U., van, d., V, Colin, E.M. & van der Cammen, T.J. (2008). Higher serum vitamin D3 levels are associated with better cognitive test performance in patients with Alzheimer's disease. *Dement Geriatr Cogn Disord* Vol.25, No.6, (2008), pp. 539-543

Page, M.M., Richardson, J., Wiens, B.E., Tiedtke, E., Peters, C.W., Faure, P.A., Burness, G. & Stuart, J.A. (2010). Antioxidant enzyme activities are not broadly correlated with longevity in 14 vertebrate endotherm species. *Age (Dordr)* Vol.32, No.2, (June 2010), pp. 255-270

Pak, J.W., Herbst, A., Bua, E., Gokey, N., McKenzie, D. & Aiken, J.M. (2003). Mitochondrial DNA mutations as a fundamental mechanism in physiological declines associated with aging. *Aging Cell* Vol.2, No.1, (February 2003), pp. 1-7

Pamplona, R. (2011). Mitochondrial DNA damage and animal longevity: insights from comparative studies. *J Aging Res* Vol.2011, (2011), pp. 807108

Pamplona, R. & Barja, G. (2011). An evolutionary comparative scan for longevity-related oxidative stress resistance mechanisms in homeotherms. *Biogerontology* (July 2011)

Pandi-Perumal, S.R., Trakht, I., Srinivasan, V., Spence, D.W., Maestroni, G.J., Zisapel, N. & Cardinali, D.P. (2008). Physiological effects of melatonin: role of melatonin receptors and signal transduction pathways. *Prog Neurobiol* Vol.85, No.3, (July 2008), pp. 335-353

Pascua, P., Camello-Almaraz, C., Camello, P.J., Martin-Cano, F., Vara, E., Tresguerres, J. & Pozo, M.J. (2011). Melatonin, and to a lesser extent growth hormone, restores colonic smooth muscle physiology in old rats. *J Pineal Res* (May 2011)

Pearl R (1928). *The rate of living* Alfred A Knopf, Inc., New York.

Pearson, K.J., Baur, J.A., Lewis, K.N., Peshkin, L., Price, N.L., Labinskyy, N., Swindell, W.R., Kamara, D., Minor, R.K., Perez, E., Jamieson, H.A., Zhang, Y., Dunn, S.R., Sharma, K., Pleshko, N., Woollett, L.A., Csiszar, A., Ikeno, Y., Le, C.D., Elliott, P.J., Becker, K.G., Navas, P., Ingram, D.K., Wolf, N.S., Ungvari, Z., Sinclair, D.A. & de, C.R. (2008). Resveratrol delays age-related deterioration and mimics transcriptional aspects of dietary restriction without extending life span. *Cell Metab* Vol.8, No.2, (August 2008), pp. 157-168

Perez, V.I., Bokov, A., Van, R.H., Mele, J., Ran, Q., Ikeno, Y. & Richardson, A. (2009). Is the oxidative stress theory of aging dead? *Biochim Biophys Acta* Vol.1790, No.10, (October 2009), pp. 1005-1014

Pham, D.Q. & Plakogiannis, R. (2005). Vitamin E supplementation in cardiovascular disease and cancer prevention: Part 1. *Ann Pharmacother* Vol.39, No.11, (November 2005), pp. 1870-1878

Pozo, M.J., Gomez-Pinilla, P.J., Camello-Almaraz, C., Martin-Cano, F.E., Pascua, P., Rol, M.A., cuna-Castroviejo, D. & Camello, P.J. (2010). Melatonin, a potential therapeutic agent for smooth muscle-related pathological conditions and aging. *Curr Med Chem* Vol.17, No.34, (2010), pp. 4150-4165

Rebrin, I., Zicker, S., Wedekind, K.J., Paetau-Robinson, I., Packer, L. & Sohal, R.S. (2005). Effect of antioxidant-enriched diets on glutathione redox status in tissue homogenates and mitochondria of the senescence-accelerated mouse. *Free Radic Biol Med* Vol.39, No.4, (August 2005), pp. 549-557

Regulska, M., Leskiewicz, M., Budziszewska, B., Kutner, A., Basta-Kaim, A., Kubera, M., Jaworska-Feil, L. & Lason, W. (2006). Involvement of PI3-K in neuroprotective effects of the 1,25-dihydroxyvitamin D3 analogue - PRI-2191. *Pharmacol Rep* Vol.58, No.6, (November 2006), pp. 900-907

Reid, M.E., Duffield-Lillico, A.J., Garland, L., Turnbull, B.W., Clark, L.C. & Marshall, J.R. (2002). Selenium supplementation and lung cancer incidence: an update of the nutritional prevention of cancer trial. *Cancer Epidemiol Biomarkers Prev* Vol.11, No.11, (November 2002), pp. 1285-1291

Rickman, A.D., Williamson, D.A., Martin, C.K., Gilhooly, C.H., Stein, R.I., Bales, C.W., Roberts, S. & Das, S.K. (2011). The CALERIE Study: Design and methods of an innovative 25% caloric restriction intervention. *Contemp Clin Trials* (July 2011)

Rose, G., Dato, S., Altomare, K., Bellizzi, D., Garasto, S., Greco, V., Passarino, G., Feraco, E., Mari, V., Barbi, C., BonaFe, M., Franceschi, C., Tan, Q., Boiko, S., Yashin, A.I. & De, B.G. (2003). Variability of the SIRT3 gene, human silent information regulator Sir2 homologue, and survivorship in the elderly. *Exp Gerontol* Vol.38, No.10, (October 2003), pp. 1065-1070

Rudman, D. (1985). Growth hormone, body composition, and aging. *J Am Geriatr Soc* Vol.33, No.11, (November 1985), pp. 800-807

Sanz, A., Caro, P., Sanchez, J.G. & Barja, G. (2006a). Effect of lipid restriction on mitochondrial free radical production and oxidative DNA damage. *Ann N Y Acad Sci* Vol.1067, (May 2006a), pp. 200-209

Sanz, A., Gomez, J., Caro, P. & Barja, G. (2006b). Carbohydrate restriction does not change mitochondrial free radical generation and oxidative DNA damage. *J Bioenerg Biomembr* Vol.38, No.5-6, (December 2006b), pp. 327-333

Schleithoff, S.S., Zittermann, A., Tenderich, G., Berthold, H.K., Stehle, P. & Koerfer, R. (2006). Vitamin D supplementation improves cytokine profiles in patients with congestive heart failure: a double-blind, randomized, placebo-controlled trial. *Am J Clin Nutr* Vol.83, No.4, (April 2006), pp. 754-759

Schriner, S.E., Linford, N.J., Martin, G.M., Treuting, P., Ogburn, C.E., Emond, M., Coskun, P.E., Ladiges, W., Wolf, N., Van, R.H., Wallace, D.C. & Rabinovitch, P.S. (2005). Extension of murine life span by overexpression of catalase targeted to mitochondria. *Science* Vol.308, No.5730, (June 2005), pp. 1909-1911

Selesniemi, K., Lee, H.J. & Tilly, J.L. (2008). Moderate caloric restriction initiated in rodents during adulthood sustains function of the female reproductive axis into advanced chronological age. *Aging Cell* Vol.7, No.5, (October 2008), pp. 622-629

Selman, C., Lingard, S., Choudhury, A.I., Batterham, R.L., Claret, M., Clements, M., Ramadani, F., Okkenhaug, K., Schuster, E., Blanc, E., Piper, M.D., Al-Qassab, H., Speakman, J.R., Carmignac, D., Robinson, I.C., Thornton, J.M., Gems, D., Partridge, L. & Withers, D.J. (2008). Evidence for lifespan extension and delayed age-related biomarkers in insulin receptor substrate 1 null mice. *FASEB J* Vol.22, No.3, (March 2008), pp. 807-818

Selman, C., Tullet, J.M., Wieser, D., Irvine, E., Lingard, S.J., Choudhury, A.I., Claret, M., Al-Qassab, H., Carmignac, D., Ramadani, F., Woods, A., Robinson, I.C., Schuster, E., Batterham, R.L., Kozma, S.C., Thomas, G., Carling, D., Okkenhaug, K., Thornton, J.M., Partridge, L., Gems, D. & Withers, D.J. (2009). Ribosomal protein S6 kinase 1 signaling regulates mammalian life span. *Science* Vol.326, No.5949, (October 2009), pp. 140-144

Sharp, Z.D. & Richardson, A. (2011). Aging and cancer: can mTOR inhibitors kill two birds with one drug? *Target Oncol* Vol.6, No.1, (March 2011), pp. 41-51

Sheppard, M.C. (2005). GH and mortality in acromegaly. *J Endocrinol Invest* Vol.28, No.11 Suppl International, (2005), pp. 75-77

Singer, C., Tractenberg, R.E., Kaye, J., Schafer, K., Gamst, A., Grundman, M., Thomas, R. & Thal, L.J. (2003). A multicenter, placebo-controlled trial of melatonin for sleep disturbance in Alzheimer's disease. *Sleep* Vol.26, No.7, (Nov. 2003), pp. 893-901

Skulachev, V.P. (2004). Mitochondria, reactive oxygen species and longevity: some lessons from the Barja group. *Aging Cell* Vol.3, No.1, (February 2004), pp. 17-19

Sohal, R.S., Svensson, I. & Brunk, U.T. (1990). Hydrogen peroxide production by liver mitochondria in different species. *Mech Ageing Dev* Vol.53, No.3, (April 1990), pp. 209-215

Speakman, J.R. (2005). Correlations between physiology and lifespan:two widely ignored problems with comparative studies. *Aging Cell* Vol.4, No.4, (Aug.2005), pp. 167-175

Speakman, J.R. & Hambly, C. (2007). Starving for life: what animal studies can and cannot tell us about the use of caloric restriction to prolong human lifespan. *J Nutr* Vol.137, No.4, (April 2007), pp. 1078-1086

Speakman, J.R. & Mitchell, S.E. (2011). Caloric restriction. *Mol Aspects Med* (August 2011)

Speakman, J.R. & Selman, C. (2011). The free-radical damage theory: Accumulating evidence against a simple link of oxidative stress to ageing and lifespan. *Bioessays* Vol.33, No.4, (April 2011), pp. 255-259

Spindler, S.R. (2011). Review of the literature and suggestions for the design of rodent survival studies for the identification of compounds that increase health and life span. *Age (Dordr)* (March 2011)

Stolzenberg-Solomon, R.Z. (2009). Vitamin D and pancreatic cancer. *Ann Epidemiol* Vol.19, No.2, (February 2009), pp. 89-95

Suh, Y., Atzmon, G., Cho, M.O., Hwang, D., Liu, B., Leahy, D.J., Barzilai, N. & Cohen, P. (2008). Functionally significant insulin-like growth factor I receptor mutations in centenarians. *Proc Natl Acad Sci U S A* Vol.105, No.9, (March 2008), pp. 3438-3442

Sundaresan, N.R., Gupta, M., Kim, G., Rajamohan, S.B., Isbatan, A. & Gupta, M.P. (2009). Sirt3 blocks the cardiac hypertrophic response by augmenting Foxo3a-dependent antioxidant defense mechanisms in mice. *J Clin Invest* Vol.119, No.9, (September 2009), pp. 2758-2771

Takala, J., Ruokonen, E., Webster, N.R., Nielsen, M.S., Zandstra, D.F., Vundelinckx, G. & Hinds, C.J. (1999). Increased mortality associated with growth hormone treatment in critically ill adults. *N Engl J Med* Vol.341, No.11, (September 1999), pp. 785-792

Tapia, P.C. (2006). Sublethal mitochondrial stress with an attendant stoichiometric augmentation of reactive oxygen species may precipitate many of the beneficial alterations in cellular physiology produced by caloric restriction, intermittent fasting, exercise and dietary phytonutrients: "Mitohormesis" for health and vitality. *Med Hypotheses* Vol.66, No.4, (2006), pp. 832-843

Thomas, M.L., Armbrecht, H.J. & Forte, L.R. (1984). Effects of long-term vitamin D deficiency and response to vitamin D repletion in the mature and aging male and female rat. *Mech Ageing Dev* Vol.25, No.1-2, (April 1984), pp. 161-175

Trifunovic, A., Hansson, A., Wredenberg, A., Rovio, A.T., Dufour, E., Khvorostov, I., Spelbrink, J.N., Wibom, R., Jacobs, H.T. & Larsson, N.G. (2005). Somatic mtDNA mutations cause aging phenotypes without affecting reactive oxygen species production. *Proc Natl Acad Sci U S A* Vol.102, No.50, (Dec.2005), pp. 17993-17998

Utiger, R.D. (1998). The need for more vitamin D. *N Engl J Med* Vol.338, No.12, (March 1998), pp. 828-829

van Geijlswijk, I.M., Korzilius, H.P. & Smits, M.G. (2010). The use of exogenous melatonin in delayed sleep phase disorder: a meta-analysis. *Sleep* Vol.33, No.12, (December 2010), pp. 1605-1614

Vazquez-Martin, A., Oliveras-Ferraros, C. & Menendez, J.A. (2009). The antidiabetic drug metformin suppresses HER2 (erbB-2) oncoprotein overexpression via inhibition of the mTOR effector p70S6K1 in human breast carcinoma cells. *Cell Cycle* Vol.8, No.1, (January 2009), pp. 88-96

Veldhuis, J.D., Liem, A.Y., South, S., Weltman, A., Weltman, J., Clemmons, D.A., Abbott, R., Mulligan, T., Johnson, M.L., Pincus, S. & . (1995). Differential impact of age, sex steroid hormones, and obesity on basal versus pulsatile growth hormone secretion in men as assessed in an ultrasensitive chemiluminescence assay. *J Clin Endocrinol Metab* Vol.80, No.11, (November 1995), pp. 3209-3222

Vendelbo, M.H. & Nair, K.S. (2011). Mitochondrial longevity pathways. *Biochim Biophys Acta* Vol.1813, No.4, (April 2011), pp. 634-644

Viña, J., Lloret, A., Orti, R. & Alonso, D. (2004). Molecular bases of the treatment of Alzheimer's disease with antioxidants: prevention of oxidative stress. *Mol Aspects Med* Vol.25, No.1-2, (February 2004), pp. 117-123

Wade, A.G., Ford, I., Crawford, G., McConnachie, A., Nir, T., Laudon, M. & Zisapel, N. (2010). Nightly treatment of primary insomnia with prolonged release melatonin for 6 months: a randomized placebo controlled trial on age and endogenous melatonin as predictors of efficacy and safety. *BMC Med* Vol.8, (2010), pp. 51

Wang, Y., Liang, Y. & Vanhoutte, P.M. (2011). SIRT1 and AMPK in regulating mammalian senescence: a critical review and a working model. *FEBS Lett* Vol.585, No.7, (April 2011), pp. 986-994

Willcox, B.J., Donlon, T.A., He, Q., Chen, R., Grove, J.S., Yano, K., Masaki, K.H., Willcox, D.C., Rodriguez, B. & Curb, J.D. (2008). FOXO3A genotype is strongly associated with human longevity. *Proc Natl Acad Sci U S A* Vol.105, No.37, (September 2008), pp. 13987-13992

Xiang, L. & He, G. (2011). Caloric restriction and antiaging effects. *Ann Nutr Metab* Vol.58, No.1, (2011), pp. 42-48

Yakes, F.M. & Van, H.B. (1997). Mitochondrial DNA damage is more extensive and persists longer than nuclear DNA damage in human cells following oxidative stress. *Proc Natl Acad Sci U S A* Vol.94, No.2, (January 1997), pp. 514-519

Yamamoto, H., Schoonjans, K. & Auwerx, J. (2007). Sirtuin functions in health and disease. *Mol Endocrinol* Vol.21, No.8, (August 2007), pp. 1745-1755

Yamamoto, M., Clark, J.D., Pastor, J.V., Gurnani, P., Nandi, A., Kurosu, H., Miyoshi, M., Ogawa, Y., Castrillon, D.H., Rosenblatt, K.P. & Kuro-o M (2005). Regulation of oxidative stress by the anti-aging hormone klotho. *J Biol Chem* Vol.280, No.45, (November 2005), pp. 38029-38034

Ylikomi, T., Laaksi, I., Lou, Y.R., Martikainen, P., Miettinen, S., Pennanen, P., Purmonen, S., Syvala, H., Vienonen, A. & Tuohimaa, P. (2002). Antiproliferative action of vitamin D. *Vitam Horm* Vol.64, (2002), pp. 357-406

Zittermann, A., Schleithoff, S. & Koerfer, R.(2005). Putting cardiovascular disease and vitamin D insufficiency into perspective.*Br J Nutr* Vol.94,No.4,(Oct.2005), pp.483-492

2

Pharmacology of Hormone Replacement Therapy in Menopause

Adela Voican et al.*
¹*Universitatea de Medicina din Craiova (AV,LN)*,
²*Univ Paris-Sud, Faculté de Médecine Paris-Sud UMR-S693, Le Kremlin Bicêtre,*
¹*Romania*
²*France*

1. Introduction

Menopause represents the final stage of the continuous process of reproductive aging in a woman's life, marking the end of her fertility. According to the World Health Organization (WHO), the natural menopause is defined *as the permanent cessation of menstruation resulting from the loss of ovarian follicular activity* (WHO Report, 1996). Preceded by endocrine and menstrual cycle changes described as "menopausal transition", natural menopause occurs at an average age of approximately 51 years, although a high inter-individual variability is supported by results from epidemiological studies. However, occurrence of menopause outside the estimated normal age interval (45-55 years) is associated with increased morbidity, either when a late or on the contrary, a premature cessation of menstruation appears. A late menopause implies a longer exposure to estrogens and a possible increased risk for breast (Colditz, 1993; Kelsey & Bernstein, 1996) and endometrial cancer (Dossus et al., 2010; McPherson et al., 1996) or for venous thromboembolism (Simon et al., 2006). On the other hand, women entering menopause earlier are facing a hypo-estrogenic state for a longer period compared to women undergoing normal menopause. That is the case for about 1% of women, which are confronted with the diagnosis of primary ovarian insufficiency (POI). POI is defined by the presence of amenorrhea associated with elevated follicle-stimulating hormone (FSH) levels in the menopausal range in women younger than 40 years (Bachelot et al., 2009). Women facing a premature cessation of the ovarian function were shown to be at increased risk for premature death, cardiovascular disease, neurologic disease, mood disorders, osteoporosis or psychosexual dysfunction (Shuster et al., 2010). As the main rationale for these disorders was linked to hormonal changes, maintaining a certain level of ovarian steroids for a given period of time arose as an essential condition for conserving life quality in women (Wilson, [1966]). Accentuated by the increasing life span, researches related to menopause and its treatment have provided scientific community with an increased body of data during the last decades. However, different aspects regarding the benefit/risk balance or the ideal doses and routes of administration of hormone replacement therapy (HRT) in menopausal women remain uncertain (Grodstein et al., 1997; Rossouw et al., 2002).

* Bruno Francou, Liliana Novac, Nathalie Chabbert-Buffet, Marianne Canonico, Geri Meduri,
Marc Lombes, Pierre-Yves Scarabin, Jacques Young, Anne Guiochon-Mantel and Jérôme Bouligand
Univ Paris-Sud, France

In this context, our paper addresses various issues related to steroid hormone substitution, ranging from the basic pharmacology of sex steroids to their clinical use in HRT and subsequent benefits and risks.

2. Sex steroids

2.1 Natural oestrogens and progestogens

During a woman's reproductive lifetime, sex steroids (Oestrogens and Progestogens - the two main classes of female steroids) result mainly from the process of ovarian steroidogenesis and only small amounts are being secreted by the peripheral compartments (e.g. adrenals, adipose tissue). This characteristic is maintained until menopause, when subsequent to a decline in ovarian synthesis, sex steroid plasmatic levels rely only to the less significant amounts produced peripherally. In the particular case of pregnant women, the pivotal role for steroid secretion shifts from ovaries to placenta.

Ovarian secretion of sex steroids during reproductive age follows a monthly cyclic evolution under the control of pituitary gonadotropins (Figure 1A). This precise central control of the ovarian function depends on the coordinated pulsatile secretions of the hypothalamic GnRH (Bouligand et al., 2009) and of pituitary gonadotropins. The decrease in sex steroids levels in menopause abolishes the normal negative feedback at the hypothalamus and pituitary glands, resulting in an over-secretion of gonadotropins, especially FSH (Figure 1B). The pharmacological basis of hormone replacement therapy is to compensate the decrease of estradiol production by ovaries in order to limit the adverse events due to sex steroids deficiency.

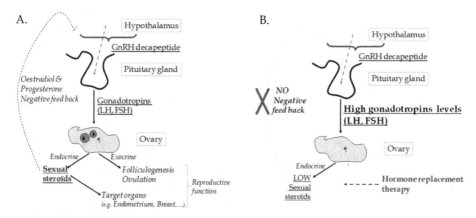

Fig. 1. The Hypothalamic-Pituitary-Gonadal (HPG) axis in women. A. Characteristics of HPG axis during the reproductive age. B. Changes in HPG axis following menopause.

Among the three forms of **natural circulating oestrogens** (i.e. estradiol, estriol and estrone, Figure 2), the main biological effect is exerted by estradiol, with a potency of approximately ten times that of estrone (Coldham et al., 1997; Van den Belt et al., 2004), while estriol exhibits the weakest estrogenic activity. In the second class of female sex steroids, **progesterone** represents the most important component, with significantly higher secreted levels than 17-hydroxyprogesterone, the other naturally occurring progestogen (Figure 2).

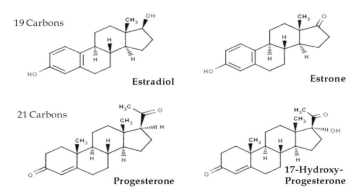

Fig. 2. Chemical Structure of Natural Sex Steroids

2.2 Mechanisms of action of sex steroids

The mechanisms by which oestrogen and progesterone exert their effects are complex (Figure 3A), and involve both classic pathways of hormone gene transcription through their cognate receptors, as well as "non-genomic" actions, the latter being characterized by significantly faster response rates (e.g. seconds, minutes).

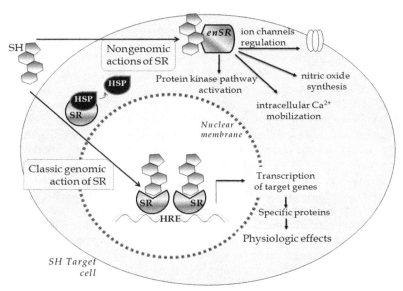

SH: steroid hormones (oestrogen, progesterone) ; SR: steroid receptor (ER, PR) ; enSR: extranuclear steroid receptors ; HSP: heat shock proteins ; HRE: hormone response elements.

Fig. 3.a. Sex steroids mechanism of action

Oestradiol and progesterone receptors (ERs and PRs respectively) belong to the large family of nuclear receptors (NRs), sharing several structural features (Loosfelt et al., 1986) and acting as transcriptional factors in a ligand dependent manner (For review, (Edwards, 2005).

Two major forms have been identified for each of the two types of ovarian steroid receptor, namely ERα and ERβ (Kuiper et al., 1996; Walter et al., 1985), and PR-A and PR-B respectively (Conneely et al., 1989; Huckaby et al., 1987; Kastner et al., 1990; Khan et al., 2011) (Figure 3B).

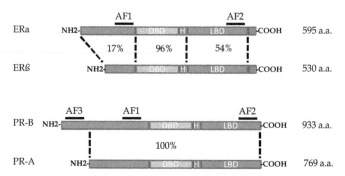

LBD: ligand binding domain; DBD: DNA binding domain; AF: transcription activation domain (AF-1, AF-2, AF-3); H: Hinge region, a.a. : amino-acids. The percentages indicate the amino acid identity between domains of ERα and ERβ and between A and B forms of PR.

Fig. 3.b. Domain structures of estrogen (ER) and progesterone (PR) receptors.

Most of ERs and PRs are constitutively localized in the nucleus in the absence of their ligands (Welshons et al., 1985), and nuclear localization signals have been described in the hinge region (Guiochon-Mantel et al., 1989; Picard et al., 1990). Due to their lipophilic nature, steroids will easily cross the cell membrane and bind to specific receptors, resulting in hormone-receptor complexes. Prior to ligand binding, receptors are inactive and associate protein complexes, among which the heat shock proteins (hsp) play important roles (e.g. hsp 90, hsp 70)(Pratt & Toft, 1997). But in the presence of their ligands, receptors undergo conformational changes with subsequent release of the associated protein complexes and bind to specific DNA sequences (hormone-response elements) from the promoter regions of target genes. The expression of target genes is thus modulated after interaction with various coregulators (Rosenfeld & Glass, 2001; Amazit et al., 2011). ERs and PRs bind DNA as dimers and have the ability to form both homodimers and heterodimers (ER$_{\alpha/\beta}$, PR$_{A/B}$ respectively)(Cowley et al., 1997; Leonhardt et al., 1998). Furthermore, the complexity of oestrogen and progesterone actions is enhanced by the growing body of evidence supporting the non-genomic mechanisms of steroid hormones action (Hammes & Levin, 2007; Levin, 2011; Losel & Wehling, 2003). These rapid effects may not be explained by the classic pathway and involve a variety of signalling events, such as the activation of various kinases, ion channels regulation and intracellular calcium mobilization or nitric oxide synthesis (Edwards, 2005; Madak-Erdogan et al., 2008). Responsible for generating these effects may be either membrane forms of classically ERs and PRs or alternative unrelated molecules (Wendler et al., 2010).

2.3 Physiological effects

Oestrogens and progestogens main effects concern the **reproductive organs**, initiating and supporting their development and functionality. Secondary sex characteristics are under the close control of gonadal steroids. During the reproductive lifetime of a woman, oestrogens dictate the proliferation of the uterine endometrium and the development of endometrial glands, while progesterone promotes secretory changes of the endometrium, in a process of preparation of the ideal milieu for implantation of the fertilized ovum. In the **breast,** oestrogens promote the development of the stromal and ductal systems together with fat deposition at this level, and progesterone induces the development of the secretory units of the breast, causing alveolar cells to proliferate.

Although the reproductive system represents the principal target for sex steroids, their effects are far from being limited only to this system. **Bone health,** for instance, is greatly influenced by oestrogens levels, as they play an important role in the process of bone remodelling. Under their action, skeletal resorption is diminished due to a decreased osteoclastic activity and by consequence, bone formation is promoted. Furthermore, a **cardioprotective** role exerted by ovarian steroids was inferred due to the significantly lower rates of cardiovascular diseases manifested by women prior to menopause compared to men and the cancelation of these gender differences following menopause. Several **metabolic effects** are also described, oestrogens slightly increasing the metabolic rate, promoting deposition of the fat in subcutaneous tissue and changing lipoprotein profiles by increasing HDL and decreasing LDL cholesterol (Edwards, 2005; Guyton & Hall, c2006).

3. Menopause principal consequences

Given the multitude of physiological effects exerted by sex steroids in women, it is not surprising that the hormonal changes related to menopause have been linked to a wide spectrum of symptoms and disorders. The most frequent menopausal symptoms include vasomotor disorders (e.g. hot flashes, night sweets), urogenital atrophy (e.g. vaginal dryness, urinary symptoms), or psychological disturbances (e.g. sleep disturbances, forgetfulness, mood changes or depression), all of which may seriously impact on women's quality of life. Decreased oestrogen levels in menopause result in an altered bone structure with reduced bone mineral density (BMD) and increased risk for subsequent fractures. Postmenopausal women, compared to the premenopausal period, are also more prone to develop cardiovascular disease (CVD), which represents the leading cause of death in women. Furthermore, the increased risk of dementia and Alzheimer disease in postmenopausal women was also partially attributed to endogenous oestradiol depletion (Yaffe et al., 2007).

If the aforementioned effects are present in women undergoing natural menopause, the magnitude of these consequences is even higher in POI women and the dimension of each long-term effect may vary in relation to the exact cause of POI and to the rapidity of apparition of the oestrogen deficit (e.g. women undergoing surgical oophorectomy will face a sudden decrease in steroids levels compared to women experiencing a spontaneous POI) (Maclaran et al., 2010). All-cause mortality rates in women appear to be associated with age at menopause, women entering menopause before 40 years having mortality rates twice as the ones seen in the 50-54 years group (Snowdon et al., 1989). Studies on the cardiovascular risk in POI demonstrated that several risk factors for CVD are influenced by a premature occurence of menopause (e.g. alteration of lipid profiles (Knauff et al., 2008), decreased insulin sensitivity(Corrigan et al., 2006) or the presence of metabolic syndrome (Eshtiaghi et al., 2010)). Moreover, the impaired endothelial function found in women with POI, precursor of more severe vascular abnormalities, was improved by hormonal replacement, further supporting the role of steroids in normal cardiovascular function (Kalantaridou et al., 2004). POI patients present with low BMD, which seems to be greatly influenced by the accelerated bone loss during the first 4-5 years of menopause (Amarante et al., 2011; Anasti et al., 1998; Gallagher, 2007; Uygur et al., 2005; van Der Voort et al., 2003), and hence having an increased risk of fractures compared to their peers who underwent a physiological menopause. Finally, an increased risk for cognitive impairment, dementia and Parkinson disease, inversely proportional with age at menopause, was reported in premature menopausal women following oophorectomy (Rocca et al., 2007, 2008).

4. Hormone replacement therapy

4.1 Basis for the hormone replacement therapy in menopause

When an installed hormonal deficiency generates symptoms in an individual, disturbing its well-being, it is expected that by adjusting the deficit, an improvement or even an offset of the symptoms should be reached (Wilson, [1966]). That was the hypothesis guiding clinicians decisions about substitution of ovarian steroids in menopause. Hormone replacement therapy (HRT) has been a common practice during the last decades, being initially used for both treatment of symptoms and prevention of chronic medical conditions related to menopause (e.g. heart and bone diseases). But 2002, the year when the first results from a large randomized and placebo-controlled trial (the Women Health Initiative – WHI) were published, marked a major change in both clinicians and patients perception towards the use of HRT(Rossouw et al., 2002). Conducted with the aim of evaluating HRT major benefits and risks, WHI results contradicted previous observational studies and showed an increased risk for cardiovascular events together with that of breast cancer rates in the studied population. Even if this resulted in a significant reduction in the use of HRT worldwide (Hersh et al., 2004; Lagro-Janssen et al., 2010; MacLennan et al., 2004), it represented also the subject to some major controversies. One major debate is the legitimacy of applying these conclusions to all women, when most of the women concerned by HRT prescription belong to the 50-54 years age group while participants in the WHI study had an average age of 63 years and a high body mass index. Thus, following the release of the first WHI report, various studies intended to better evaluate the real risks and benefits associated with HRT were conducted. The resulting body of evidence has led to the necessity of periodic revision of the existing recommendations and statements in this field (North American Menopause Society (NAMS) position statement, 2010; Santen et al., 2010; Sturdee et al., 2011).

4.2 Current recommendations

Current recommendations specify that HRT use should be restricted mainly to moderate or severe menopausal symptoms alleviation. It should not be used as a mean of chronic disease prevention and it is advisable to restrict treatment administration to the shortest period and the lowest dosage possible to control symptoms effectively. Nevertheless, in selected cases, HRT may be used to treat or to reduce the risk of diseases (e.g. osteoporosis). This involves HRT use *in prevention of further bone loss and/or reduction of osteoporotic fracture in menopausal women when alternate therapies are not appropriate or cause side effects* (NAMS position statement, 2010) or for *women younger than 60 years, with an increased risk of fracture* (Sturdee et al., 2011). In the particular case of women diagnosed with POI, HRT is recommended at least until the median age of natural menopause is reached (NAMS position statement, 2010).

4.3 Hormone replacement therapy regimens

4.3.1 Oestrogens and progestins in HRT

HRT comprises a variety of regimens, compounds, dosages and routes of administration. In most women, excepting hysterectomized patients, menopausal treatment requires preparations combining oestrogens with a progestin, the latter being used mainly to balance oestrogen's effects on the endometrium and to avoid endometrial hyperplasia and an increased risk of secondary carcinoma. This combination therapy may be administrated either in a sequential cyclic regimen or in a continuous one. The sequential regimen involves the alternation of a pure oestrogenic period to an oestro-progestative one, leading to withdrawal bleeding when the progestin administration is discontinued. This regimen is commonly administrated with a monthly cyclicity including at least 10 days of progestin treatment. Quarterly regimens are also available, involving progestin administration every 3 months, although in this case the risk for endometrial hyperplasia needs further evaluation. The continuous combined treatment implies the administration of both compounds on a daily basis and uses lower doses of progestin compared to the sequential regimen. This constitutes an option especially in older women not desiring a monthly withdrawal bleeding, even if uterine bleeding with unpredictable onset may not be excluded particularly during the first administrations (Doren, 2000; Ylikorkala & Rozenberg, 2000). Available formulations for the estrogens and progestins in HRT and their commonly used doses are listed in Table 1.

4.3.2 Other therapeutic options

Androgens are thought to play a role in maintaining a normal libido and sexual function in postmenopausal women and to potentially prevent the decline of bone quality, muscular force and cognitive function. Thus, after exclusion of other possible causes, androgen therapy represents an option for menopausal women with hypoactive sexual desire disorder undergoing concomitant oestrogen treatment, especially in those who have suffered a surgical menopause (Davis et al., 2008).

Tibolone is a synthetic compound with mixed oestrogenic, progestogenic and androgenic activities, representing an alternative to conventional HRT (Lazovic et al., 2008). It represents an efficient option for vasomotor symptoms alleviation or prevention of BMD loss in menopausal women (Gallagher et al., 2001; Swanson et al., 2006).

Another possible option in menopausal therapy refers to the **selective oestrogen receptor modulators (SERMs)**. These are pharmacologic agents characterised by variable oestrogen activity, acting as oestrogen agonists in some tissues while in other tissues they exert oestrogen antagonist effects. Examples of SERMs of interest in menopause treatment include raloxifene together with novel molecules like bazedoxifene, lasofoxifene or ospemifene.

Route	Oestrogens	Dosage
Oral	Conjugated estrogens (conjugated equine oestrogens)	0.625 mg
	Micronized 17 beta oestradiol	1, 2 mg
	Oestradiol valerate	1, 2 mg
	Estropipate (piperazine estrone sulphate)	0.75, 1.5, 3 mg
Transdermal	17 beta oestradiol (patch)	25, 37.5, 50, 75, 100 µg/day
	Oestradiol (gel)	1 mg/ 1g
Subcutaneous	Oestradiol (implant)	20, 50, 100 mg
Vaginal	Estriol (gel)	1mg/g
	Estradiol (tabs)	25µg
	Progestins	
Oral	Norethisterone acetate	0.5, 1 mg
	Medroxyprogesterone acetate	2.5, 5 mg
	Chlormadinone acetate	2, 5, 10 mg
	Drospirenone	2 mg
	Dydrogesterone	5, 10 mg
	Nomogestrol acetate	3.75, 5 mg
	Promegestone	0.125, 0.25, 0.5 mg
	Micronized progesterone	100, 200 mg
Transdermal	Levonorgestrel	7, 10µg/24h
Intrauterine	Levonorgestrel intrauterine device	20 µg/24h

Table 1. Commonly used oestrogens and progestins

4.4 Primary ovarian insufficiency: Particular requirements

Current publications highlight the lack of specifically designed HRT regimens for women with POI and the fact that existing observations from studies conducted on older women undergoing natural menopause should not be extrapolated to the much younger category of POI women. In the absence of a consensus regarding the ideal hormonal replacement regimen for women facing a premature cessation of the ovarian function, the oestro-progestative substitution commonly involves either HRT or combined oral contraceptive pills (COCP) prescription. Even if the use of the latter may be associated with a lower emotional impact for these patients, being perceived less as a treatment, it must be underlined that COCP standard preparations contain synthetic steroids in higher doses than the ones required for physiologic hormonal replacement in POI (Nelson et al., 2005). There is an urgent need to develop evidence-based guidelines relying on solid research in order to optimize the care of this group of women (Panay & Kalu, 2009).

4.5 Benefit versus risk of hormonal replacement therapy based 1 on the reviews of clinical studies

Despite the wide agreement that hormonal substitution remains the most effective option for the alleviation of menopausal symptoms, a careful evaluation of the benefit-risk balance is however essential prior to prescribing a HRT regimen because of its associated risks (Santen et al., 2010). The principal benefits and risks related to HRT in the light of recent evidences are further discussed in this paragraph.

The **cardiovascular events** represent the first cause of mortality in postmenopausal women and constituted a major subject of controversy regarding the use of HRT, an uncertainty accentuated by the discrepant results between randomised controlled trials (RCTs) (Hulley et al., 1998; Rossouw et al., 2002; Vickers et al., 2007) and observational studies (Bush et al., 1987; Grodstein et al., 1997; Stampfer et al., 1991). Initially, as expected from the physiological functions of oestrogens, several observational studies suggested a protective role of HRT on the cardiovascular system. Contrary to these observations, the WHI, a randomised, placebo-controlled trial, failed to validate the cardioprotective effect of HRT. The primary outcome of this study was related to the effects of menopausal substitution on the cardiovascular function and breast cancer risk, participants receiving either conjugated equine estrogens (CEE) alone (0.625mg/day) if hysterectomised (Anderson et al., 2004) or 0.625mg/day CEE in combination with 2.5mg/day medroxyprogesterone acetate (MPA) if they presented with an intact uterus (Rossouw et al., 2002). In an attempt to explain the disparity between these results the "timing hypothesis" arose as a possible answer, supported by differences between women enrolled in this study and those participating in observational studies (Grodstein et al., 2003). Thus, while the former included women more than a decade away from the onset of menopause, in the latter HRT was usually initiated shortly after menopause. Animal studies supported this hypothesis and demonstrated that the positive cardiovascular effects of hormonal substitution are inversely correlated with the delay of initiating the treatment (Clarkson, 2007). Several analysis, including some of the WHI subgroup data, tested the timing hypothesis and showed a trends towards a decreased risk in women younger and closer to menopause (Rossouw et al., 2007; Salpeter et al., 2006). Trials addressing specifically the effects of HRT in younger women (e.g. Kronos EarlyEstrogen Prevention Study (KEEPS) (Harman et al., 2005), Early Versus Late Intervention Trial With Estradiol (ELITE, NCT00114517) are currently under way and their results will probably shed a better light on these controversial facts.

Venous thromboembolism (VTE) is one of the major harmful effects of hormone therapy use among postmenopausal women (Olie et al., 2010). A recent meta-analysis on the risk of VTE in women using HRT indicated an increased risk by twofold to threefold when oral oestrogens were administrated (the combined relative risk (RR) from both trials and observational studies of 1.9 and confidence interval (CI) of 1.3 to 2.3, with a higher risk within the first year of treatment (Canonico, Plu-Bureau et al., 2008). When VTE risk was analysed in women receiving transdermal oestrogen, there was a combined RR of 1.0 (CI, 0.9 - 1.1). The impact of the route of administration on VTE risk and the recent pharmacogenetic studies providing support for the implication of the first pass effect in these different outcomes are detailed in chapter 5.

Musculoskeletal effects. Both observational studies (Cauley et al., 1995; Grodstein, Stampfer et al., 1999; Kiel et al., 1987) and RCTs (Cauley et al., 2003; Jackson et al., 2006; Lindsay et al., 2005) have proven HRT efficacy in reducing bone loss in menopausal women. Additionally, this positive effect appears to be present even when lower doses of oestrogen are used (Lindsay et al., 2005). However, rapidly after its discontinuation the protective effect on BMD is no longer evident. A recent study, evaluating hip fracture incidence after HRT cessation in a large cohort of 80.955 postmenopausal women, reported a significantly increased risk of hip fracture within only two years following HRT cessation compared to women who continued using HRT (Karim et al., 2011).

HRT and cancer risks. There is a large body of studies investigating the association between HRT and the risk for various types of cancer, primarily those hormone-dependent and particularly **breast cancer**. Breast cancer was one of the reasons for the premature discontinuation after 5.2 years of follow-up of the arm receiving combined HRT in the WHI trial, as the increased risk in breast cancer exceeded the stopping boundary for this adverse effect (RR 1.26; 95% CI 1.00-1.59) (Rossouw et al., 2002). Contrary to these findings, in the oestrogen-only group the relative risk was inferior compared to the control group (RR 0.77, 95% CI 0.57–1.06) (Anderson et al., 2004), suggesting that in addition to oestrogen, progestins have also a role in breast cancer pathophysiology. The risk of developing breast cancer increases with longer duration of HRT use (Beral, 2003; Fournier et al., 2008). One meta-analysis assessing the impact of HRT on the risk of invasive breast cancer in epidemiological studies and RCTs reported an increased annual risk for breast cancer varying between 0-9% in the case of E+P regimens and 0–3% in oestrogen-only administration (Greiser et al., 2005).

Although the risk of CHD was reported to increase when HRT is started a long time after the onset of menopause, the reverse situation seems to apply in the case of breast cancer. Data from the WHI trial supported this so called "gap time hypothesis" and reported an increased risk for breast cancer when HRT is started less than 5 years after the onset of menopause in both E (with a RR of 1.12 versus 0.58 when HRT was initiated less than 5 and respectively more than 5 years from menopause in women without a prior HRT use, or a relative risk (RR) of 1.00 versus 0.77 in women with prior HRT use) and E+P arms (with a RR of 1.77 versus 0.99 when HRT was initiated less than 5 and respectively more than 5 years from menopause in women without a prior HRT use, or a RR of 2.06 versus 1.30 in women with prior HRT use)(Prentice et al., 2009). The fact that ER positive breast tumours in postmenopausal women, but not in premenopausal ones, respond to treatment with high-dose oestrogen further supports this hypothesis and suggests that the decline in oestrogen levels associated with menopause may sensitize breast cancer cells to the proapoptotic effects of estrogen (Taylor & Manson, 2011).

Endometrial cancer (EC) constitutes another adverse effect linked to HRT use. The most common form of EC, the endometrioid (type I) variant, is generally hormonally responsive and women with an unbalanced oestrogen exposure are at increased risk for this form of EC. No risk increase was reported in women using a continuous combined HRT regimen, while the use of sequential HRT resulted in different risk profiles according to the duration of treatment (Jaakkola et al., 2011). Thus, when used for less than 5 years, the sequential E+P regimen showed a decreased risk for EC (RR 0.67, 95% CI 0.52-0.86), while continuing treatment after 5 years resulted in an increased risk for EC (RR 1.11,

95%CI 0.87-1.41 for the 5-10 years interval and RR 1.38, 95%CI 1.15-1.66 for an use exceeding 10 years).

Several studies reported an increased risk for **ovarian cancer** in women using HRT (Beral et al., 2007; Morch et al., 2009), with a stronger association in the case of unopposed oestrogen administration (Hildebrand et al., 2010). However, due to the small excess risk, the overall benefit-risk balance in HRT appears not to be significantly influenced by these results (Taylor & Manson, 2011).

Colorectal cancer. Observational studies have suggested an association between the use of HRT and a reduced incidence in colorectal cancer (Grodstein, Newcomb et al., 1999), an observation also validated by data from the E+P arm from the WHI trial (Chlebowski et al., 2004). However, despite a reduced overall rate, poor prognosis forms of colon cancer were diagnosed more frequently in women receiving HRT than in the placebo group. In contrast to the group receiving E+P, the reduced incidence of colorectal cancer was not found in the oestrogen-alone arm of WHI (Ritenbaugh et al., 2008). The relation between colorectal cancer and hormone exposure is further complicated by recent evidences suggesting that a greater endogenous estrogen exposure may increase the risk of colorectal cancer in postmenopausal women (Clendenen et al., 2009; Zervoudakis et al., 2011).

Finally, results from several studies comprising those of WHI (Chlebowski et al., 2009) have led to the inclusion of **lung cancer** on the list of potential adverse effects of HRT, although a neutral effect of HRT on lung cancer risk (Ayeni & Robinson, 2009) or even lower risks (Rodriguez et al., 2008) have been reported by others. Post-hoc analysis of WHI showed than even if the incidence of lung cancer in women using HRT did not increase, the number of death from lung cancer was significantly higher (in particular deaths from non-small-cell lung cancer) in women receiving combined HRT (Chlebowski et al., 2009), contrary to the use of oestrogen alone where the death rates were similar to the control group (Chlebowski et al., 2010).

The effect of HRT on a variety of conditions (e.g. mood disturbances, neurocognitive impairment, gallbladder disease, immune disorders, etc) have also been investigated. However, as either current evidences are insufficient or their impact on the overall benefit-risk balance is not significant, we will not detail them.

Particularities of the HRT benefit-risk balance in POI patients. Available results from studies evaluating HRT effects, especially its risks, do not address particularly the population of POI patients, but rather there is a tendency to apply to this group an extrapolation of findings from natural menopause, although there are evident differences in the HRT benefit-risk ratio between the two populations.

Cardiovascular and breast cancer risks, the two main adverse effects related to HRT use, need a special consideration in the context of women diagnosed with POI. First, the "timing hypothesis" for cardiovascular effects of HRT suggest a clear trend towards cardiovascular benefits in young women using HRT and hence, it is possible that the benefits in the younger POI patients might be even greater (Panay & Fenton, 2008). Secondly, the breast cancer risk profile differs in women undergoing a premature menopause compared to the general population. A younger age at menopause is protective against breast cancer regardless of whether the menopause was natural or surgical (Hulka & Moorman, 2008).

Thus, POI patients should be informed that results from reports on HRT associated breast cancer do not necessarily apply to their case, in which treatment is intended to provide the hormones that should be physiologically present at their age (Maclaran & Panay, 2011).

These particularities of the HRT risk profile in women facing a premature cessation of the ovarian function, together with the beneficial bone effects (Farquhar et al., 2009), support the current recommendations regarding the need for HRT substitution until the average age of natural menopause (Vujovic et al., 2010).

5. Pharmacology of hormone replacement therapy

The pharmacology of hormone replacement therapy is of a particular interest given the complex benefit/risk balance and the importance of this treatment for women health. As illustrated in previous paragraphs, there is a wide diversity of drugs and protocols proposed for HRT. Our analysis will be limited to the pharmacology of the natural sex steroid 17β-estradiol.

5.1 The route of oestradiol administration (oral versus transdermal) highlights the hepatic first pass effect

Oral oestradiol is commonly used by women receiving HRT, being seen as a convenient and inexpensive option. In turn, following oral administration, oestradiol is subject to the first-pass effect, a term that encompasses the metabolic changes underwent by a drug before it reaches systemic circulation. This results in the use of higher doses of oestradiol (~ 1,5 mg/day) compared to parenteral routes (patch ~ 50μg/24h). Moreover, subsequent to the various metabolic changes suffered by oestrogens once absorbed in the intestinal tract, a specific profile of oestradiol metabolites and oestrogen-dependent serum parameters with particular pathophysiological implications will appear, widely different from what is observed after the use of transdermal oestradiol where the first-pass effect is avoided.

The oestradiol metabolism pathway (Raftogianis et al., 2000) is outlined in Figure 4. Rapidly after the intestinal absorption, part of oral oestradiol is converted to oestrone, a reversible reaction catalysed by 17β-hydroxysteroid-dehydrogenase (HSD), and the conversion may continue towards their inactive conjugates (i.e. sulfates and glucuronides). Subsequent to this process, the oestrone/ oestradiol ratio resulting from oral administration is significantly higher (approximately 5:1) than the one observed following transdermal administration (approximately 1:1, which is similar to the physiologic ratio found in premenopausal women)(Kuhl, 2005). Contrary to the aforementioned transformations, further phase I reactions (oxidation reactions catalysed by cytochrome P450 (CYP) enzymes) are no more reversible. The final steps in oestrogen metabolism involve the process of detoxification under the action of phase II enzymes.

The first pass effect of oestradiol results in various biological consequences (De Lignieres et al., 1986). For instance, a well known effect attributed to hepatic first pass is the decrease of IGF-1 after oral oestradiol, whereas no significant change was observed with transdermal oestrogens (Sonnet et al., 2007). Furthermore, an increased synthesis of blood coagulation factors (Caine et al., 1992) and resistance to activated protein C (Oger et al., 2003) constitute another important consequences which are directly implicated in VTE pathophysiology, one of the major adverse events of oral oestrogens.

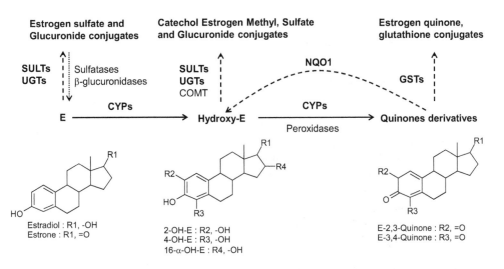

Various isoforms of cytochromes P450s (CYP3A, CYP1A and CYP1B families) activate estrogens during phase-1 metabolism. Oxidative metabolites, such as hydroxyestradiol and quinone derivatives, are conjugated by various phase-2 enzymes. The expression of several of these enzymes (SULTs, UGTs, GSTs and NQO1) is regulated by Nrf2. E: estradiol or estrone; CYPs: cytochrome P450s; UGTs: UDP-glucuronosyltransferase; COMT: catechol-o-methyltransferase; GSTs: glutathione S-transferases; NQO1: NAD(P)H dehydrogenase, quinone 1. Phase-1 metabolism is represented by horizontal arrows. Phase-2 metabolism is represented by vertical arrows (dashed).

Fig. 4. Oestrogens hepatic metabolism

5.2 Pharmacokinetic of oral *versus* transdermal oestrogens

The pharmacokinetics of exogenous estrogens is complex and most efficacy studies of transdermal *versus* oral oestrogens have not included the measurement of oestrogens concentrations. The oral route of oestradiol administration is easy and convenient, however the hormone is extensively metabolized in the gut and the liver leading to first-pass effect and, as previously mentioned, to a high estrone/oestradiol ratio (Kuhl, 2005). On the other hand, transdermal 17β-oestradiol is well absorbed through the epidermis and produces higher parent oestrogens serum concentrations and lower metabolites ratios because it bypasses the liver. Moreover, owing to a very low bioavailability [0.1 – 12%] of oral micronized 17β-oestradiol (O'Connell, 1995), higher doses are needed for the oral route compared to transdermal administration (O'Connell, 1995; Powers et al., 1985).

Pharmacokinetic profiles of transdermal and oral oestradiol are very different with oral administration producing fluctuant concentrations compared to the more constant levels achieved with transdermal formulations (Kopper et al., 2009). Interestingly, there is no pharmacokinetic/pharmacodynamic relationship between serum levels and positive effects of oestradiol treatment. It has been clearly shown that serum level after transdermal oestradiol does not predict the outcome when treating hot flushes (Steingold et al., 1985). The precise oestradiol and oestrone concentrations required to prevent bone loss and cardiovascular disease after either oral or transdermal oestrogen administration are also unknown (O'Connell, 1995).

5.3 Venous thromboembolism risk and HRT

As previously mentioned, VTE represents one of the main adverse effects of HRT in postmenopausal women (Canonico, Plu-Bureau et al., 2008; Cushman et al., 2004). Yet, while oral oestrogen was associated with a significantly increased risk for VTE, this was not observed in women treated with transdermal oestrogen (Canonico et al., 2010; Canonico et al., 2007; Olie et al., 2010; Scarabin et al., 2003; Straczek et al., 2005). An explanation for the distinct VTE risk profile following the two routes of administration involves the first-pass effect of oestrogen. This was shown to affect the synthesis of various oestrogen-dependent hepatic serum factors (Kuhl, 2005), including coagulation and fibrinolysis factors, resulting in blood coagulation activation (Scarabin et al., 1997; Vehkavaara et al., 2001), increased thrombin generation (Scarabin et al., 2011) or induction of resistance to activated protein C (Hemelaar et al., 2006; Oger et al., 2003). However, the precise mechanisms by which these changes occur are still unclear.

5.4 Pharmacogenetics: Genetics factors predisposing to venous thromboembolism (VTE) after oral oestradiol

Straczek et al. investigated the impact of the route of oestrogen administration on the association between a prothrombotic mutation (factor V Leiden or prothrombin G20210A mutation) and VTE risk. This study confirms the increase risk of VTE due to oral 17β-oestradiol in women presenting a genetic predisposition to VTE (Straczek et al., 2005). On the other hand, we have recently suggested that the hepatic metabolism of oestrogen may modulate the risk of VTE either through an increased phase I metabolism or through a decreased phase II metabolism. To address this important question, we have tested genetic polymorphisms capable to modulate oestradiol phase I or phase II liver metabolism. These polymorphisms do not increase the risk of VTE in the absence of HRT. First, we have demonstrated that increased expression of CYP3A5, a phase I enzyme of particular interest in oestrogen liver metabolism, in women carrying the CYP3A5*1 allele, is associated with a higher risk of VTE during oral oestrogen administration (RR 14.5; CI 2.8 - 73.9), without observing the same interaction in women receiving transdermal oestrogen (Canonico, Bouaziz et al., 2008). Further, we have investigated the association between VTE and nuclear factor (erythroid-derived 2)-like 2 (NFE2L2) polymorphisms (Bouligand et al., 2011). NFE2L2 gene encodes for a transcription factor also known as Nrf2 (NF-E2 related factor 2), essential for both maintenance and induction of phase II metabolism (Thimmulappa et al., 2002). One functional polymorphism (rs6721961) from the promoter region of NFE2L2 was described to be associated with an impaired auto-induction of this transcription factor (Marzec et al., 2007). The presence of this polymorphism may subsequently alter the expression of phase II genes, including those essential for the detoxification of oestrogen metabolites (see Figure 5) (Raftogianis et al., 2000). Our post-hoc analysis of the ESTHER Study (Canonico et al., 2007; Scarabin et al., 2003; Straczek et al., 2005) demonstrated the association between VTE risk and the NFE2L2 polymorphism (i.e. rs672196) in oral oestrogen users (RR 17.9; CI 3.7 – 85.7).

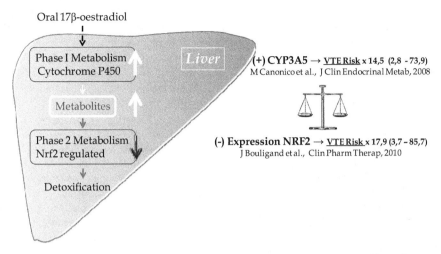

Fig. 5. Genetic polymorphisms modulating liver metabolism and first pass effect of oestrogens.

These pharmacogenetic studies provide new insights suggesting that liver metabolism of oestrogens may be implicated in the pathophysiology of VTE among women using HRT with oral oestrogen therapy. This original finding deserves further investigations in largest and independent series of women receiving oral 17β-oestradiol as well as other oestrogens with different metabolic pathways, not only to treat postmenopausal symptoms but also for contraception. Taking into account the proportion of women using exogenous hormone therapy, these new results may have important clinical implications to improve the stratification of thrombotic risk and identify new groups at high risk.

6. Conclusion

The increasing life expectancy observed during the last century, without an equivalent change in the average age of menopause, resulted in an increased number of women facing the effects of low ovarian steroids for a longer period of time. Thus, the high interest towards therapeutic options capable to alleviate menopausal symptoms and the extensive research in this field are not surprisingly. Despite the current controversies summarised here which encompass HRT use, further researches will likely improve therapeutic outcomes. In this context, pharmacogenetics studies play a key role in fulfilling the aim of providing patients with an individualised therapy which will reduce risks and improve benefits related to HRT.

7. References

Amarante, F., Vilodre, L. C., Maturana, M. A.& Spritzer, P. M. (2011). Women with primary ovarian insufficiency have lower bone mineral density. *Braz J Med Biol Res*, Vol. 44, No. 1, (Jan 2011), pp. 78-83.

Amazit, L., Roseau, A., Khan, J. A., Chauchereau, A., Tyagi, R. K., Loosfelt, H., Leclerc, P., Lombes, M.& Guiochon-Mantel, A. (2011). Ligand-dependent degradation of SRC-1 is pivotal for progesterone receptor transcriptional activity. *Mol Endocrinol*, Vol. 25, No. 3, (Mar 2011), pp. 394-408.

Anasti, J. N., Kalantaridou, S. N., Kimzey, L. M., Defensor, R. A.& Nelson, L. M. (1998). Bone loss in young women with karyotypically normal spontaneous premature ovarian failure. *Obstet Gynecol*, Vol. 91, No. 1, (Jan 1998), pp. 12-15.

Anderson, G. L., Limacher, M., Assaf, A. R., Bassford, T., Beresford, S. A., Black, H., Bonds, D., Brunner, R., Brzyski, R., Caan, B., Chlebowski, R., Curb, D., Gass, M., Hays, J., Heiss, G., Hendrix, S., Howard, B. V., Hsia, J., Hubbell, A., Jackson, R., Johnson, K. C., Judd, H., Kotchen, J. M., Kuller, L., LaCroix, A. Z., Lane, D., Langer, R. D., Lasser, N., Lewis, C. E., Manson, J., Margolis, K., Ockene, J., O'Sullivan, M. J., Phillips, L., Prentice, R. L., Ritenbaugh, C., Robbins, J., Rossouw, J. E., Sarto, G., Stefanick, M. L., Van Horn, L., Wactawski-Wende, J., Wallace, R.& Wassertheil-Smoller, S. (2004). Effects of conjugated equine estrogen in postmenopausal women with hysterectomy: the Women's Health Initiative randomized controlled trial. *JAMA*, Vol. 291, No. 14, (Apr 2004), pp. 1701-1712.

Ayeni, O.& Robinson, A. (2009). Hormone replacement therapy and outcomes for women with non-small-cell lung cancer: can an association be confirmed? *Curr Oncol*, Vol. 16, No. 3, (May 2009), pp. 21-25.

Bachelot, A., Rouxel, A., Massin, N., Dulon, J., Courtillot, C., Matuchansky, C., Badachi, Y., Fortin, A., Paniel, B., Lecuru, F., Lefrere-Belda, M. A., Constancis, E., Thibault, E., Meduri, G., Guiochon-Mantel, A., Misrahi, M., Kuttenn, F.& Touraine, P. (2009). Phenotyping and genetic studies of 357 consecutive patients presenting with premature ovarian failure. *Eur J Endocrinol*, Vol. 161, No. 1, (Jul 2009), pp. 179-187.

Beral, V. (2003). Breast cancer and hormone-replacement therapy in the Million Women Study. *Lancet*, Vol. 362, No. 9382, (Aug 2003), pp. 419-427.

Beral, V., Bull, D., Green, J.& Reeves, G. (2007). Ovarian cancer and hormone replacement therapy in the Million Women Study. *Lancet*, Vol. 369, No. 9574, (May 2007), pp. 1703-1710.

Bouligand, J., Cabaret, O., Canonico, M., Verstuyft, C., Dubert, L., Becquemont, L., Guiochon-Mantel, A.& Scarabin, P. Y. (2011). Effect of NFE2L2 genetic polymorphism on the association between oral estrogen therapy and the risk of venous thromboembolism in postmenopausal women. *Clin Pharmacol Ther*, Vol. 89, No. 1, (Jan 2011), pp. 60-64.

Bouligand, J., Ghervan, C., Tello, J. A., Brailly-Tabard, S., Salenave, S., Chanson, P., Lombes, M., Millar, R. P., Guiochon-Mantel, A.& Young, J. (2009). Isolated familial hypogonadotropic hypogonadism and a GNRH1 mutation. *N Engl J Med*, Vol. 360, No. 26, (Jun 2009), pp. 2742-2748.

Bush, T. L., Barrett-Connor, E., Cowan, L. D., Criqui, M. H., Wallace, R. B., Suchindran, C. M., Tyroler, H. A.& Rifkind, B. M. (1987). Cardiovascular mortality and noncontraceptive use of estrogen in women: results from the Lipid Research Clinics Program Follow-up Study. *Circulation*, Vol. 75, No. 6, (Jun 1987), pp. 1102-1109.

Caine, Y. G., Bauer, K. A., Barzegar, S., ten Cate, H., Sacks, F. M., Walsh, B. W., Schiff, I.& Rosenberg, R. D. (1992). Coagulation activation following estrogen administration to postmenopausal women. *Thromb Haemost*, Vol. 68, No. 4, (Oct 1992), pp. 392-395.

Canonico, M., Bouaziz, E., Carcaillon, L., Verstuyft, C., Guiochon-Mantel, A., Becquemont, L.& Scarabin, P. Y. (2008). Synergism between oral estrogen therapy and cytochrome P450 3A5*1 allele on the risk of venous thromboembolism among postmenopausal women. *J Clin Endocrinol Metab,* Vol. 93, No. 8, (Aug 2008), pp. 3082-3087.

Canonico, M., Fournier, A., Carcaillon, L., Olie, V., Plu-Bureau, G., Oger, E., Mesrine, S., Boutron-Ruault, M. C., Clavel-Chapelon, F.& Scarabin, P. Y. (2010). Postmenopausal hormone therapy and risk of idiopathic venous thromboembolism: results from the E3N cohort study. *Arterioscler Thromb Vasc Biol,* Vol. 30, No. 2, (Feb 2010), pp. 340-345.

Canonico, M., Oger, E., Plu-Bureau, G., Conard, J., Meyer, G., Levesque, H., Trillot, N., Barrellier, M. T., Wahl, D., Emmerich, J.& Scarabin, P. Y. (2007). Hormone therapy and venous thromboembolism among postmenopausal women: impact of the route of estrogen administration and progestogens: the ESTHER study. *Circulation,* Vol. 115, No. 7, (Feb 2007), pp. 840-845.

Canonico, M., Plu-Bureau, G., Lowe, G. D.& Scarabin, P. Y. (2008). Hormone replacement therapy and risk of venous thromboembolism in postmenopausal women: systematic review and meta-analysis. *BMJ,* Vol. 336, No. 7655, (May 2008), pp. 1227-1231.

Cauley, J. A., Robbins, J., Chen, Z., Cummings, S. R., Jackson, R. D., LaCroix, A. Z., LeBoff, M., Lewis, C. E., McGowan, J., Neuner, J., Pettinger, M., Stefanick, M. L., Wactawski-Wende, J.& Watts, N. B. (2003). Effects of estrogen plus progestin on risk of fracture and bone mineral density: the Women's Health Initiative randomized trial. *JAMA,* Vol. 290, No. 13, (Oct 2003), pp. 1729-1738.

Cauley, J. A., Seeley, D. G., Ensrud, K., Ettinger, B., Black, D.& Cummings, S. R. (1995). Estrogen replacement therapy and fractures in older women. Study of Osteoporotic Fractures Research Group. *Ann Intern Med,* Vol. 122, No. 1, (Jan 1995), pp. 9-16.

Chlebowski, R. T., Anderson, G. L., Manson, J. E., Schwartz, A. G., Wakelee, H., Gass, M., Rodabough, R. J., Johnson, K. C., Wactawski-Wende, J., Kotchen, J. M., Ockene, J. K., O'Sullivan, M. J., Hubbell, F. A., Chien, J. W., Chen, C.& Stefanick, M. L. (2010). Lung cancer among postmenopausal women treated with estrogen alone in the women's health initiative randomized trial. *J Natl Cancer Inst,* Vol. 102, No. 18, (Sep 2010), pp. 1413-1421.

Chlebowski, R. T., Schwartz, A. G., Wakelee, H., Anderson, G. L., Stefanick, M. L., Manson, J. E., Rodabough, R. J., Chien, J. W., Wactawski-Wende, J., Gass, M., Kotchen, J. M., Johnson, K. C., O'Sullivan, M. J., Ockene, J. K., Chen, C.& Hubbell, F. A. (2009). Oestrogen plus progestin and lung cancer in postmenopausal women (Women's Health Initiative trial): a post-hoc analysis of a randomised controlled trial. *Lancet,* Vol. 374, No. 9697, (Oct 2009), pp. 1243-1251.

Chlebowski, R. T., Wactawski-Wende, J., Ritenbaugh, C., Hubbell, F. A., Ascensao, J., Rodabough, R. J., Rosenberg, C. A., Taylor, V. M., Harris, R., Chen, C., Adams-Campbell, L. L.& White, E. (2004). Estrogen plus progestin and colorectal cancer in postmenopausal women. *N Engl J Med,* Vol. 350, No. 10, (Mar 2004), pp. 991-1004.

Clarkson, T. B. (2007). Estrogen effects on arteries vary with stage of reproductive life and extent of subclinical atherosclerosis progression. *Menopause,* Vol. 14, No. 3 Pt 1, (May-Jun 2007), pp. 373-384.

Clendenen, T. V., Koenig, K. L., Shore, R. E., Levitz, M., Arslan, A. A.& Zeleniuch-Jacquotte, A. (2009). Postmenopausal levels of endogenous sex hormones and risk of colorectal cancer. *Cancer Epidemiol Biomarkers Prev*, Vol. 18, No. 1, (Jan 2009), pp. 275-281.

Coldham, N. G., Dave, M., Sivapathasundaram, S., McDonnell, D. P., Connor, C.& Sauer, M. J. (1997). Evaluation of a recombinant yeast cell estrogen screening assay. *Environ Health Perspect*, Vol. 105, No. 7, (Jul 1997), pp. 734-742.

Colditz, G. A. (1993). Epidemiology of breast cancer. Findings from the nurses' health study. *Cancer*, Vol. 71, No. 4 Suppl, (Feb 1993), pp. 1480-1489.

Conneely, O. M., Kettelberger, D. M., Tsai, M. J., Schrader, W. T.& O'Malley, B. W. (1989). The chicken progesterone receptor A and B isoforms are products of an alternate translation initiation event. *J Biol Chem*, Vol. 264, No. 24, (Aug 1989), pp. 14062-14064.

Corrigan, E. C., Nelson, L. M., Bakalov, V. K., Yanovski, J. A., Vanderhoof, V. H., Yanoff, L. B.& Bondy, C. A. (2006). Effects of ovarian failure and X-chromosome deletion on body composition and insulin sensitivity in young women. *Menopause*, Vol. 13, No. 6, (Nov-Dec 2006), pp. 911-916.

Cowley, S. M., Hoare, S., Mosselman, S.& Parker, M. G. (1997). Estrogen receptors alpha and beta form heterodimers on DNA. *J Biol Chem*, Vol. 272, No. 32, (Aug 1997), pp. 19858-19862.

Cushman, M., Kuller, L. H., Prentice, R., Rodabough, R. J., Psaty, B. M., Stafford, R. S., Sidney, S.& Rosendaal, F. R. (2004). Estrogen plus progestin and risk of venous thrombosis. *JAMA*, Vol. 292, No. 13, (Oct 2004), pp. 1573-1580.

Davis, S. R., Moreau, M., Kroll, R., Bouchard, C., Panay, N., Gass, M., Braunstein, G. D., Hirschberg, A. L., Rodenberg, C., Pack, S., Koch, H., Moufarege, A.& Studd, J. (2008). Testosterone for low libido in postmenopausal women not taking estrogen. *N Engl J Med*, Vol. 359, No. 19, (Nov 2008), pp. 2005-2017.

De Lignieres, B., Basdevant, A., Thomas, G., Thalabard, J. C., Mercier-Bodard, C., Conard, J., Guyene, T. T., Mairon, N., Corvol, P., Guy-Grand, B.& et al. (1986). Biological effects of estradiol-17 beta in postmenopausal women: oral versus percutaneous administration. *J Clin Endocrinol Metab*, Vol. 62, No. 3, (Mar 1986), pp. 536-541.

Doren, M. (2000). Hormonal replacement regimens and bleeding. *Maturitas*, Vol. 34 Suppl 1, (Jan 2000), pp. S17-23.

Dossus, L., Allen, N., Kaaks, R., Bakken, K., Lund, E., Tjonneland, A., Olsen, A., Overvad, K., Clavel-Chapelon, F., Fournier, A., Chabbert-Buffet, N., Boeing, H., Schutze, M., Trichopoulou, A., Trichopoulos, D., Lagiou, P., Palli, D., Krogh, V., Tumino, R., Vineis, P., Mattiello, A., Bueno-de-Mesquita, H. B., Onland-Moret, N. C., Peeters, P. H., Dumeaux, V., Redondo, M. L., Duell, E., Sanchez-Cantalejo, E., Arriola, L., Chirlaque, M. D., Ardanaz, E., Manjer, J., Borgquist, S., Lukanova, A., Lundin, E., Khaw, K. T., Wareham, N., Key, T., Chajes, V., Rinaldi, S., Slimani, N., Mouw, T., Gallo, V.& Riboli, E. (2010). Reproductive risk factors and endometrial cancer: the European Prospective Investigation into Cancer and Nutrition. *Int J Cancer*, Vol. 127, No. 2, (Jul 2010), pp. 442-451.

Edwards, D. P. (2005). Regulation of signal transduction pathways by estrogen and progesterone. *Annu Rev Physiol*, Vol. 67, pp. 335-376.

Eshtiaghi, R., Esteghamati, A.& Nakhjavani, M. (2010). Menopause is an independent predictor of metabolic syndrome in Iranian women. *Maturitas*, Vol. 65, No. 3, (Mar 2010), pp. 262-266.

Farquhar, C., Marjoribanks, J., Lethaby, A., Suckling, J. A.& Lamberts, Q. (2009). Long term hormone therapy for perimenopausal and postmenopausal women. *Cochrane Database Syst Rev*, No. 2, pp. CD004143.

Fournier, A., Fabre, A., Mesrine, S., Boutron-Ruault, M. C., Berrino, F.& Clavel-Chapelon, F. (2008). Use of different postmenopausal hormone therapies and risk of histology- and hormone receptor-defined invasive breast cancer. *J Clin Oncol*, Vol. 26, No. 8, (Mar 2008), pp. 1260-1268.

Gallagher, J. C. (2007). Effect of early menopause on bone mineral density and fractures. *Menopause*, Vol. 14, No. 3 Pt 2, (May-Jun 2007), pp. 567-571.

Gallagher, J. C., Baylink, D. J., Freeman, R.& McClung, M. (2001). Prevention of bone loss with tibolone in postmenopausal women: results of two randomized, double-blind, placebo-controlled, dose-finding studies. *J Clin Endocrinol Metab*, Vol. 86, No. 10, (Oct 2001), pp. 4717-4726.

Greiser, C. M., Greiser, E. M.& Doren, M. (2005). Menopausal hormone therapy and risk of breast cancer: a meta-analysis of epidemiological studies and randomized controlled trials. *Hum Reprod Update*, Vol. 11, No. 6, (Nov-Dec 2005), pp. 561-573.

Grodstein, F., Clarkson, T. B.& Manson, J. E. (2003). Understanding the divergent data on postmenopausal hormone therapy. *N Engl J Med*, Vol. 348, No. 7, (Feb 2003), pp. 645-650.

Grodstein, F., Newcomb, P. A.& Stampfer, M. J. (1999). Postmenopausal hormone therapy and the risk of colorectal cancer: a review and meta-analysis. *Am J Med*, Vol. 106, No. 5, (May 1999), pp. 574-582.

Grodstein, F., Stampfer, M. J., Colditz, G. A., Willett, W. C., Manson, J. E., Joffe, M., Rosner, B., Fuchs, C., Hankinson, S. E., Hunter, D. J., Hennekens, C. H.& Speizer, F. E. (1997). Postmenopausal hormone therapy and mortality. *N Engl J Med*, Vol. 336, No. 25, (Jun 1997), pp. 1769-1775.

Grodstein, F., Stampfer, M. J., Falkeborn, M., Naessen, T.& Persson, I. (1999). Postmenopausal hormone therapy and risk of cardiovascular disease and hip fracture in a cohort of Swedish women. *Epidemiology*, Vol. 10, No. 5, (Sep 1999), pp. 476-480.

Guiochon-Mantel, A., Loosfelt, H., Lescop, P., Sar, S., Atger, M., Perrot-Applanat, M.& Milgrom, E. (1989). Mechanisms of nuclear localization of the progesterone receptor: evidence for interaction between monomers. *Cell*, Vol. 57, No. 7, (Jun 1989), pp. 1147-1154.

Guyton, A. C.& Hall, J. E. (c2006). *Textbook of medical physiology*, Elsevier Saunders, 0721602401, Philadelphia.

Hammes, S. R.& Levin, E. R. (2007). Extranuclear steroid receptors: nature and actions. *Endocr Rev*, Vol. 28, No. 7, (Dec 2007), pp. 726-741.

Harman, S. M., Brinton, E. A., Cedars, M., Lobo, R., Manson, J. E., Merriam, G. R., Miller, V. M., Naftolin, F.& Santoro, N. (2005). KEEPS: The Kronos Early Estrogen Prevention Study. *Climacteric*, Vol. 8, No. 1, (Mar 2005), pp. 3-12.

Hemelaar, M., Rosing, J., Kenemans, P., Thomassen, M. C., Braat, D. D.& van der Mooren, M. J. (2006). Less effect of intranasal than oral hormone therapy on factors associated with venous thrombosis risk in healthy postmenopausal women. *Arterioscler Thromb Vasc Biol*, Vol. 26, No. 7, (Jul 2006), pp. 1660-1666.

Hersh, A. L., Stefanick, M. L.& Stafford, R. S. (2004). National use of postmenopausal hormone therapy: annual trends and response to recent evidence. *JAMA*, Vol. 291, No. 1, (Jan 2004), pp. 47-53.

Hildebrand, J. S., Gapstur, S. M., Feigelson, H. S., Teras, L. R., Thun, M. J.& Patel, A. V. (2010). Postmenopausal hormone use and incident ovarian cancer: Associations differ by regimen. *Int J Cancer*, Vol. 127, No. 12, (Dec 2010), pp. 2928-2935.

Huckaby, C. S., Conneely, O. M., Beattie, W. G., Dobson, A. D., Tsai, M. J.& O'Malley, B. W. (1987). Structure of the chromosomal chicken progesterone receptor gene. *Proc Natl Acad Sci U S A*, Vol. 84, No. 23, (Dec 1987), pp. 8380-8384.

Hulka, B. S.& Moorman, P. G. (2008). Breast cancer: hormones and other risk factors. *Maturitas*, Vol. 61, No. 1-2, (Sep-Oct 2008), pp. 203-213; discussion 213.

Hulley, S., Grady, D., Bush, T., Furberg, C., Herrington, D., Riggs, B.& Vittinghoff, E. (1998). Randomized trial of estrogen plus progestin for secondary prevention of coronary heart disease in postmenopausal women. Heart and Estrogen/progestin Replacement Study (HERS) Research Group. *JAMA*, Vol. 280, No. 7, (Aug 1998), pp. 605-613.

Jaakkola, S., Lyytinen, H. K., Dyba, T., Ylikorkala, O.& Pukkala, E. (2011). Endometrial cancer associated with various forms of postmenopausal hormone therapy: a case control study. *Int J Cancer*, Vol. 128, No. 7, (Apr 2011), pp. 1644-1651.

Jackson, R. D., Wactawski-Wende, J., LaCroix, A. Z., Pettinger, M., Yood, R. A., Watts, N. B., Robbins, J. A., Lewis, C. E., Beresford, S. A., Ko, M. G., Naughton, M. J., Satterfield, S.& Bassford, T. (2006). Effects of conjugated equine estrogen on risk of fractures and BMD in postmenopausal women with hysterectomy: results from the women's health initiative randomized trial. *J Bone Miner Res*, Vol. 21, No. 6, (Jun 2006), pp. 817-828.

Kalantaridou, S. N., Naka, K. K., Papanikolaou, E., Kazakos, N., Kravariti, M., Calis, K. A., Paraskevaidis, E. A., Sideris, D. A., Tsatsoulis, A., Chrousos, G. P.& Michalis, L. K. (2004). Impaired endothelial function in young women with premature ovarian failure: normalization with hormone therapy. *J Clin Endocrinol Metab*, Vol. 89, No. 8, (Aug 2004), pp. 3907-3913.

Karim, R., Dell, R. M., Greene, D. F., Mack, W. J., Gallagher, J. C.& Hodis, H. N. (2011). Hip fracture in postmenopausal women after cessation of hormone therapy: results from a prospective study in a large health management organization. *Menopause*, (Jul 2011).

Kastner, P., Krust, A., Turcotte, B., Stropp, U., Tora, L., Gronemeyer, H.& Chambon, P. (1990). Two distinct estrogen-regulated promoters generate transcripts encoding the two functionally different human progesterone receptor forms A and B. *EMBO J*, Vol. 9, No. 5, (May 1990), pp. 1603-1614.

Kelsey, J. L.& Bernstein, L. (1996). Epidemiology and prevention of breast cancer. *Annu Rev Public Health*, Vol. 17, pp. 47-67.

Khan, J. A., Amazit, L., Bellance, C., Guiochon-Mantel, A., Lombes, M.& Loosfelt, H. (2011). p38 and p42/44 MAPKs Differentially Regulate Progesterone Receptor A and B Isoform Stabilization. *Mol Endocrinol*, (Aug 2011).doi:10.1210/me.2011-1042

Kiel, D. P., Felson, D. T., Anderson, J. J., Wilson, P. W.& Moskowitz, M. A. (1987). Hip fracture and the use of estrogens in postmenopausal women. The Framingham Study. *N Engl J Med,* Vol. 317, No. 19, (Nov 1987), pp. 1169-1174.

Knauff, E. A., Westerveld, H. E., Goverde, A. J., Eijkemans, M. J., Valkenburg, O., van Santbrink, E. J., Fauser, B. C.& van der Schouw, Y. T. (2008). Lipid profile of women with premature ovarian failure. *Menopause,* Vol. 15, No. 5, (Sep-Oct 2008), pp. 919-923.

Kopper, N. W., Gudeman, J.& Thompson, D. J. (2009). Transdermal hormone therapy in postmenopausal women: a review of metabolic effects and drug delivery technologies. *Drug Des Devel Ther,* Vol. 2, pp. 193-202.

Kuhl, H. (2005). Pharmacology of estrogens and progestogens: influence of different routes of administration. *Climacteric,* Vol. 8 Suppl 1, (Aug 2005), pp. 3-63.

Kuiper, G. G., Enmark, E., Pelto-Huikko, M., Nilsson, S.& Gustafsson, J. A. (1996). Cloning of a novel receptor expressed in rat prostate and ovary. *Proc Natl Acad Sci U S A,* Vol. 93, No. 12, (Jun 1996), pp. 5925-5930.

Lagro-Janssen, A., Knufing, M. W., Schreurs, L.& van Weel, C. (2010). Significant fall in hormone replacement therapy prescription in general practice. *Fam Pract,* Vol. 27, No. 4, (Aug 2010), pp. 424-429.

Lazovic, G., Radivojevic, U.& Marinkovic, J. (2008). Tibolone: the way to beat many a postmenopausal ailments. *Expert Opin Pharmacother,* Vol. 9, No. 6, (Apr 2008), pp. 1039-1047.

Leonhardt, S. A., Altmann, M.& Edwards, D. P. (1998). Agonist and antagonists induce homodimerization and mixed ligand heterodimerization of human progesterone receptors in vivo by a mammalian two-hybrid assay. *Mol Endocrinol,* Vol. 12, No. 12, (Dec 1998), pp. 1914-1930.

Levin, E. R. (2011). Minireview: Extranuclear steroid receptors: roles in modulation of cell functions. *Mol Endocrinol,* Vol. 25, No. 3, (Mar 2011), pp. 377-384.

Lindsay, R., Gallagher, J. C., Kleerekoper, M.& Pickar, J. H. (2005). Bone response to treatment with lower doses of conjugated estrogens with and without medroxyprogesterone acetate in early postmenopausal women. *Osteoporos Int,* Vol. 16, No. 4, (Apr 2005), pp. 372-379.

Loosfelt, H., Atger, M., Misrahi, M., Guiochon-Mantel, A., Meriel, C., Logeat, F., Benarous, R.& Milgrom, E. (1986). Cloning and sequence analysis of rabbit progesterone-receptor complementary DNA. *Proc Natl Acad Sci U S A,* Vol. 83, No. 23, (Dec 1986), pp. 9045-9049.

Losel, R.& Wehling, M. (2003). Nongenomic actions of steroid hormones. *Nat Rev Mol Cell Biol,* Vol. 4, No. 1, (Jan 2003), pp. 46-56.

Maclaran, K., Horner, E.& Panay, N. (2010). Premature ovarian failure: long-term sequelae. *Menopause Int,* Vol. 16, No. 1, (Mar 2010), pp. 38-41.

Maclaran, K.& Panay, N. (2011). Premature ovarian failure. *J Fam Plann Reprod Health Care,* Vol. 37, No. 1, (Jan 2011), pp. 35-42.

MacLennan, A. H., Taylor, A. W.& Wilson, D. H. (2004). Hormone therapy use after the Women's Health Initiative. *Climacteric,* Vol. 7, No. 2, (Jun 2004), pp. 138-142.

Madak-Erdogan, Z., Kieser, K. J., Kim, S. H., Komm, B., Katzenellenbogen, J. A.& Katzenellenbogen, B. S. (2008). Nuclear and extranuclear pathway inputs in the regulation of global gene expression by estrogen receptors. *Mol Endocrinol,* Vol. 22, No. 9, (Sep 2008), pp. 2116-2127.

Marzec, J. M., Christie, J. D., Reddy, S. P., Jedlicka, A. E., Vuong, H., Lanken, P. N., Aplenc, R., Yamamoto, T., Yamamoto, M., Cho, H. Y.& Kleeberger, S. R. (2007). Functional polymorphisms in the transcription factor NRF2 in humans increase the risk of acute lung injury. *FASEB J,* Vol. 21, No. 9, (Jul 2007), pp. 2237-2246.

McPherson, C. P., Sellers, T. A., Potter, J. D., Bostick, R. M.& Folsom, A. R. (1996). Reproductive factors and risk of endometrial cancer. The Iowa Women's Health Study. *Am J Epidemiol,* Vol. 143, No. 12, (Jun 1996), pp. 1195-1202.

Morch, L. S., Lokkegaard, E., Andreasen, A. H., Kruger-Kjaer, S.& Lidegaard, O. (2009). Hormone therapy and ovarian cancer. *JAMA,* Vol. 302, No. 3, (Jul 2009), pp. 298-305.

Nelson, L. M., Covington, S. N.& Rebar, R. W. (2005). An update: spontaneous premature ovarian failure is not an early menopause. *Fertil Steril,* Vol. 83, No. 5, (May 2005), pp. 1327-1332.

North American Menopause Society. Estrogen and progestogen use in postmenopausal women: 2010 position statement of The North American Menopause Society. (2010). *Menopause,* Vol. 17, No. 2, (Mar 2010), pp. 242-255.

O'Connell, M. B. (1995). Pharmacokinetic and pharmacologic variation between different estrogen products. *J Clin Pharmacol,* Vol. 35, No. 9 Suppl, (Sep 1995), pp. 18S-24S.

Oger, E., Alhenc-Gelas, M., Lacut, K., Blouch, M. T., Roudaut, N., Kerlan, V., Collet, M., Abgrall, J. F., Aiach, M., Scarabin, P. Y.& Mottier, D. (2003). Differential effects of oral and transdermal estrogen/progesterone regimens on sensitivity to activated protein C among postmenopausal women: a randomized trial. *Arterioscler Thromb Vasc Biol,* Vol. 23, No. 9, (Sep 2003), pp. 1671-1676.

Olie, V., Canonico, M.& Scarabin, P. Y. (2010). Risk of venous thrombosis with oral versus transdermal estrogen therapy among postmenopausal women. *Curr Opin Hematol,* Vol. 17, No. 5, (Sep 2010), pp. 457-463.

Panay, N.& Fenton, A. (2008). Premature ovarian failure: a growing concern. *Climacteric,* Vol. 11, No. 1, (Feb 2008), pp. 1-3.

Panay, N.& Kalu, E. (2009). Management of premature ovarian failure. *Best Pract Res Clin Obstet Gynaecol,* Vol. 23, No. 1, (Feb 2009), pp. 129-140.

Picard, D., Kumar, V., Chambon, P.& Yamamoto, K. R. (1990). Signal transduction by steroid hormones: nuclear localization is differentially regulated in estrogen and glucocorticoid receptors. *Cell Regul,* Vol. 1, No. 3, (Feb 1990), pp. 291-299.

Powers, M. S., Schenkel, L., Darley, P. E., Good, W. R., Balestra, J. C.& Place, V. A. (1985). Pharmacokinetics and pharmacodynamics of transdermal dosage forms of 17 beta-estradiol: comparison with conventional oral estrogens used for hormone replacement. *Am J Obstet Gynecol,* Vol. 152, No. 8, (Aug 1985), pp. 1099-1106.

Pratt, W. B.& Toft, D. O. (1997). Steroid receptor interactions with heat shock protein and immunophilin chaperones. *Endocr Rev,* Vol. 18, No. 3, (Jun 1997), pp. 306-360.

Prentice, R. L., Manson, J. E., Langer, R. D., Anderson, G. L., Pettinger, M., Jackson, R. D., Johnson, K. C., Kuller, L. H., Lane, D. S., Wactawski-Wende, J., Brzyski, R., Allison, M., Ockene, J., Sarto, G.& Rossouw, J. E. (2009). Benefits and risks of postmenopausal hormone therapy when it is initiated soon after menopause. *Am J Epidemiol,* Vol. 170, No. 1, (Jul 2009), pp. 12-23.

Raftogianis, R., Creveling, C., Weinshilboum, R.& Weisz, J. (2000). Estrogen metabolism by conjugation. *J Natl Cancer Inst Monogr*, No. 27, pp. 113-124.

Ritenbaugh, C., Stanford, J. L., Wu, L., Shikany, J. M., Schoen, R. E., Stefanick, M. L., Taylor, V., Garland, C., Frank, G., Lane, D., Mason, E., McNeeley, S. G., Ascensao, J.& Chlebowski, R. T. (2008). Conjugated equine estrogens and colorectal cancer incidence and survival: the Women's Health Initiative randomized clinical trial. *Cancer Epidemiol Biomarkers Prev*, Vol. 17, No. 10, (Oct 2008), pp. 2609-2618.

Rocca, W. A., Bower, J. H., Maraganore, D. M., Ahlskog, J. E., Grossardt, B. R., de Andrade, M.& Melton, L. J., 3rd. (2007). Increased risk of cognitive impairment or dementia in women who underwent oophorectomy before menopause. *Neurology*, Vol. 69, No. 11, (Sep 2007), pp. 1074-1083.

Rocca, W. A., Bower, J. H., Maraganore, D. M., Ahlskog, J. E., Grossardt, B. R., de Andrade, M.& Melton, L. J., 3rd. (2008). Increased risk of parkinsonism in women who underwent oophorectomy before menopause. *Neurology*, Vol. 70, No. 3, (Jan 2008), pp. 200-209.

Rodriguez, C., Spencer Feigelson, H., Deka, A., Patel, A. V., Jacobs, E. J., Thun, M. J.& Calle, E. E. (2008). Postmenopausal hormone therapy and lung cancer risk in the cancer prevention study II nutrition cohort. *Cancer Epidemiol Biomarkers Prev*, Vol. 17, No. 3, (Mar 2008), pp. 655-660.

Rosenfeld, M. G.& Glass, C. K. (2001). Coregulator codes of transcriptional regulation by nuclear receptors. *J Biol Chem*, Vol. 276, No. 40, (Oct 2001), pp. 36865-36868.

Rossouw, J. E., Anderson, G. L., Prentice, R. L., LaCroix, A. Z., Kooperberg, C., Stefanick, M. L., Jackson, R. D., Beresford, S. A., Howard, B. V., Johnson, K. C., Kotchen, J. M.& Ockene, J. (2002). Risks and benefits of estrogen plus progestin in healthy postmenopausal women: principal results From the Women's Health Initiative randomized controlled trial. *JAMA*, Vol. 288, No. 3, (Jul 2002), pp. 321-333.

Rossouw, J. E., Prentice, R. L., Manson, J. E., Wu, L., Barad, D., Barnabei, V. M., Ko, M., LaCroix, A. Z., Margolis, K. L.& Stefanick, M. L. (2007). Postmenopausal hormone therapy and risk of cardiovascular disease by age and years since menopause. *JAMA*, Vol. 297, No. 13, (Apr 2007), pp. 1465-1477.

Salpeter, S. R., Walsh, J. M., Greyber, E.& Salpeter, E. E. (2006). Brief report: Coronary heart disease events associated with hormone therapy in younger and older women. A meta-analysis. *J Gen Intern Med*, Vol. 21, No. 4, (Apr 2006), pp. 363-366.

Santen, R. J., Allred, D. C., Ardoin, S. P., Archer, D. F., Boyd, N., Braunstein, G. D., Burger, H. G., Colditz, G. A., Davis, S. R., Gambacciani, M., Gower, B. A., Henderson, V. W., Jarjour, W. N., Karas, R. H., Kleerekoper, M., Lobo, R. A., Manson, J. E., Marsden, J., Martin, K. A., Martin, L., Pinkerton, J. V., Rubinow, D. R., Teede, H., Thiboutot, D. M.& Utian, W. H. (2010). Postmenopausal hormone therapy: an Endocrine Society scientific statement. *J Clin Endocrinol Metab*, Vol. 95, No. 7 Suppl 1, (Jul 2010), pp. s1-s66.

Scarabin, P. Y., Alhenc-Gelas, M., Plu-Bureau, G., Taisne, P., Agher, R.& Aiach, M. (1997). Effects of oral and transdermal estrogen/progesterone regimens on blood coagulation and fibrinolysis in postmenopausal women. A randomized controlled trial. *Arterioscler Thromb Vasc Biol*, Vol. 17, No. 11, (Nov 1997), pp. 3071-3078.

Scarabin, P. Y., Hemker, H. C., Clement, C., Soisson, V.& Alhenc-Gelas, M. (2011). Increased thrombin generation among postmenopausal women using hormone therapy:

importance of the route of estrogen administration and progestogens. *Menopause,* Vol. 18, No. 8, (Aug 2011), pp. 873-879.

Scarabin, P. Y., Oger, E.& Plu-Bureau, G. (2003). Differential association of oral and transdermal oestrogen-replacement therapy with venous thromboembolism risk. *Lancet,* Vol. 362, No. 9382, (Aug 2003), pp. 428-432.

Shuster, L. T., Rhodes, D. J., Gostout, B. S., Grossardt, B. R.& Rocca, W. A. (2010). Premature menopause or early menopause: long-term health consequences. *Maturitas,* Vol. 65, No. 2, (Feb 2010), pp. 161-166.

Simon, T., Beau Yon de Jonage-Canonico, M., Oger, E., Wahl, D., Conard, J., Meyer, G., Emmerich, J., Barrellier, M. T., Guiraud, A.& Scarabin, P. Y. (2006). Indicators of lifetime endogenous estrogen exposure and risk of venous thromboembolism. *J Thromb Haemost,* Vol. 4, No. 1, (Jan 2006), pp. 71-76.

Snowdon, D. A., Kane, R. L., Beeson, W. L., Burke, G. L., Sprafka, J. M., Potter, J., Iso, H., Jacobs, D. R., Jr.& Phillips, R. L. (1989). Is early natural menopause a biologic marker of health and aging? *Am J Public Health,* Vol. 79, No. 6, (Jun 1989), pp. 709-714.

Sonnet, E., Lacut, K., Roudaut, N., Mottier, D., Kerlan, V.& Oger, E. (2007). Effects of the route of oestrogen administration on IGF-1 and IGFBP-3 in healthy postmenopausal women: results from a randomized placebo-controlled study. *Clin Endocrinol (Oxf),* Vol. 66, No. 5, (May 2007), pp. 626-631.

Stampfer, M. J., Colditz, G. A., Willett, W. C., Manson, J. E., Rosner, B., Speizer, F. E.& Hennekens, C. H. (1991). Postmenopausal estrogen therapy and cardiovascular disease. Ten-year follow-up from the nurses' health study. *N Engl J Med,* Vol. 325, No. 11, (Sep 1991), pp. 756-762.

Steingold, K. A., Laufer, L., Chetkowski, R. J., DeFazio, J. D., Matt, D. W., Meldrum, D. R.& Judd, H. L. (1985). Treatment of hot flashes with transdermal estradiol administration. *J Clin Endocrinol Metab,* Vol. 61, No. 4, (Oct 1985), pp. 627-632.

Straczek, C., Oger, E., Yon de Jonage-Canonico, M. B., Plu-Bureau, G., Conard, J., Meyer, G., Alhenc-Gelas, M., Levesque, H., Trillot, N., Barrellier, M. T., Wahl, D., Emmerich, J.& Scarabin, P. Y. (2005). Prothrombotic mutations, hormone therapy, and venous thromboembolism among postmenopausal women: impact of the route of estrogen administration. *Circulation,* Vol. 112, No. 22, (Nov 2005), pp. 3495-3500.

Sturdee, D. W., Pines, A., Archer, D. F., Baber, R. J., Barlow, D., Birkhauser, M. H., Brincat, M., Cardozo, L., de Villiers, T. J., Gambacciani, M., Gompel, A. A., Henderson, V. W., Kluft, C., Lobo, R. A., MacLennan, A. H., Marsden, J., Nappi, R. E., Panay, N., Pickar, J. H., Robinson, D., Simon, J., Sitruk-Ware, R. L.& Stevenson, J. C. (2011). Updated IMS recommendations on postmenopausal hormone therapy and preventive strategies for midlife health. *Climacteric,* Vol. 14, No. 3, (Jun 2011), pp. 302-320.

Swanson, S. G., Drosman, S., Helmond, F. A.& Stathopoulos, V. M. (2006). Tibolone for the treatment of moderate to severe vasomotor symptoms and genital atrophy in postmenopausal women: a multicenter, randomized, double-blind, placebo-controlled study. *Menopause,* Vol. 13, No. 6, (Nov-Dec 2006), pp. 917-925.

Taylor, H. S.& Manson, J. E. (2011). Update in hormone therapy use in menopause. *J Clin Endocrinol Metab,* Vol. 96, No. 2, (Feb 2011), pp. 255-264.

Thimmulappa, R. K., Mai, K. H., Srisuma, S., Kensler, T. W., Yamamoto, M.& Biswal, S. (2002). Identification of Nrf2-regulated genes induced by the chemopreventive agent sulforaphane by oligonucleotide microarray. *Cancer Res,* Vol. 62, No. 18, (Sep 2002), pp. 5196-5203.

Uygur, D., Sengul, O., Bayar, D., Erdinc, S., Batioglu, S.& Mollamahmutoglu, L. (2005). Bone loss in young women with premature ovarian failure. *Arch Gynecol Obstet,* Vol. 273, No. 1, (Nov 2005), pp. 17-19.

Van den Belt, K., Berckmans, P., Vangenechten, C., Verheyen, R.& Witters, H. (2004). Comparative study on the in vitro/in vivo estrogenic potencies of 17beta-estradiol, estrone, 17alpha-ethynylestradiol and nonylphenol. *Aquat Toxicol,* Vol. 66, No. 2, (Feb 2004), pp. 183-195.

van Der Voort, D. J., van Der Weijer, P. H.& Barentsen, R. (2003). Early menopause: increased fracture risk at older age. *Osteoporos Int,* Vol. 14, No. 6, (Jul 2003), pp. 525-530.

Vehkavaara, S., Silveira, A., Hakala-Ala-Pietila, T., Virkamaki, A., Hovatta, O., Hamsten, A., Taskinen, M. R.& Yki-Jarvinen, H. (2001). Effects of oral and transdermal estrogen replacement therapy on markers of coagulation, fibrinolysis, inflammation and serum lipids and lipoproteins in postmenopausal women. *Thromb Haemost,* Vol. 85, No. 4, (Apr 2001), pp. 619-625.

Vickers, M. R., MacLennan, A. H., Lawton, B., Ford, D., Martin, J., Meredith, S. K., DeStavola, B. L., Rose, S., Dowell, A., Wilkes, H. C., Darbyshire, J. H.& Meade, T. W. (2007). Main morbidities recorded in the women's international study of long duration oestrogen after menopause (WISDOM): a randomised controlled trial of hormone replacement therapy in postmenopausal women. *BMJ,* Vol. 335, No. 7613, (Aug 2007), pp. 239.

Vujovic, S., Brincat, M., Erel, T., Gambacciani, M., Lambrinoudaki, I., Moen, M. H., Schenck-Gustafsson, K., Tremollieres, F., Rozenberg, S.& Rees, M. (2010). EMAS position statement: Managing women with premature ovarian failure. *Maturitas,* Vol. 67, No. 1, (Sep 2010), pp. 91-93.

Walter, P., Green, S., Greene, G., Krust, A., Bornert, J. M., Jeltsch, J. M., Staub, A., Jensen, E., Scrace, G., Waterfield, M.& et al. (1985). Cloning of the human estrogen receptor cDNA. *Proc Natl Acad Sci U S A,* Vol. 82, No. 23, (Dec 1985), pp. 7889-7893.

Welshons, W. V., Krummel, B. M.& Gorski, J. (1985). Nuclear localization of unoccupied receptors for glucocorticoids, estrogens, and progesterone in GH3 cells. *Endocrinology,* Vol. 117, No. 5, (Nov 1985), pp. 2140-2147.

Wendler, A., Baldi, E., Harvey, B. J., Nadal, A., Norman, A.& Wehling, M. (2010). Position paper: Rapid responses to steroids: current status and future prospects. *Eur J Endocrinol,* Vol. 162, No. 5, (May 2010), pp. 825-830.

WHO Report. Research on the menopause in the 1990s. Report of a WHO Scientific Group. (1996). *World Health Organ Tech Rep Ser,* Vol. 866, pp. 1-107.

Wilson, R. A. ([1966]). *Feminine forever,* M. Evans; distributed in association with Lippincott, New York.

Yaffe, K., Barnes, D., Lindquist, K., Cauley, J., Simonsick, E. M., Penninx, B., Satterfield, S., Harris, T.& Cummings, S. R. (2007). Endogenous sex hormone levels and risk of cognitive decline in an older biracial cohort. *Neurobiol Aging,* Vol. 28, No. 2, (Feb 2007), pp. 171-178.

Ylikorkala, O.& Rozenberg, S. (2000). Efficacy and tolerability of fully transdermal hormone replacement in sequential or continuous therapy at two doses of progestogen in postmenopausal women. *Maturitas,* Vol. 37, No. 2, (Dec 2000), pp. 83-93.

Zervoudakis, A., Strickler, H. D., Park, Y., Xue, X., Hollenbeck, A., Schatzkin, A.& Gunter, M. J. (2011). Reproductive history and risk of colorectal cancer in postmenopausal women. *J Natl Cancer Inst,* Vol. 103, No. 10, (May 2011), pp. 826-834.

3

Pharmacological Neuromodulation in Autism Spectrum Disorders

Bill J. Duke
Child Psychopharmacology Institute
USA

1. Introduction

This chapter will examine pharmacological approaches to neuromodulation in Autism Spectrum Disorders (ASD), pharmacological clinical trials and pharmacological strategies on the horizon.

Drugs used in autism target neuromodulation at different neuronal sites. Those utilizing anti-convulsant, neurolepic, anti-depressant, stimulant, cholinesterase inhibitors, anxiolytics, mood stabilizers and other pharmacological interventions in autism do so for a variety of purposes. Each of these classes of drugs will be examined relative to their proposed neuromodulatory actions as they relate to the Autism Spectrum Disorder population.

Children with ASD demonstrate deficits in 1) social interaction, 2) verbal and nonverbal communication, and 3) repetitive behaviors or interests. Many have unusual sensory responses. Symptoms range from mild to severe and present with individual uniqueness and complexity. Some aspects of learning may seem exceptional while others may lag. These children reflect a mix of communication, social, and behavioral patterns that are individual but fit into the overall diagnosis of ASD. Aggression, irritability and/or self-injury in children with autistic spectrum disorders often meet the threshold indicating pharmacological intervention.

Autism Spectrum Disorders have been shown to be related to complex combinations of environmental, neurological, immunological, and genetic factors. In addition to strong genetic links, environmental factors such as infection and drug exposure during pregnancy, perinatal hypoxia, postnatal infections and metabolic disorders have each been implicated in autistic populations. Summarizing an earlier Centers for Disease Control and Prevention Study (CDC) with subsequent major studies on autism prevalence, the CDC estimates 2-6 per 1,000 (from 1 in 500 to 1 in 150) children have an ASD. The risk is 3-4 times higher in males than females (Rice 2006)(CDC 2011).

The pathogenetic components and biological endophenotypes in autism spectrum disorders were described by Sacco and colleagues as: Circadian & Sensory Dysfunction; Immune Dysfunction; Neurodevelopmental Delay; and Stereotypic Behavior (Sacco R, et al 2010).

The heterogeneity of Autism Spectrum Disorders has resulted in many genes being studied that are thought to have an impact on the development of the pathological characteristics associated with Autism Spectrum Disorder (Greer PL, et al 2010). The developmental neurobiology of ASD is incrementally illuminated at the cutting edges of science. The permutations of mutations and epigenetic effects in ASD are both daunting yet increasingly identifiable targets for pharmacologic intervention. Clinical necessity and clincial trials drive discoveries for therapeutic interventions until stem cell or genetic solutions arrive.

Some states or effects seen in ASD may be responsive to developmental interventions while others may not. As we know, prompt thyroid replacement in a hypothyroid infant will generally allow normative intellectual development and prevent developmental disability. An example of variation of developmental impact is a mutation in MECP2, which encodes the epigenetic regulator methyl-CpG-binding protein 2 and is associated with Rett Syndrome. A recent study asked the question whether providing MeCP2 function exclusively during early post-natal life might prevent or mitigate disease in adult animals. Re-expression of MeCP2 in symptomatic mice rescued several features of the disease. The investigators argue "...the temporal association of disease with the postnatal period of development may be unrelated to any 'developmental' or stage restricted function of MeCP2, at least in mouse models." They concluded that "...therapies for RTT, like MeCP2 function must be continuously maintained" (McGraw, et al 2011).

Genetic-environment interactions in ASD that continue to be investigated include: parental age; maternal genotype; maternal-fetal immunoreactivity; in vitro fertilization; maternal ingestion of drugs; toxic chemicals in the environment during pregnancy; and maternal illnesses during pregnancy such as maternal diabetes or infections (Hallmayer J, 2011) . Recent studies are consistent with a fetal programming hypothesis of ASD that considers environmental risk factors that affect the fetal environment and interact with genetic variants (Szatmari 2011). The pathogenic potential of dysregulated states may further stress developmentally vulnerable neurodevelopment (Duke, B. , 2008).

As these genes and interacting effects become better characterized therapeutic strategies can be developed (Buxbaum 2009) (Levy et al, 2011)(Sanders et al, 2011)(Gilman et al, 2011). These genes include those involved in the patterning of the central nervous system; those that govern biochemical pathways; those responsible for the development of dendrites and synapses; and, genes associated with the immune system and autoimmune disorders (Ashwood et al, 2006) (Careaga M et al, 2010).

Neuroimaging studies further enlighten our theoretical models and techniques such as diffusion tensor imaging (DTI) have gained prominence as a means of assessing brain development (Isaacson & Provenzale, 2011). Studies of emotional perception demonstrated that while listening to either happy or sad music, individuals with ASD activated cortical and subcortical brain regions known to be involved in emotion processing and reward. The investigators, using functional magnetic resonance imaging compared ASD participants with neurotypical individuals and found ASD individuals had decreased brain activity in the premotor area and in the left anterior insula, especially in response to happy music excerpts. Their findings illuminate our understanding of the neurobiological correlates of preserved and altered emotional processing in ASD (Caria A, et al 2011).

Other imaging studies have found: diminished gray matter within the hypothalamus in autism disorder and suggest this is a potential link to hormonal effects (Kurth F, et al 2011); elevated repetitive and stereotyped behavior (RSB) associated with decreased volumes in several brain regions: left thalamus, right globus pallidus, left and right putamen, right striatum and a trend for left globus pallidus and left striatum within the ASD group (Estes A, et al 2011); alterations in frontal lobe tracts and corpus callosum in young children with autism spectrum disorder (Kumar A, et al 2010); and, revealed pervasive microstructural abnormalities (Groen WB, et al 2011).

As our theoretical constructs are tested and enriched clinical scientists are poised to learn exponentially as treatment response databases and measurement methods and systems are further developed. We are ready to experience an evolution and fusion of medical arts strengthened by scientific methods and information technology.

Psychopharmacological treatment guidelines for very young children suggest that children with persistent moderate to severe symptoms and impairment, despite psychotherapeutic interventions, may be better served by carefully monitored medication trials than by continuing ineffective treatments (Gleason MM, et al 2007).

The treatment of children with ASD has challenges that are also present in the treatment of many mood disorders and in schizophrenia. In Stephen Stahl's text, Essential Psychopharmacology (Stahl 2010), he deconstructs the syndrome of schizophrenia into five symptom dimensions: Positive and Negative symptoms, aggression, affect and cognition. These symptom dimensions are also relevant to children with ASD and many children with mood disorders. Individual presentations and variability of treatment response can be managed by enlisting the parents to be observers utilizing defined measurements.

Multiple medications have utility in ASD treatment and are sometimes used in combination. Thoughtful utilization and management of medications can offer children with autism spectrum disorders significiant reductions of impairment. Each of the medications used, as true with any medication, has varying degrees and potential related to benefits, risk and limitations. Although the antipsychotic risperidone has been demonstrated as effective in reducing serious behavioral problems, it shares adverse neurological and metabolic risks with other typical and atypical antipsychotic agents. Nevertheless, risperidone has demonstrated efficacy at relatively low doses and treatment monitoring can assist in managing risks when substantial benefit is possible.

Antidepressants have been reported as helpful for some with ASD, particularly related to repetitive or obsessive compulsive behaviors, however, studies reviewing off-label uses of anti-depressants have also reported adverse effects of increased agitation, behavioral activation and sleep disturbance. If we consider these findings as evidence suggesting antidepressants, in some, perturb inhibitory- excitatory neuronal balance or, in a broad sense, contribute to central nervous system hyperarousal, it follows that such effects could contribute to pathogenesis rather than decrease the allostatic load. This does not suggest that anti-depressant medications can't be helpful. It is recognized that in many cases antidepressants are helpful; however, vigilance for signs of disinhibition or other dysregulation is prudent.

Known stimulant benefits include increased ability to sustain attention, reduced motoric hyperactivity and reduced impulsivity. Adverse effects associated with stimulants include dysphoric responses, sleep disturbances and appetite supression.

Anticonvulsants have demonstrated their place in the treatment regimen of many children with ASD and approximately twenty percent of those with ASD are thought to have a seizure disorder (Tuchman & Cuccaro, 2011). Benefits can include seizure control and mood stabilization while adverse effects can include cognitive dulling. When anticonvulsants are useful, cognitive dulling can often be managed by anticonvulsant selection and dosing.

Current pharmacological interventions in autism spectrum disorders are essentially directed at reducing cognitive and behavioral impairments. Treatment studies have demonstrated little observable benefit to core deficits of ASD, however, the argument is made that, in addition to the practical benefits of reducing behavioral and cognitive impairments, symptom reduction is a reflection of more efficient neural processing and development.

Effective impairment reduction often allows children to remain in a family home, function in a school setting, optimize reponsiveness to behavioral and educational methods and, generally, function more normally than would otherwise be possible. Those of us who treat children who will otherwise be excluded from normal environments appreciate the importance and complexity of these interventions. The greater promise of pharmacological interventions is their potential, through early intervention, to inhibit or reduce the development of pathological and pathogenic endophenotypes.

2. Conceptualization of clinical hypotheses, treatment strategies and measurement of treatment response

Physicians and clinician- scientists are humbled distinguishing among nosological categories in the context of the diverse and complex treatment circumstances presented by those significantly impaired within the spectrum of autism disorders.

Treatment decisions are based on symptom profiles, types and severity of impairment, risk-benefit calculations, potential treatments available and clinical hypotheses related to the nature of the disorder. Unlike elegantly designed experiments with exquisitely defined variables and thoughtful control of confounding variables, those suffering functional and qualitative impairment present with inherent experimental limitations. Despite these limitations, the application of scientific principles related to individual measurement and monitoring of treatment response provides a platform from which to assess treatment response and dynamically test clinical hypotheses.

The deconstruction of psychiatric syndromes into symptoms is described as a way to establish a diagnosis, deconstruct the condition into its symptoms, match the symptoms to a hypothetically malfunctioning circuit and consider the collection of neurotransmitters and neuromodulators known to regulate the circuit. "Next, one can match each symptom to a hypothetically malfunctioning circuit and – with knowledge of the neurotransmitters regulating that circuit and drugs acting on those neurotransmitters – choose a therapeutic agent to reduce that symptom. If such a strategy proves unsuccessful, it is possible that adding or switching to another agent acting on another neurotransmitter in that circuit can be effective. Repeating this strategy for each symptom can result in remission of all symptoms in many patients." (Stahl, 2010)

Knowledge gained in the study of abnormal circuitry in mood disorders, schizophrenia and other neuropsychiatric and neurological conditions provide models by which treatment responses and clinical hypotheses can be tested. Whether the symptoms are hyperkinetic movement disorders or hyperactive mesolimbic systems, pharmacological strategies can inform and interact with the rapidly developing basic and translational sciences. Dysregulation of neuronal inhibition and excitability appears as a common theme among many disorders.

Consideration of the pathological developmental aspects of autism spectrum disorders provokes the possibility that altering disease progression may rescue or support improved functional neurodevelopmental outcomes. In a broad statement regarding psychiatric disorders that supports that potential, Stephen Stahl remarks, "It may also be possible to prevent disease recurrence and progression to treatment resistance by treating not only symptoms but also inefficient brain circuits that are asymptomatic. Failing to do so may allow 'diabolical learning' where circuits run amok, become more efficient in learning how to mediate symptoms, and are therefore more difficult to treat." (Stahl, 2010, p. 274)

The lessons and theoretical models related to pharmacological interventions in other neurological and psychiatric syndromes can be applied to treatment conceptualizations with the autistic spectrum disordered as well. For example, constructs investigated with antiepileptic drugs (AED) can also be considered within the neural circuitry issues involved in Autism Spectrum Disorders.

"Several pathophysiological mechanisms inducing a neuronal excitability seems to be involved in an imbalance of both GABAergic and glutamatergic neurotransmissions and therefore could be similar in epilepsy and hyperkinetic movement disorders. The main targets for the action of the AEDs include enhancement of GABAergic inhibition, decreased glutamatergic excitation, modulation of voltage-gated sodium and calcium channels, and effects on intracellular signaling pathways. All of these mechanisms are of importance in controlling neuronal excitability in different ways." (Siniscalchi, Gallelli & De Sarro, 2010)

When pharmacological interventions are applied, secondary to their clinical intent, they serve as probes of endophenotypic neural functioning and circuitry states revealing response to particular pharmacodynamic and pharmacokinetic profiles. The classes of antipsychotic drugs considered to be atypical are described by Schwartz with such considerations in mind.

"The second generation antipsychotics are clearly delineated in the treatment of psychosis and mania and share similar mechanisms of action to achieve these results: dopamine-2 receptor antagonism for efficacy and serotonin-2a receptor antagonism for EPS tolerability. From here, each agent has a unique pharmacodynamic and pharmacokinetic profile where some agents carry more, or less antidepressant, anxiolytic, or hypnotic profiles. Choosing an agent and dosing it in low, middle, or high ranges may result in differential effectiveness and tolerability" (Schwartz & Stahl, 2011).

We are further humbled by the incomplete pharmacodynamic and pharmacokinetic profiles of the drugs we employ. Many of the drugs and compounds used have poorly understood neuromodulary effects in addition to known receptor specific actions. Nevertheless, contributions to our knowledge continue to further characterize and define drugs as well as continue to discover relationships of enviromental effects and immunological response. Researchers, for example, have recently shown the inhibitory effects of some antidepressants as well as some typical/atypical antipsychotics on the release of inflammatory cytokines and free radicals from activated microglia, which the investigators state have been discovered to cause synaptic pathology, a decrease in neurogenesis, and white matter abnormalities found in the brains of patients with psychiatric disorders. (Monji A, 2011). We operate with limited visibility that is increased by clinical experience and science.

Despite the complexity and challenges of ASD, potential for early interventions are supported by animal research. An example is the recent demonstration that autism risk genes differentially impact cortical development (Eagleson K, et al 2011). The demonstrations of these risk genes and their interaction with various states, illustrate animal models that may further elucidate pathogenic developmental processes. The role of glutamate (Hamberger A, et al 1992), serotonin (Levitt P, 2011) and sigma 1 ligands (Yagasaki Y, et al 2006) have each demonstrated potential importance in modulating glutamatergic and other developmentally critical signaling processes.

In autism spectrum disorders as well as in other neurological and neurodegenerative disorders, discoveries in developmental neurobiology and genetics will continue to provide increasingly sophisticated models in which interventions of developmentally specific neuropathogenic processes can be assessed and clinical hypotheses considered and tested. Coinciding are increasingly sophisticated objective measures that will allow greater definition of treatment response characteristics and endophenotypic response profiles. Applications related to treatment response measurement and management utilizing on-line observational and other measurements related to eye, facial, voice, reaction time consistency, sleep and activity are currently being studied and developed at the Child Psychopharmacolgy Institute.

3. Registered clinical trials (NIH- USA) in autism spectrum disorders

We can learn a great deal from the current foci of pharmacological interventions in ASD by reviewing clinical trials that have been conducted and those that are current.

	Frequency	Percent
Drug Studies	151	53.5
Behavioral Studies	43	15.2
Dietary Studies	18	6.4
Device or Procedure Studies	5	1.8
Obervational and Other Studies	65	23.0
Total	282	100.0

Table 1. ASD Study Types- NIH Registrations of Record July 2011

Drug Classes Used In Autism Spectrum Disorder Clinical Trials
Antidepressant
Stimulant
Anticonvulsant
Antipsychotic
NMDA Antagonists And Glutamatergic
Antibacterial Anti-Infective
Immunomodulator
Hyperbaric Oxygen
Hormone Or Enzyme Factors
Adrenergic
Anti-Hypertensive
Diruretic
Opioid Antagonist
Anti-Oxidants
Hypoglycemic Agents
Supplements
GABA B Recepter Agonist
Trichuris Suis Ova
Antidote Heavy Metal
Ampa Receptor Modulator
Anxioytic

Table 2. Drug Classes Used in Autism Spectrum Disorder July 2011 NIH

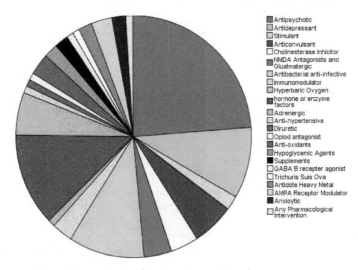

Fig. 1. Spectrum of Drug Classes in Autism Spectrum Disorders

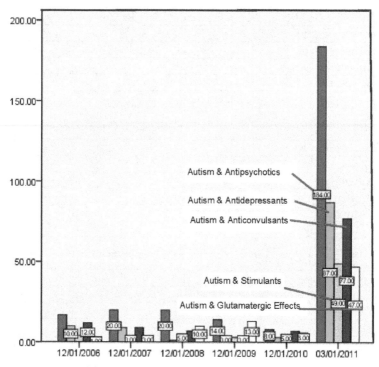

Fig. 2. NLM Clinical Trial Reviews 2006 to 2011

Table 3 displays a sampling of drugs in clinical trials and their generally proposed actions.

Antipsychotic Drugs
Risperidone is a selective blocker of dopamine d2 receptors and serotonin 5-ht2 receptors that acts as an atypical antipsychotic agent.
Aripiprazole has both presynaptic dopamine autoreceptor agonistic activity and postsynaptic D2 receptor antagonistic activity; use associated with hyperglycemia. It can also be described as a Dopamine Partial Agonist.
Ziprasidone -antipsychotic-A benzisothiazoylpiperazine derivative; has combined dopamine and serotonin receptor antagonist activity; structurally related to tiospirone.
Zyprexa (olanzapine) has combined dopamine and serotonin receptor antagonist activity.
Antidepressant Drugs
Fluoxetine: serotonin specific uptake inhibitor
Citalopram serotonin specific uptake inhibitor. The drug is also effective in reducing ethanol uptake in alcoholics and is used in depressed patients who also suffer from tardive dyskinesia
The SSRI fluvoxamine is not only an inhibitor of SERT, but also acts at sigma receptors, perhaps as a sigma-1 agonist, with some preclinical evidence that fluvoxamine can improve PCP-induced cognitive deficits
Atomoxetine: norepinephrine selective reuptake inhibitor.

Anticonvulsant Drugs
Divalproex sodium: A fatty acid with anticonvulsant properties used in the treatment of epilepsy. The mechanisms of its therapeutic actions are not well understood. It may act by increasing gamma-aminobutyric acid levels in the brain.
Riluzole: A glutamate antagonist (receptors, glutamate) used as an anticonvulsant (anticonvulsants) and to prolong the survival of patients with amyotrophic lateral sclerosis.
Lamotrigine,Sodium Valproate, or Carbamazepine: Anticonvulsants
Stimulant Drugs
Methylphenidate is a racemic mixture comprised of the d- and l-threo enantiomers. The d-threo enantiomer is more pharmacologically active than the l-threo enantiomer. Methylphenidate HCl is a central nervous system (CNS) stimulant.
Methylphenidate transdermal system: Methylphenidate HCl is a central nervous system (CNS) stimulant.
Choline and Cholinesterase Inhibitors
Choline: Precursor to Acetylcholine
Donepezil: Current theories on the pathogenesis attribute some symptoms to a deficiency of cholinergic neurotransmission. Donepezil hydrochloride is postulated to exert its therapeutic effect by inhibiting AChe boosting the availability of ACh.
Drugs with Glutaminergic Effects, AMPA Modulators and NMDA Antagonists
Acamprosate is a derivative of the amino acid taurine and, like alcohol, reduces excitatory glutamate neurotransmission and enhances inhibitory GABA neurotransmission
Memantine: a weak NMDA antagonist. Persistent activation of central nervous system N-methyl-D-aspartate (NMDA) receptors by the excitatory amino acid glutamate has been hypothesized to contribute to the symptomatology of Alzheimer's disease.
Dextromethorphan and quinidine sulfate (Nuedexta): NMDA antagonist; Sigma 1 agonist; binds to SERT; proposed neuromodulator.
Hormones
Oxytocin: A nonapeptide hormone released from the neurohypophysis (pituitary gland, posterior). it differs from vasopressin by two amino acids at residues 3 and 8.
Vasopressin
Anti-infective-Anti-bacterial-Immunomodulators
N Acetylcysteine N-acetyl derivative of cysteine. It is used as a mucolytic agent to reduce the viscosity of mucous secretions. It has also been shown to have antiviral effects in patients with HIV due to inhibition of viral stimulation by reactive oxygen.
Cycloserine Antibiotic substance produced by Streptomyces garyphalus.
Sapropterin: reduces blood phenylalanine (Phe) levels in patients with hyperphenylalaninemia (HPA) due to tetrahydrobiopterin- (BH4-) responsive Phenylketonuria (PKU). Proposed Neuroprotective and neurotransmitter effects.
Mecobalamin: a study (PMID: 20406575) demonstrated a progressive decrease of sciatic nerve IGF-1 mRNA and peptide contents, and peripheral nerve dysfunction in the saline-treated diabetics over 12 weeks in contrast to the normal control non-diabetics.

Table 3. Sampling of Drugs in ASD Clinical Trials and Their Generally Proposed Actions

Study of Aripiprazole to Treat Children and Adolescents With Autism	Phase II	The Clinical Global impression (CGI) Improvement Scale.; The Irritability subscale of the Aberrant Behavior Checklist (ABC); The Clinical Global Impression Severity Scale.
A Study of Aripiprazole in Children and Adolescents With Aspergers and Pervasive Developmental Disorder.	Phase II	The Clinical Global impression(CGI) Improvement Scale.; The Irritability subscale of the Aberrant Behavior Checklist (ABC); The Clinical Global Impression Severity Scale.;CY-BOCS (Children's Yale-Brown Obsessive Compulsive Scale)
Study of Aripiprazole in the Treatment of Serious Behavioral Problems in Children and Adolescents With Autistic Disorder (AD)	Phase III	Number of Participants With Serious Adverse Events (SAEs), Treatment-Emergent Adverse Events (AEs), Deaths, AEs Leading to Discontinuation, Extra Pyramidal Syndrome (EPS)-Related AEs; Mean Change From Baseline in Total Simpson-Angus Scale (SAS)
Aripiprazole in Children With Autism: A Pilot Study	Phase II	Clinical Global Impressions; Children's Psychiatric Rating Scale
An Open-Label Trial of Aripiprazole in Autism Spectrum Disorders	Phase II	Clinical Global Impressions-Improvement; Aberrant Behavior Checklist-Irritability subscale
Pilot Study of the Effect of Aripiprazole Treatment in Autism Spectrum Disorders on Functional Magnetic Resonance Imaging (fMRI) Activation Patterns and Symptoms	Phase IV	RBS-R (Repetitive Behavior Scale - Revised); CY-BOCS (Children's Yale-Brown Obsessive Compulsive Scale)
OPT - Phase IV Long Term Maintenance Study of Aripiprazole for the Treatment of Irritability Associated With Autistic Disorder	Phase IV	Time from randomization to relapse; Mean change from end of Phase 1 to Week 16 endpoint (LOCF) on the Aberrant Behavior Checklist - Irritability Subscale; Mean Clinical Global Impression - Improvement scale score at Week 16 endpoint (LOCF)
Study of Aripiprazole in the Treatment of Children and Adolescents With Autistic Disorder (AD)	Phase III	Mean Change (Week 8 - Baseline) in the Autistic Behavior Checklist (ABC) Irritability Subscale Score; Mean Clinical Global Impressions Improvement Scale (CGI-I) Score; Number of Participants With Response at Week 8; Mean Change (Week 8 - Baseline)
Study of Aripiprazole in the Treatment of Children and Adolescents With Autistic Disorder (AD)	Phase III	Mean Change (Week 8 - Baseline) in the Autistic Behavior Checklist (ABC) Irritability Subscale Score; Mean Clinical Global Impressions Improvement Scale (CGI-I) Score; Number of Participants With Response at Week 8; Mean Change (Week 8 - Baseline)

Evaluating the Effectiveness of Aripiprazole and D-Cycloserine to Treat Symptoms Associated With Autism	Phase III	Aberrant Behavior Checklist (ABC) Irritability Subscale; Clinical Global Impression (CGI) Scale; ABC Subscales; Vineland Maladaptive Behavior Subscales; A modified version of the Compulsion Subscale of the Children's Yale-Brown Obsessive Compulsive Scale.
Efficacy of Aripiprazole Versus Placebo in the Reduction of Aggressive and Aberrant Behavior in Autistic Children	Phase I	Clinical Global Impression Improvement (CGI-AD); Aberrant Behavior Checklist; Abnormal Involuntary Movement Scale (AIMS)
Long-Term Olanzapine Treatment in Children With Autism	Phase II Phase III	Children's Psychiatric Rating Scale; Aberrant Behavior Checklist; Clinical Global Impressions; Treatment Emergent Symptoms Scale; Olanzapine Untoward Effects Checklist; Abnormal Involuntary Movement Scale; Neurological Rating Scale

Table 4. Antipsychotic Clinical Trials, Trial Phase and Outcome Measures (Continued on table 5)

A Controlled Study of Olanzapine in Children With Autism	Phase II	Children's Psychiatric Rating Scale; Clinical Global Impressions; Abberant Behavior Checklist; Treatment Emergent Symptoms Scale; Olanzapine Untoward Effects Checklist; Abnormal Involuntary Movement Scale; Neurological Rating Scale
Study of Paliperidone ER in Adolescents and Young Adults With Autism	Phase III	The IrritablIrritibility subscale of the Aberrant Behavior Checklist (ABC) will be used as the caregiver-rated primary outcome measure. The Clinical Global Impression- Improvement(CGI-I) will be included as a primary outcome measure
A Study of the Effectiveness and Safety of Two Doses of Risperidone in the Treatment of Children and Adolescents With Autistic Disorder	Phase IV	Allocation: Randomized; Endpoint Classification: Safety/Efficacy Study; Intervention Model: Parallel Assignment; Masking: Double Blind (Subject, Caregiver, Investigator); Primary Purpose: Treatment
A Study of the Effectiveness and Safety of Risperidone Versus Placebo in the Treatment of Children With Autistic Disorder and Other Pervasive Developmental Disorders (PDD)	Phase III	Change in the Irritability Subscale of the Aberrant Behavior Checklist (ABC) and other ABC subscales at end of treatment compared with baseline; Change from baseline to end of treatment in Nisonger Child Behavior Rating Form (N-CBRF), Visual Analogue Scale

Pharmacogenomics in Autism Treatment	Phase II Phase III	ABC and CGI; ABC
Treatment of Autism in Children and Adolescents	Phase III	
Risperidone Pharmacokinetics in Children With Pervasive Developmental Disorder (PDD)	Phase I	Quantify tVariability of clearance and volume of distribution among AE rating, weight gain and ABC responder status; Exploratory analysis will be performed to examine the relationship of other factors to risperidone and metabolite concentrations.
Pharmacogenetics of Risperidone in Children With Pervasive Developmental Disorder (PDD)	Phase I	
Comparison of Applied Behavioral Analysis (ABA) Versus ABA and Risperidone		
RUPP PI PDD: Drug and Behavioral Therapy for Children With Pervasive Developmental Disorders		Home Situations Questionnaire; Vineland Daily Living Skills Scale; Irritability subscale-Aberrant Behavioral Checklist; Clinical Global Impressions-Improvement (CGI-I)
Risperidone Treatment In Children With Autism Spectrum Disorder And High Levels Of Repetitive Behavior	Phase II	Aberrant Behavior Checklist
Ziprasidone in Children With Autism: A Pilot Study	Phase II	Clinical Global Impressions; Children's Psychiatric Rating Scale
An Observational Study to Evaluate the Safety and the Effects of Risperidone Compared With Other Atypical Antipsychotic Drugs on the Growth and Sexual Maturation in Children		To comparZ-scores for height, age at current Tanner stage, and prolactin-related adverse events between patients exposed to risperidone and patients exposed to other atypical antipsychotic drugs.; Assess the prolactin value and risk of hyperprolactine

Table 5. Antipsychotic Clinical Trials, Trial Phase and Outcome Measures (Continued)

Citalopram for Children With Autism and Repetitive Behavior (STAART Study 1)	Phase II	Clinical Global Improvement; Safety Monitoring Uniform Research Form (SMURF); Children's Yale-Brown Obsessive-Compulsive Scale (CYBOCS); Repetitive Behavior Scale-Revised (RBS-R); Parent Chief Complaint; Aberrant Behavior Checklist;
Functional MRI Evaluation of the Effect of Citalopram in Autism Spectrum Disorders	PhaseI	Functional Magnetic Resonance Imaging; Clinicians Global Improvement Scale; Childrens Yale- Brown Obsessive Compulsive Scale
Randomized Study of Fluoxetine in Children and Adolescents With Autism	Phase I	
Study of Fluoxetine in Adults With Autistic Disorder	PhaseI	
Extended Management and Measurement of Autism	Phase III	Safety Outcomes: Laboratory determinations, Urine drugs of abuse tests,Vital Signs,Physical Examinations, Adverse Events/Serious Adverse Events, Clinical Global Impression of Severity (CGI-S AD)
Fluoxetine Essay in Children With Autism	Phase II	Subscores of Autism Diagnostic Interview (ADI-R)at each visit of the protocol (LECOUTER et RUTTER, 1989); Sides effect scale (FSEC); Aberrant Behavior Checklist (Aman et al., 1985); Clinical Global Impressions (CGI) severity and improvement.
Study of Fluoxetine in Autism	Phase III	The percentage change from baseline to the endpoint visit for the CYBOCS-PDD score; The time and dose related course of therapeutic effects; The inter-relationship between these effects in the context of global clinical changes; The indirect effect.
Effectiveness of Early Intervention With Fluoxetine in Enhancing Developmental Processes in Children With Autism (STAART Study 2)	Phase III	Feasibility and safety of conducting placebo control trial of fluoxetine; Side effect and drop out evaluation
Fluvoxamine and Sertraline in Childhood Autism - Does SSRI Therapy Improve Behaviour and/or Mood?	Phase III	The severity of the autistic child's behaviour or condition (assessed by parents); Weight and vital signs; Blood count and liver function studies
Mirtazapine Treatment of Anxiety in Children and Adolescents With Pervasive Developmental Disorders	Phase III	Pediatric Anxiety Rating Scale (PARS); Clinical Global Impressions (CGI)

Table 6. Antidepressant Clinical Trials, Trial Phase and Outcome Measures

Methylphenidate for Attention Deficit Hyperactivity Disorder and Autism in Children	Phase III	Conners' Teacher Rating Scale-Revised (CTRS-R); Continuous Performance Test (CPT); Matching Familiar Figures Test (MFFT); Speeded Classification Task (SCT); Delay of Gratification Task (DOG); Conners' Parent Rating Scale (CPRS)-Short Form;
A Pilot Study of Daytrana TM in Children With Autism Co-Morbid for Attention Deficit Hyperactivity Disorder (ADHD) Symptoms	Phase III	Determine if Daytrana is safe and well-tolerated by children with Autism co-morbid for ADHD; Determine if Daytrana is effective in both school and home

Table 7. Stimulant Clinical Trials, Trial Phase and Outcome Measures

Divalproex Sodium ER vs Placebo in Childhood/Adolescent Autism valproex Sodium vs. Placebo in Childhood/Adolescent Autism	Phase II	Clinical Global Impression-Improvement; Aberrant Behavior Checklist Clinical Global Impression-Improvement; Aberrant Behavior Checklist; Clinical Global Impression-Improvement; Aberrant Behavior Checklist
Divalproex Sodium ER in Adult Autism	Phase IV	
A Study of Divalproex Sodium in Children With ASD and Epileptiform EEG	Phase II	epileptiform EEG discharges; Improvement in behavior
Oxcarbazepine Versus Placebo in Childhood Autism	1	Vineland Adaptive Behavior Scales; Aberrant Behavior Checklist; Clinical Global Impression Improvement Scale; Autism Diagnostic Observation Schedule
Riluzole to Treat Child and Adolescent Obsessive-Compulsive Disorder With or Without Autism Spectrum Disorders	Phase II	Reduction of 30% or more in Children's Yale-Brown Obsessive-Compulsive Scale (CY-BOCS) and Repetitive Behavior Scale; Much/Very much improved on Clinical Global Impressions - Improvement score (CGI-I)
Valproate Response in Aggressive Autistic Adolescents	Phase III	

Table 8. Anticonvulsant Clinical Trials, Trial Phase and Outcome Measures

Treatment With Acetyl-Choline Esterase Inhibitors in Children With Autism Spectrum Disorders	Phase IV	Core autistic symptoms (ATEC); Side effects and adverse events questionnaire; Linguistic performance (CELF-4); Adaptive functioning (Vineland-II); Co-morbid behaviors (CSI-4 questionnaire); Executive functions (BRIEF) questionnaire
Drug Treatment for Autism	Phase II	Cognitive Assessment
The Effect of Donepezil on REM Sleep in Children With Autism	Phase II	The primary outcome measure of this protocol is to determine if donepezil can increase the percentage of time that subjects with autism spend in REM sleep.; A secondary aim of this protocol is to examine changes in functional outcome, including cognitive.
Galantamine Versus Placebo in Childhood Autism	Phase III	Autism Diagnostic Observation Schedule-Generic (ADOS-G)- Change from Baseline to Final Visit; Clinical Global Impression Improvement (CGI)- Change from Baseline to Final Visit; Aberrant Behavior Checklist (ABC) (hyperactivity/irritability sections).

Table 9. AcetylCholine Esterase Inhibitors Clinical Trials, Trial Phase and Outcome Measures

An Open Label Extension Study of STX209 in Subjects With Autism Spectrum Disorders	Phase II	Irritability subscale of the Aberrant Behavior Checklist
Study of Arbaclofen for the Treatment of Social Withdrawal in Subjects With Autism Spectrum Disorders	Phase II	Aberrant Behavior Checklist-Social Withdrawal Subscale
Open-Label Study of the Safety and Tolerability of STX209 in Subjects With Autism Spectrum Disorders	Phase II	Adverse events; Irritability Subscale of the Aberrant Behavior Checklist, Community Version

Table 10. Immunomodulator Clinical Trials, Trial Phase and Outcome Measures

Open-Label Extension Study of Kuvan for Autism	Phase II Phase III	Clinical Global Impressions Scale; Vineland Adaptive Behavior Scale; Clinical Global Impression: Severity; Children's Yale Brown Obsessive Compulsive Scale; Parental Global Assessment; Preschool Language Scale; Connor's Preschool ADHD question
Intranasal Oxytocin for the Treatment of Autism Spectrum Disorders	Phase II	Change from Baseline to week 12 on the Diagnostic Analysis of Nonverbal Accuracy (DANVA2); Change from Baseline to week 12 on the Social Responsivity Scale (SRS); Change from Baseline to week 12 on the Clinical Global Impressions Scale - Improvement
Intranasal Oxytocin in the Treatment of Autism	Phase II	Clinical Global Impressions Scale (CGI); Diagnostic Analysis of Nonverbal Accuracy, Adult Paralanguage Test (DANVA2-AP); Repetitive Behavior Scale (RBS); Event Contingent Reporting; Yale-Brown Obsessive-Compulsive Scale (YBOCS); Social Responsiveness.
An fMRI Study of the Effect of Intravenous Oxytocin vs. Placebo on Response Inhibition and Face Processing in Autism	Phase I	
A Study of Oxytocin in Children and Adolescents With Autistic Disorder	Phase II	Tolerability of Oxytocin Nasal Spray; Biomarkers; Feasibility; Acceptability of Oxytocin Nasal Spray
Brain Imaging Study of Adults With Autism Spectrum Disorders	Phase I	Changes in brain activations; Performance scores and reaction time on behavioral tasks.
Study of Glutathione, Vitamin C and Cysteine in Children With Autism and Severe Behavior Problems	Phase I	Improvement in both developmental skills and behavior with either glutathione or glutathione, Vitamin C and N-acetylcysteine therapy as compared to placebo therapy. Subjects will also be monitored using clinical and laboratory safety parameters.
Synthetic Human Secretin in Children With Autism	Phase III	
Synthetic Human Secretin in Children With Autism and Gastrointestinal Dysfunction	Phase III	

Sapropterin as a Treatment for Autistic Disorder	Phase II	Clinical Global Impression -- Improvement (CGI-I) Scale; Preschool Language Scale (PLS); Vineland Adaptive Behavior Scale-II; Children's Yale Brown Obsessive Compulsive Scale (C-YBOCS); Connor's Preschool ADHD questionnaire; Adverse Events Scale
Secretin for the Treatment of Autism	Phase III	
The Effects of Oxytocin on Complex Social Cognition in Autism Spectrum Disorders	Phase I	Empathic accuracy performance; fmri BOLD response during empathic accuracy task
Cholesterol in ASD: Characterization and Treatment	Phase I Phase II	Behavioral Changes

Table 11. Hormone or Related Clinical Trials, Trial Phase and Outcome Measures

A Study of Atomoxetine for Attention Deficit and Hyperactive/Impulsive Behaviour Problems in Children With ASD
Atomoxetine and Parent Management Training in Treating Children With Autism and Symptoms of Attention Deficit Disorder With Hyperactivity
Effectiveness of Atomoxetine in Treating ADHD Symptoms in Children and Adolescents With Autism
Atomoxetine Versus Placebo for Symptoms of Attention-Deficit/Hyperactivity Disorder (ADHD) in Children and Adolescents With Autism Spectrum Disorder
Atomoxetine, Placebo and Parent Management Training in Autism
Efficiency of Bumetanide in Autistic Children
Early Pharmacotherapy Aimed at Neuroplasticity in Autism : Safety and Efficacy
Buspirone in the Treatment of 2-6 Year Old Children With Autistic Disorder
A Trial of CM-AT in Children With Autism- Open Label Extension Study
A Trial of CM-AT in Children With Autism
Effects of CX516 on Functioning in Fragile X Syndrome and Autism
Mercury Chelation to Treat Autism
Dimercaptosuccinic Acid (DMSA) Treatment of Children With Autism and Heavy Metal Toxicity
Trial of Low-Dose Naltrexone for Children With Pervasive Developmental Disorder (PDD)
A Pilot Trial of Mecamylamine for the Treatment of Autism
Treatment of Sleep Problems in Children With Autism Spectrum Disorder With Melatonin

| An Open-label Trial of Metformin for Weight Control of Pediatric Patients on Antipsychotic Medications. |
| Efficacy Study of Subcutaneous Methyl-B12 in Children With Autism |
| Methylphenidate in Children and Adolescents With Pervasive Developmental Disorders |
| Omega-3 Fatty Acids Monotherapy in Children and Adolescents With Autism Spectrum Disorders |
| Evaluation and Treatment of Copper/Zinc Imbalance in Children With Autism |
| Dose Finding Study of Pioglitazone in Children With Autism Spectrum Disorders (ASD) |
| Transcranial Magnetic Stimulation (TMS) Measures of Plasticity and Excitatory/Inhibitory Ratio as Biomarkers: R-baclofen Effects in Normal Volunteers |
| Melatonin for Sleep in Children With Autism |
| Trichuris Suis Ova Adult Autism Symptom Domains |
| Multidimensional Measurement of Psychopharmacological Treatment Response * CPI |

Table 12. Other Clinical Trials

4. Pharmacological strategies in autism spectrum disorders

Treatment monitoring and treatment response measurement provide methods by which treatment strategies may be assessed, tested and dynamically applied to the treatment process. Two examples are presented. The first illustrates the longitudinal measurement of risperidone response and the second illustrates a treatment review and re-conceptualization of treatment strategy.

The first case is an actigraphic, psychometric and observational study of risperidone response in a six year old autism spectrum disordered child with Kabuki Syndrome. It provides an illustration of circadian and behavioral disturbances in a child, and the utility of single subject repeated actigraphic, psychometric and observational measurements of treatment response (Duke, 2010).

Actigraphic measurements, such as those used in the following case, are not necessary to obtain meaningful treatment response data, although additional measurements, such as actigraphic data, are helpful.

The non-invasive nature of watch-like actigraphy devices (Rispironics Actiwatch) is particularly attractive for use in pediatric populations. Meaningful treatment response measurements are obtained when actigraphic data is combined with psychometric and observational repeated measurements.

This case study includes baseline and repeated psychological, observational and actigraphic measurements that were initiated prior to treatment with risperidone and repeated throughout the treatment process.

Actigraphic measurements provide a basis by which to measure sleep and sleep onset latency as well as periods of mobility and immobility. In this case the actigraphic device was programmed to record activity every thirty seconds.

Actigraphic measurements were made utilizing a watch-like actigraphic device with an 11 day baseline actigraphic measurement period and continued measurements that included the initiation of a pharmacological intervention for 6 days, followed by a planned adjustment to b.i.d. dosing that was measured for an additional 4 days. This initial actigraphic study resulted in over 65,000 measurements of activity. Repeated observations continued throughout the treatment period and actigraphic studies were repeated after 23 months of risperidone treatment.

The measurement methods included the Personality Inventory for Children (PIC) an objective multidimensional measurement of affect, behavior, ability and family function. The PIC was administered prior to treatment with risperidone and repeated after 23 months of treatment. The PIC serves as both an actuarial pre-treatment diagnostic tool as well as a post-treatment repeated measurement indicating treatment and developmentally associated change (Duke, B., 1991).

Observational methods were employed throughout the treatment process. A primary observer (The Child's Mother) was trained to report symptom percentages present since previous observations utilizing the operationally defined and observer defined items of the Systematic Observation Scale™ (Duke, B., 1990) throughout the treatment process. The Systematic Observation Scale™ utilizes single-subject repeated measurements. Symptoms and issues of interest are defined and a variety of frequency and sampling methods can be applied. The Systematic Observation Scale was designed so Primary Observers (parents, guardians, self observers or others) can make pre-treatment and subsequent observations to track, document and evaluate symptom variation over the course of an illness. The measurement utilized is the percentage of time the symptom is observed by the primary observer since the previous observation.

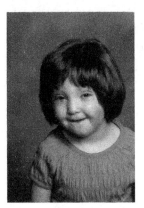

Fig. 3. The child's parents kindly consented to the use of this photograph.

The actigraphic study was designed to select a child anticipating a psychopharmacological intervention.

The study was reviewed and approved by the Child Psychopharmacology Institute Institutional Review Board and was registered with the National Institutes of Health Protocol Registration System (NCT00723580) as a non-randomized, single subject, case study clinical trial.

The Study Investigator's DSM-IV diagnoses were:

- Axis I
- 299.80 Pervasive Developmental Disorder Not Otherwise Specified
- 314.01 Attention-Deficit Hyperactivity Disorder
- 327.30 Circadian Rhythm Sleep Disorder (unspecified type)
- Axis II
- 317 Mild Mental Retardation
- Axis III
- Kabuki Syndrome*
- Hearing Impairment

The child's impulsivity and inability to sleep represented a significant symptom and risk factors. She frequently moved about restlessly until 5:00 AM and would often sleep (or partially sleep) with her eyes open. She had frequent infections and had been previously stimulated by diphenylhydramine, over-sedated on clonidine and had mood destabilization when tried on mirtazapine. The child's diagnosis of Kabuki Syndrome had been previously established by a geneticist at the Mayo Clinic. The child presented with severe impulsivity, psychomotor acceleration, severe insomnia and obsessive compulsive behaviors that included touching objects to the whites of her eyes (these behaviors occurred multiple times an hour). An MLL2 mutation has been verified in this child. It has recently been reported that Kabuki Syndrome is caused by mutations in MLL2, a gene that encodes a Trithorax-group histone methyltransferase, a protein important in the epigenetic control of active chromatin states (Hannibal et, al, 2011).

Dr. Niikawa and Dr. Kuroki described Kabuki Syndrome in 1981. The term was used because of the affected children's facial resemblance to the famous Kabuki actors that perform in traditional Japanese theater.

Kabuki Syndrome is rare and diagnosis is complicated by the diverse spectrum of characteristics. Arched eyebrows, thick eyelashes, eversion of the lateral lower lid and long palpebral fissures contribute to the resemblance. Skeletal and dermatological abnormalities are common along with short stature, behavioral and pervasive developmental disorders and mild to moderate intellectual disability. Congenital heart defects and hearing impairment are often associated with the syndrome. The proportion of male to female occurrence is equal and no correlation with birth order has been found (Adam & Hudgins, 2005).

The assessment and treatment plan included a baseline biopsychosocial history, a baseline cognitive and personality assessment and the initiation of actigraphy measurements. The initial 21 day study of actigraphic measurements included an eleven day baseline prior to pharmacological interventions. The pharmacological Intervention following the medication free baseline utilized risperidone .25 mg q.h.s. initiated for seven days and then increased to twice daily dosing. Subsequent actigraphic measurements reflected the subsequent risperdal dose of .5 mg three times daily. Systematic observations continued throughout the treatment period and the personality assessment was repeated at the study end point. The established treatment goals were to: improve sleep; reduce general impairment; reduce hyperactivity; reduce impulsivity; reduce irritability and improve social functioning.

Hypotheses and Outcome Measures:

H1: Reduced percentages of primary symptoms will be associated with increased sleep during sleep periods (activity and sleep measurements). Actiwatch Communication and Sleep Analysis Instruction Manual (Respironics).

H2: Sleep quality will be reflected by reduced standard deviations of activity during sleep periods.

H3: Positive treatment response as reflected by reduced percentages of primary symptoms will be associated with decreased activity during activity periods.

H4: Reduced impulsivity will be associated with reduced standard deviations of activity during activity periods.

Outcome Measures

a.   Actigraphic Measurement of Treatment Conditions:
b.   Baseline May 12, 2008 and two additional 21 day periods between May 12, 2008 to July 14, 2010
c.   Systematic Observation Scale™ Measurements: May 7, 2008 to July 14th, 2010
d.   Personality Inventory for Children-Revised: pre-test May 2008 and post-test April 2010

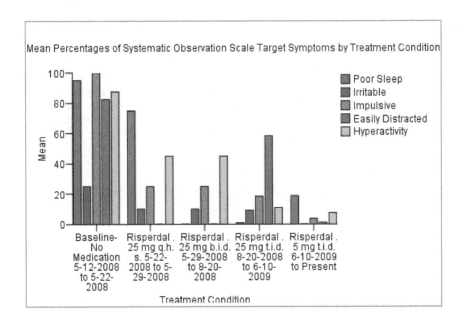

Fig. 4. Target Symptoms by Treatment Condition (BL- .25 mg - .5 mg t.i.d)

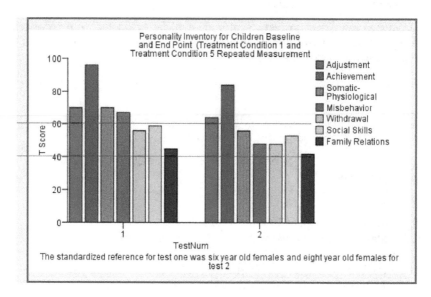

Fig. 5. Personality Inventory Pre-Test and Post-Test

Study conclusions: Sleep quantity was increased; Sleep quality was improved; Hyperactivity was reduced; Impulsivity was reduced; Significance between treatment conditions, activity and target symptoms was demonstrated.

The second case is a ten year old male who had received numerous medications over the past several years. Despite these treatments, and optimal family environment and commitment, the primary symptoms of mood instability and cognitive impairment continued. The child was receiving aripiprazole 5 mg q.a.m. and Concerta 36 mg q.a.m. Prior to the treatment review, the child had become disinhibited and severely impulsive in response to treatment with an SSRI, which was discontinued. He had also demonstrated a dose related worsening when tried on quetiapine. The quetiapine was discontinued due to associated insomnia and worsened mood and behavioral states.

At the time of the review the child presented with neurological immaturity, delayed fine motor integration, jerky saccadic eye movements and possible symptoms of partial complex seizures. The child's episodic emotional dyscontrol, attention and cognitive functioning did not appear to be, pharmacologically, optimally addressed.

DSM IV Diagnoses: Axis I:

299.80 Pervasive Developmental Disorder NOS

296.90 Mood Disorder NOS

314.01 Attention Deficit/Hyperactivity Disorder, Combined Type

307.7 Encopresis

		Sum of Squares	df	Mean Square	F	Sig.
Activity	Between Groups	4.476E8	3	1.492E8	1057.569	.000
	Within Groups	2.698E10	191235	141065.613		
	Total	2.742E10	191238			
Poor Sleep	Between Groups	16583.631	4	4145.908	10.542	.002
	Within Groups	3539.583	9	393.287		
	Total	20123.214	13			
Impulsive	Between Groups	13278.274	4	3319.568	15.707	.000
	Within Groups	1902.083	9	211.343		
	Total	15180.357	13			
Hyperactivity	Between Groups	11034.524	4	2758.631	10.994	.002
	Within Groups	2258.333	9	250.926		
	Total	13292.857	13			
Irritable	Between Groups	838.095	4	209.524	4.481	.029
	Within Groups	420.833	9	46.759		
	Total	1258.929	13			
Easily Distracted	Between Groups	14721.131	4	3680.283	4.379	.031
	Within Groups	7564.583	9	840.509		
	Total	22285.714	13			

Fig. 6. Treatment Response: Analysis of Variance

Following the treatment review the initial strategy was to add carbamazepine 200 mg ER q.p.m. x 7 days then b.i.d. Subsequent to improved emotional stability and broadly reduced symptoms the contribution of aripiprazole was assessed by a dose reduction to 2.5 mg q.a.m. for four days and subsequently replaced with risperidone .5 mg b.i.d. Plans were made to subsequently assess his stimulant treatment response as the monitoring continued. Figure 7 displays symptom percentage averages over the treatment transition.

Printable observation forms and item defintions are available and free for non-commercial use on the Child Psychopharmacology Institute website (www. ChildPsychopharmacologyInstitute.org).

5. Pharmacological protection and prevention strategies on the horizon: Glutamatergic modulation and neuroprotection

Although pharmacological interventions utilized in Autistic Spectrum Disorders are generally associated with targeting behavioral or emotional impairments, little attention has been given to the important potential of glutamatergic regulation and neuroprotection in this vulnerable population.

While a single drug has not triumphed in the treatment of autism spectrum disorders, many drugs have proven helpful to varying degrees and for various purposes. The dearth of children's pharmacological studies stand in stark contrast to wide use of pharmacological interventions in ASD children.

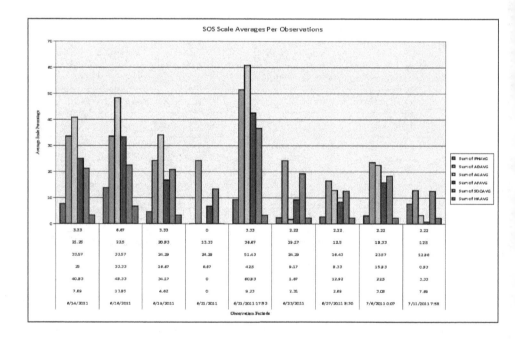

Fig. 7. Symptom Percentage Observation Scale Averages

Alternative pathways of ASD pathology being explored include the study of tetrahydrobiopterin (BH$_4$) as a novel therapeutic intervention and point to ASD children as having low levels of BH$_4$. Early studies suggest low BH$_4$ levels during development have devastating consequences on the central nervous system leading to or potentiating the neuropathology of ASD (Frye, et al, 2010). These studies are promising and may suggest a role for BH$_4$ treatment or treatment augmentation in the ASD population.

It is proposed that pharmacological approaches with neuroprotective characteristics have potential to reduce the dynamic pathogenic states that are likely occurring in highly symptomatic young children who are in developmentally critical stages of neural patterning and maturation. In a manner similar to the example provided regarding atypical antipsychotics, drugs will increasingly be chosen based on their particular characteristics or used together for separate or synergistic effects.

Arriving at a full understanding of these approaches will take further studies that consider the potential for unwanted effects. The Frye study, for example, noted that based on seven studies in which 451 patients with autism were treated with sapropterin (synthetic BH_4) that ninety-seven (21.5%) experienced adverse effects for which a causal relationship with the study drug could not be ruled out. The most frequently reported adverse effects were sleep disorders, excitement, hyperkinesia, enuresis and diarrhea. It will be important to learn if sapropterin's benefits are primarily from developmentally critical neuroprotective effects and/or effects on neurotransmitters. It will also be important to determine if indiscriminate neurotransmitter potentiation in dysregulated neurons and circuits are being reflected in the adverse effect profile that some demonstrate.

Synaptic molecules are important targets for protective treatments, to slow disease progression and preserve cognitive and functional abilities by preserving synaptic structure and function. Glutamate receptors and post synaptic density proteins play a central role in excitatory synaptic plasticity. Synaptic dysregulation may contribute to brain disorders present in those with Autism Spectrum Disorders by preventing appropriate synaptic signaling and plasticity.

The NMDA receptor is fundamental to excitatory synaptic plasticity and neurological diseases. Synaptic loss is a pathologic correlate of cognitive decline. Synaptic dysfunction is evident long before synapses and neurons are lost. The synapse constitutes an important target for treatments to slow progression and preserve cognitive and functional abilities in these diseases. (van Spronsen & Hoogenraad, 2010)

5.1 Excitotoxity and glutamatergic activity

Current hypotheses propose excessive glutamate activity can lead to excitotoxicity interfering with normal neurodevelopment in schizophrenia. Similarly, these effects may be involved in the neurodevelopment in ASD. The excitotoxicity is hypothesized to continue and is linked to disease progression in schizophrenia ultimately resulting in pathologically functioning NMDA glutamate receptors. These hypotheses are consistent with those that identify the final common pathway of many neuropsychiatric diseases as synaptic pathology.

While the future promises biomarkers, RNAi strategies, stem cell transplantation and other genetic treatments, arresting and/or reducing developmental pathogenic potential by discovering and developing methods of effecting glutamatergic regulation by NMDA antagonism or other methods is a worthy, if not urgent, treatment goal for Autism Spectrum Disordered children. Blocking or moderating excessive glutamate neurotransmission with NMDA antagonists may prevent or mitigate damage, maladaptive neurodevelopment or neurodegenerative processes.

Some NMDA antagonists appear to be neuromodulators that reduce the excitotoxicity effects of dysregulated circuits and support dendritic health, long term potentiation and neural plasticity. Such treatments may one day provide preventative pharmacological interventions as well as those that can reduce impairment and improve functioning.

Two NMDA antagonists are particuilarly interesting candidates for therapeutic potential in the ASD population, memantine and dextromethorphan/quinidine (Duke & Kaye, 2010).

Memantine, as an augmenting agent, demonstrated significant improvements in open-label use for language function, social behavior, and self-stimulatory behaviors, although self-stimulatory behaviors comparatively improved to a lesser degree. Chronic use so far appears to have no serious side effects (Chez MG, et al 2007).

Dextromethorphan/quinidine (DM/Q) shares the attributes of being an uncompetitive NMDA antagonist with memantine, however, importantly; DM/Q is a sigma 1 agonist and binds to SERT. Binding data comparing memantine with DM/Q demonstrate the presence of Sigma 1 and SERT binding in DM/Q but not in memantine (Werling, et al 2007).

One of the characteristics that suggests DM/Q might have therapeutic potential in ASD is its efficacy in pseudobulbar affect (PBA). The efficacy and safety of dextromethorphan and quinidine was demonstrated in clinical trials of late stage neurological conditions (amyotrophic lateral Sclerosis and Multiple Sclerosis) demonstrating reductions of emotional lability and improvements in sleep. These findings suggest that the pharmacological characteristics of DM/Q may, at some level rescue synaptic signaling and may have the potential to affect neurodevelopmental trajectory in dysregulated developing nervous systems such as those with Autism Spectrum Disorders.

AVP-923 was approved by the FDA in 2010 as Nuedexta™ the first and only treatment for Pseudobulbar Affect (PBA). This is an important therapeutic for those suffering the debilitating effects of pseudobulbar affect. The efficacy in reducing dysregulated and involuntary congruent and incongruent emotional expressions is a significant achievement. Why is DM/Q (Nuedexta) effective in PBA? That, of course, is unknown, but PBA is often considered the result of connectivity and neural circuitry failures and ASD is known to have signaling and connectivity pathologies. Emotional lability is often associated with behavioral dyscontrol, irritibility, assaultive and raging behaviors that prompt pharmacological intervention in children with ASD.

NMDA antagonists may offer a therapeutic pathway through modulation or regulation of dysregulated glutamatergic processes. The potential of DM/Q (Nuedexta) in ASD, particularly in the early developmental stages of the illness, to rescue and support synaptic function is worthy of further study.

Although the mechanism of action of DM/Q is not fully characterized, its unique properties as an NMDA receptor antagonist and as a Sigma 1 receptor agonist appear to convey effects of both neuroprotection and neuromodulation. Future studies will help us determine if these unique characteristics will lead to improved outcomes for those with autism spectrum disorders.

6. Conclusion

The distress, irritability and emotional lability often seen in Autism Spectrum Disorders may be a reflection of pathological glutamatergic functioning or otherwise dysregulated circuits relative to inhibitory-excitatory balance. When sustained, these symptoms demonstrate potential for pathological development of abnormal neural circuits capable of dysregulation through neural synchronicity and state dependent effects on genetic expression. Within the framework of this hypothesis the neural plasticity and critical periods, present in developing brains, place them at particular risk.

We currently have drugs and compounds that have the ability to reduce impairment and improve functioning in many with ASD when used, monitored and managed thoughtfully. Early pharmacological intervention related to severe emotional lability, irritability and dysregulated circuits may also reduce the pathogenic potential and reduce or prevent the development or maintenance of pathological processes.

7. Acknowledgement

As a faculty member of the Child Psychopharmacology Institute and as a consultant for Avanir Pharmaceuticals I wish to express my gratitude to my colleagues Randall Kaye, M.D., MPH, R. Dennis Staton, Ph.D., M.D. and Scott Siegert, Pharm.D. for their collegial support and expertise.

8. References

Adam, MP & Hudgins, L. "Kabuki Syndrome: A Review." Clin Genet, 2005: Mar;67(3):209-19.

Ashwood, P., Wills S., and Van de Water, J. "The immune response in autism: a new frontier for autism research." *Journal of Leukocyte Biology*, 2006 : Volume 80, July.

Buxbaum, JD. "Multiple rare variants in the etiology of autism spectrum disorders." *Dialogues Clin Neurosci.*, 2009: 11(1)35-43.

Careaga M, Van de Water J, Ashwood P. "Immune dysfunction in autism: a pathway to treatment." *Neurotherapeutics*, 2010 : Jul;7(3) 283-92.

Caria A, Venuti P, & de Falco S. "Functional and Dysfunctional Brain Circuits Underlying Emotional Processing of Music in Autism Spectrum Disorders." *Cereb Cortex*, 2011: May 6. CDC. *Autism Spectrum Disorders.* August 1, 2011. http://www.cdc.gov/ncbddd/autism/research.html (accessed August 1, 2011).

Chez MG, Burton Q, Dowling T, Chang M, Khanna P, Kramer C. "Memantine as adjunctive therapy in children diagnosed with autistic spectrum disorders: an observation of initial clinical response and maintenance tolerability." *J Child Neurol.* , 2007: May;22(5):574-9.

Duke, B. & Kaye, R. "Breaking Pharmacological Barriers to Innovation: The Case for Assessing Dextromethorphan/Quinidine in Autistic Spectrum Disorders." *Journal of Brain Research Meeting: Emerging Neuroscience of Autism Spectrum Disorders.* San Diego: Elsevier, 2010.

Duke, B. "A 23 Month Longitudinal Actigraphic, Psychometric and Observational Study." *Journal of Brain Research Meeting: Emerging Neuroscience of Autism Spectrum Disorders.* San Diego: Elsevier, 2010. Poster.

Duke, B. "Measuring Response to Psychopharmacologic Interventions." *Proceedings of the American Psychological Association symposium, the Personality Inventory for Children: Assessment Linking Families and Schools.* San Francisco: American Psychological Association, 1991. D. Lachar, Chair.

Duke, B. "Pathogenic Effects of Central Nervous System Hyperarousal." *Medical Hypothesis,* 2008: 71: 212-217.

Duke, B.J. "Child Psychotherapy and the Scientific Method: The Systematic Observation Scale." *Proceedings of the Pacific Division, American Association For The Advancement of Science,* 1990: (9)1:21. .

Eagleson K., Campbell D., Thompson, B., Bergman, M., and Levitt, P. "The Autism Risk Genes MET and PLAUR Differentially Impact Cortical Development." *Autism Research 4:,* 2011: 68-83.

Estes A, Shaw DW, Sparks BF, Friedman S, Giedd JN, Dawson G, Bryan M, & Dager SR. "Basal ganglia morphometry and repetitive behavior in young children with autism spectrum disorder. ." *Autism Res. ,* 2011 : Jun;4(3):212-20. .

Frye, R, Huffman, L, & Elliot, G. Tetrahydrobiopterin as a novel therapeutic intervention for autism. Neurotherapeutics, 2010 July;7(3): 241-249

Gilman, S. R. et al. "Rare de novo variants associated with autism implicate a large functional network of genes involved in formation and function of synapses." *Neuron,* 2011: 70, 898–907 .

Gleason MM, Egger HL, Emslie GJ, Greenhill LL, Kowatch RA, Lieberman AF, Luby JL,. "Psychopharmacological treatment for very young children: contexts and guidelines." *J Am Acad Child Adolesc Psychiatry. 2007 Dec;46(12):1532-72.,* 2007: Dec;46(12):1532-72.

Greer PL, Hanayama R, Bloodgood BL, Mardinly AR, Lipton DM, Flavell W, Kim TK, Griffith EC, Waldon Z, Maehr R, Ploegh HL, Chowdhury S, Worley PF, Steen J, Greenberg ME. "The Angelman Syndrome protein Ube3A regulates synapse development by ubiquitinating arc. ." *Cell,* 2010: Mar 5;140(5):704-16.

Groen WB, Buitelaar JK, van der Gaag RJ & Zwiers MP. "Pervasive microstructural abnormalities in autism: a DTI study." *J Psychiatry Neurosci.,* 2011: Jan;36(1): 32-40.

Hallmayer J, Cleveland S, Torres A, Phillips J, Cohen B, Torigoe T, Miller J, Fedele A, Collins J, Smith K, Lotspeich L, Croen LA, Ozonoff S, Lajonchere C, Grether JK, Risch N. "Genetic heritability and shared environmental factors among twin pairs with autism." *Archives of General Psychiatry,* 2011: July.

Hamberger A, Gillberg C, Palm A, Hagberg B. "Elevated CSF glutamate in Rett syndrome." *Neuropediatrics,* 1992 : Aug;23(4) 212-3.

Hannibal, MC et al. "Spectrum of MLL2 (ALR) mutations in 110 cases of Kabuki syndrome." Am J Med Genet A. 2011 Jul;155A(7):1511-6.

Isaacson, J. & Provenzale, J. "Diffusion tensor imaging for evaluation of the childhood brain and pediatric white matter disorders." *Neuroimaging Clin N Am.*, 2011: Feb;21(1):179-89, ix.

Kumar A, Sundaram SK, Sivaswamy L, Behen ME, Makki MI, Ager J, Janisse J, Chugani HT, & Chugani DC. "Alterations in frontal lobe tracts and corpus callosum in young children with autism spectrum disorder." *Cereb Cortex*, 2010: Sep;20(9):2103-13.

Kurth F, Narr KL, Woods RP, O'Neill J, Alger JR, Caplan R, McCracken JT, & Toga AW. "Diminished gray matter within the hypothalamus in autism disorder: a potential link to hormonal effects?" *Biol Psychiatry*, 2011: Aug 1;70(3):278-82.

Levitt, P. "Serotonin and the Autisms." *Arch Gen Psychiatry*, 2011: Commentary.

Levy, D. et al. "Rare de novo and transmitted copy-number variation in autistic spectrum disorders." *Neuron*, 2011: 70, 886–897 .

McGraw, C., Samaco, R. & Zoghbi, H. "Adult Neural Function Requires MeCP2." *Science*, 2011: July Vol333 p186.

Monji, A. "The microglia hypothesis of psychiatric disorders." *Nihon Shinkei Seishin Yakurigaku Zasshi*, 2011 : Feb;31(1):1-8.

Rice, C. "Prevalence of Autism Spectrum Disorders --- Autism and Developmental Disabilities Monitoring Network." (CDC United States) 2006.

Sacco R, Curatolo P, Manzi B, Militerni R, Bravaccio C, Frolli A, Lenti C,Saccani M, Elia M, Reichelt KL, Pascucci T, Puglisi-Allegra S. "Principal pathogenetic components and biological endophenotypes in autism spectrum disorders." *Autism Res.*, 2010: Sep 27.

Sanders, S. J. et al. "Multiple recurrent de novo CNVs, including duplications of the 7q11.23 Williams syndrome region, are strongly associated with autism." *Neuron*, 2011: 70:863–885 .

Schwartz, T and Stahl S. "Treatment strategies for dosing the second generation antipsychotics." *CNS Neurosci Ther.*, 2011 : Apr;17(2):110-7.

Siniscalchi, A. Gallelli, L. and De Sarro, G. "Use of Antiepileptic Drugs for Hyperkinetic Movement Disorders." *Current Neuropharmacology*, 2010: 8, 359-366.

Stahl, Stephen. *Stahl's Essential Psychopharmacology Online: Neuroscientific Basis and Practical Applications.* New York: Cambridge University Press, 2010 p. 274.

Szatmari, P. "Is Autism, at Least in Part, a Disorder of Fetal Programming?" *Arch Gen Psychiatry*, 2011: July 5, 2011.

Tuchman, R. & Cuccaro, M. "Epilepsy and Autism: Neurodevlopmental Perspective." *Curr Neurol Neurosci Rep.*, 2011: Aug;11(4):428-34.

van Spronsen M, Hoogenraad CC. "Synapse pathology in psychiatric and neurologic disease." *Curr Neurol Neurosci Rep.*, 2010 : May;10(3) 207-14.

Werling, L., Keller, A., Frank, J., & Nuwayhid, S. "A comparison of the binding profiles of dextromethorphan, memantine,fluoxetine and amitriptyline: Treatment of involuntary emotional expression disorder." *Experimental Neurology*, 2007: 248–257.

Yagasaki Y, Numakawa T, Kumamaru E, Hayashi T, Su TP, Kunugi H. "Chronic antidepressants potentiate via sigma-1 receptors the brain-derived neurotrophic factor-induced signaling for glutamate release." *J Biol Chem.*, 2006: May 5;281(18):12941-9.

4

A Multi-Level Analysis of World Scientific Output in Pharmacology

Carlos Olmeda-Gómez, Ma-Antonia Ovalle-Perandones
and Antonio Perianes-Rodríguez
Carlos III University of Madrid
Spain

1. Introduction

Over the last few decades and particularly in the present economic context, the distribution of economic resources has been a concern addressed by governmental and corporate scientific policy, which has either benefitted only part of the scientific and technological community or furthered certain lines of research. The pharmaceutical industry in particular has had to confront not only this situation, but also ongoing internationalisation, supported by the relentless advances in communication technologies.

Until the nineteen eighties, industry internationalisation, in terms of R&D, was a marginal matter, not only for economics theory and business in general, but also for governments and the other organisations involved. Globalisation began to acquire importance after the mid nineteen nineties, although not all manufacturing industries have experienced the same degree of R&D internationalisation. The pharmaceutical industry, for one, pioneered this more universal approach to research and development (Noisi, 1999).

Contrary to the widely held opinion according to which R&D internatianlisation is the fruit of domestic innovation in many industries, pharmaceutical constitutes an exception. Indeed, international innovation intensifies the industry's R&D (Patel and Pavitt, 2000), whereas in other lines of business domestic innovation is the driver. In addition to internationalising its R&D, the pharmaceuticals industry has increased its research spending exponentially in recent years (Congressional Budget Office, 2006).

A number of earlier papers studied the bibilometric characteristics of the pharmacological publications generated as a result of the R&D effort in places such as the United States (Narin and Rozek, 1988), India (Kaur and Gupta, 2009; Gupta and Kaur, 2009) or the Middle East (Biglu and Omidi, 2010). Others stressed the contribution of pharmaceutical firms to scientific knowledge (Koening, 1983; McMillan and Hamilton, 2000; Rafols, et al. 2010; Perianes-Rodríguez, et al. 2011). The assessment of the international impact of scientific papers is a present, but not a new concern: it has been a frequent object of study since the nineteen eighties. The use of scientific indicators for several decades to characterise research by subject area, country or institution has confirmed that, although they have their limitations, they are the only suitable tool for scientific assessment (Braun T et al., 1985).

The purpose of this chapter is to analyse international research in "pharmacology, toxicology and pharmaceutics" (hereafter pharmacology) on the basis of the scientific papers listed in the Scopus multidisciplinary database. This primary objective is reached by answering the following questions (in the section on results). What weight does the subject area "pharmacology, toxicology and pharmaceutics" carry in world-wide science? What is the percentage contribution made by the various regions of the world to the subject area "pharmacology, toxicology and pharmaceutics"? Can certain regions be identified as leaders on that basis, as in other scientific contexts? Are emerging countries present in the field? Do the most productive countries also publish the largest number of journals? What features characterise the scientific output of companies that publish pharmacological papers?

2. Methodology

2.1 Database

The possible sources of information for scientometric research include multi-disciplinary databases such as Thomson Reuters' Web of Science, Elsevier's Scopus and resources such as Google Scholar, as well as specialised services such as Medline. These sources analyse research results in the form of scientific papers published in international journals and their subsequent citation by the rest of the scientific community.

Scopus, the Elsevier database created in 2004, lists over 18 000 journals edited by over 5 000 publishers[1]. When it first appeared, it was analysed by many authors and compared to other resources in a whole stream of papers (Fingerman, 2005; LaGuardia, 2005). It was chosen for the present study because of its broad subject area and linguistic coverage; in the understanding that world-wide scientific production is more fully represented in Scopus than in other databases (Sciverse Scopus, 2011). In addition, as a resource suitable for research conducted after 1996, it is particularly apt for a subject area such as pharmacology (Gorraiz and Schloegl, 2008).

Scopus' strong points as a source of information are reinforced by an open access, on-line tool known as SCImago Journal and Country Rank (SJR, 2007). As its name infers, this system of scientific information, drawing from Scopus contents from 1996 to 2010, ranks journals and countries using data intended for world-wide scientific assessment. The tool provides open access to both data and indicators by region or country, with international coverage. It proved to be particularly useful for the aims pursued in the present study.

2.2 Indicators

Two sets of bibliometric indicators were used in this study: one to determine the quantitative characteristics of scientific output and the other to analyse its quality, i.e., the qualitative characteristics of citations and journals (Rehn, 2007). The indicators included in each group are described below.

This study calculated the number of scientific papers published by the units analysed (world, region, country or industry) over the time span defined. All of the various possible types of papers (such as articles, reviews and notes to the editor,) were included in the *output* indicator.

---

[1] Available from http://www.info.sciverse.com/scopus/scopus-in-detail/facts/. 20/08/2011

When papers were co-authored by researchers from institutions in different countries, a complete computational approach was adopted. The growth rate, when provided, indicates the rise or decline in world-wide output in 2009 with respect to the baseline year, 1996.

A number of indicators were used to obtain an approximate view of the quality of world scientific output in the field of pharmacology. The number of *citations* received refers to the total number of times papers published by the unit analysed were cited during the period studied. This indicator provides an overview of the scientific impact of the articles published by the unit in question. The number of *citations per paper* was calculated as the mean number of citations received by all the papers published by the unit analysed in the period studied.

The *domestic citations* were separated from the total to determine the proportion of the output that was used as a reference in the same geographic area (region or country) and consequently, by simple subtraction, the proportion involving knowledge transfer to other areas. The results are shown as the percentage of the citations used for research conducted in the same geographic area. The *normalised citation* indicator is the relative number of times papers produced by a specific unit were cited, compared to the world-wide mean for papers of the same type, age and subject area.

While citations denote the subsequent use of papers once published, the *references* list the literature cited in papers published by a journal at any given time. The number of *references per paper* was found by dividing the total number of references by the number of papers published by the unit.

A country's *H-index*, in turn, specifies the number of papers (h) produced in that country and receiving at least h citation. It relates a country's scientific productivity (output) to its scientific impact (citations). The *international collaboration* indicator is the percentage of papers with author affiliations in more than one country. This indicator measures institutions' international networking capacity. In this chapter a journal's *% output in Q1* is the percentage of scientific papers published by an institution in what are classified as the most influential journals in the respective category, i.e., the periodicals in the first quartile or Q1, the upper 25 %, based on their SJR value.

Another qualitative indicator used, homonymous with the aforementioned scientific information system (SCImago Journal and Country Rank), was the *Scimago Journal Rank (SJR)*, used as an alternative to the traditional impact factor (I.F.). This indicator, which measures the visibility of the journals in the Scopus® database, is established by the SCImago[2] research team on the grounds of the well-known Google PageRank™ algorithm. It differs from the I.F. in two ways: citations are computed over 3 rather than 2 years; and article citations are weighted, with citations in more visible or prominent journals carrying greater weight than citations in lower-ranking journals (González-Pereira et al., 2009).

3. Results

3.1 World-wide science and pharmacology

World-wide scientific output, as listed in the Scopus database for the period running from 1996 to 2009, came to 21 100 138 papers. The total citations received by those papers during the

---

[2] http://www.scimago.es/. 20.08.2011

same period amounted to 217 388 448, for a mean of 10.03 citations per paper. The absolute numbers for pharmacology, as one of the 27 subject areas established by Scopus, were logically much smaller. The totals were 564 914 papers and 6 266 408 citations. The mean number of citations in pharmacology was therefore higher than the world average, at 11.09. The growth rate for this subject area was 4.76 %, reflecting the growth in its scientific output.

Figure 1 shows the percentage contribution of the Scopus subject areas to world-wide scientific output during the period studied. Medicine played a predominant role in the international scientific scenario, with a mean yearly contribution of over 20 %. Decision science and dentistry stood at the other extreme, with a mean yearly output of 0.35 %, shown on the figure as very thin lines. The mean yearly contribution of pharmacology to international scientific output in the period was 2.7 %, shown in red on the right half of the graph. When pooled, all the subject areas with relative outputs of under 4 %, which include pharmacology, earth and planet sciences, immunology and microbiology, accounted for 34.83 % of the scientific papers published world-wide.

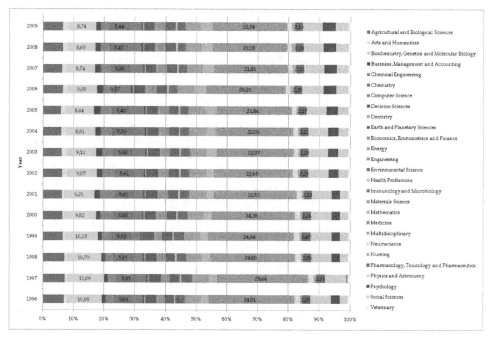

Fig. 1. World output by subject areas (%) (Scopus, 1996-2009)

3.2 Pharmacology by region

While scientific output by region is an important indicator to determine regional contributions to pharmacology, quantitative information alone is incomplete and must be supplemented with data on the impact of these papers on the scientific community. Table 1 gives the vales of some of the indicators described earlier for a number of regions, along with colour bar graphs for readier interpretation.

Region	Output	Citations	Domestic citations	%Domestic citations	Citations per paper
North America	155373	2714951	2209503	81.38	17.47
Western Europe	159512	2383236	1671534	70.14	14.94
Asia	113741	1095409	626665	57.21	9.63
Eastern Europe	21951	178157	57830	32.46	8.12
Latin America	18122	164264	78623	47.86	9.06
Pacific Region	11802	161126	45651	28.33	13.65
Middle East	10256	105817	27329	25.83	10.32
Southern Africa	2167	23987	7406	30.88	11.07
Central Africa	2035	11101	4650	41.89	5.46
Northen Africa	827	7559	1808	23.92	9.14

Table 1. Pharmacological scientific output, citations and domestic citations by region (Scopus, 1996-2009)

The behaviour of the domestic citations indicator merits comment. In North America, these citations accounted for over 80 % percent of the total. The number of domestic citations was likewise very high in Western Europe; in both regions most of the citations were found in articles published in the same country as the paper cited. Consequently, in these two regions, the large number of domestic citations led to an inordinately large number of total citations.

The regions with smaller numbers of citations also had a smaller proportion of domestic citations. In other words, their output was acknowledged primarily by other regions, while domestic citations were less frequent. The region that best illustrates this observation is Northern Africa, where only 23.92 % of the citations received were domestic.

The number of citations per paper was also highest in North America and Western Europe, with the Pacific Region ranking a close third. Central Africa's low scientific output in pharmacology was only scantly acknowledged, with only 5.46 citations per paper on average. Asia, Eastern Europe, Latin America and Northern Africa had similar citations per paper values, which ranged from 8 to 9.

The pharmacological output by regions over the period 1996 to 2009 is shown in Figure 2. The three most productive regions in that period were Western Europe (red), North America (blue) and Asia (green). Asia had a higher growth rate in the latter years of the period and was the most productive region in 2009. This rise may have been the result of greater participation in the pharmacology, particularly in countries that in those years began to adopt a very active role in the field.

3.3 Countries and pharmacology

The basic unit for the regions listed above was defined as the individual country. A total of 194 countries published pharmacological research in the period studied. The analysis conducted of their output provided greater insight into the values found for the regional indicators.

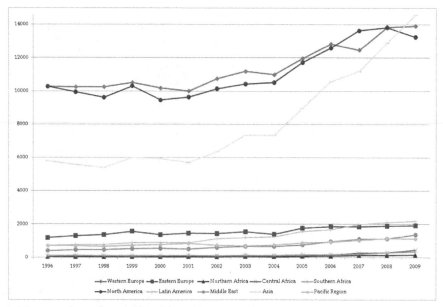

Fig. 2. Pharmacological scientific output by region (Scopus, 1996-2009)

The ten most productive countries accounted for around 71 % of world-wide pharmacological output in the period studied. These ten countries are listed in Table 2, which shows their total output in the period, the number of total and domestic citations received, the citations per paper and the H index. The list is headed by the United States, which had the largest output and number of citations, although the number per paper should be interpreted bearing in mind the impact of the large number of domestic citations identified. At 293, its H index was likewise high, indicating that 293 papers were cited in 293 other articles.

Table 3 ranks the countries whose overall data for the entire period are given in Table 2, year by year across the period. Grey shading indicates that the country changed its position from the preceding year and maroon shading that the country joined the top ten in the year in question.

The regional study showed the enormous progress in Asia in the latter years of the period. That growth was the result of greater participation in the subject area by Asian countries. Although until 2005 Japan was the second largest producer in pharmacology, from 2006 onward it was overtaken by an emerging neighbour: China. In the three earliest years China ranked tenth; in the intermediate years it gradually climbed to higher positions and finally reached second place in 2006. While still among the most productive countries, Japan's position slid, denoting its tendency to contribute less and less to pharmacological output. In the last year of the series, 2009, four of the ten most productive countries were Asian (China, India, Japan and South Korea).

The United States maintained its lead throughout the period. That leadership and Canada's contribution, from lower but still productive positions, made North America the sole region with an output comparable to Asia's in the latter years. All the other most productive countries in pharmacology were from Western Europe: United Kingdom, Germany, Italy and France, and the Netherlands and Spain in some years. Only one Latin American country was among the most productive during the period: Brazil, in 2007.

Country	Output	Citations	Domestic citations	Citations per paper	H Index
United States	154941	2516137	1221126	17.38	293
Japan	47322	543692	164265	11.38	139
United Kingdom	40531	644728	143933	16.9	195
China	36079	178269	80870	6.34	84
Germany	34443	442517	106046	13.49	157
India	23323	144862	59885	9.22	91
Italy	22593	304775	75527	14.88	128
France	21925	320578	64831	15.28	148
Canada	18667	297798	61608	17.18	143
Spain	14232	165910	41389	12.66	101

Table 2. Pharmacological scientific output, domestic citations, citations per document and H index for the 10 most productive countries (Scopus, 1996-2009)

1996	1997	1998	1999	2000	2001	2002	2003	2004	2005	2006	2007	2008	2009
USA	USA	USA	USA	USA	USA	USA	USA	USA	USA	USA	USA	USA	USA
Japan	Japan	Japan	Japan	Japan	Japan	Japan	Japan	Japan	Japan	China	China	China	China
U.K.	U.K.	U.K.	U.K.	U.K.	U.K.	U.K.	U.K.	U.K.	China	Japan	Japan	U.K.	India
Germany	Germany	Germany	Germany	Germany	Germany	Germany	Germany	Germany	U.K.	U.K.	U.K.	Japan	U.K.
France	France	France	France	France	France	Italy	China	China	Germany	Germany	Germany	India	Japan
Italy	Italy	Italy	Italy	Italy	Italy	France	France	Italy	Italy	India	India	Germany	Germany
Canada	Canada	Canada	Canada	China	China	China	Italy	France	India	Italy	Italy	Italy	Italy
Spain	Spain	Netherlands	China	Canada	Canada	Canada	Canada	Canada	France	France	France	France	France
Netherlands	Netherlands	Spain	Netherlands	Spain	Netherlands	India	India	India	Canada	Canada	Canada	Canada	Canada
China	China	China	Spain	India	Spain	Netherlands	Spain	Netherlands	Spain	Spain	Brazil	South Korea	South Korea

Table 3. Country position by output (Scopus, 1996-2009)

Figures 3 and 4 show the relationship between international collaboration and citations per paper in countries publishing at least 1 000 papers. The position occupied by the countries in each region is shown in both figures, but only Western European and North American countries are depicted in Figure 3. All the Asian, Eastern European and Latin American countries are shown in Figure 4, although only the BRIC countries (Brazil, Russia, India, China) are labelled.

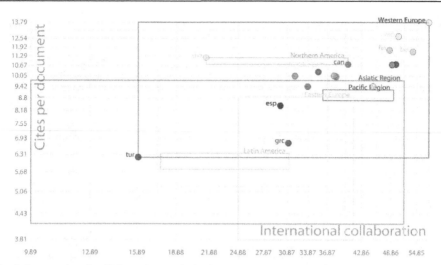

Fig. 3. International collaboration and citations per paper in North American and Western European countries (www.scimagoir.com), 2003-2009.

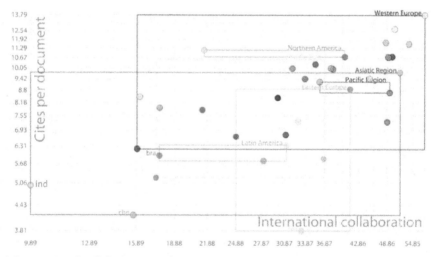

Fig. 4. International collaboration and citations per paper in BRIC countries (www.scimagoir.com), 2003-2009.

The country in Figure 3 with the smallest number of citations per paper and least intense international collaboration was Turkey. With 6.18 citations per paper and an international co-authorship percentage of 16.12, it stood at the low end of its region, Western Europe, and had lower citation values than Latin America or Eastern Europe. In Western Europe, Sweden and Belgium were the two countries both in that region and the world with the highest international collaboration indices and a mean of 12 citations per paper. Both, as well as other countries, also had higher values than the USA (in terms of international collaboration) and Canada.

Measuring their scientific status in terms of citations per paper and international collaboration values, the BRIC countries still have room for improvement. Three of those four countries were positioned very close to the origin on the graph. Of the four, only Brazil showed values close to the results recorded for Turkey.

3.4 Pharmacology in journals

The analysis of the journals that published pharmacological papers included the data for the periodicals that published at least one such paper in 2009. Under that criterion, a total of 482 journals were identified, 61 of which had been recently added to the database and consequently lacked the data needed to calculate their SJR.

Of the remaining 421 (that had published more than one paper and had an SJR index), 110 were edited in the United States, although a fair number were also published in other countries: Netherlands (87), United Kingdom (75), Germany (25), China (12), India (12), Japan (11), Spain (11), France (8), Switzerland (7) and New Zealand (6).

The remaining journals were published in a total of 33 countries, each with less than six journals.

10 top journals by SJR value	SJR	Ouput (2009)	Citations (3years)	Citations per paper (2years)	Refs	Ref per doc	Country
Annual Review of Pharmacology and Toxicology	3.56	19	1429	22.94	2367	124.58	United States
Pharmacological Reviews	3.3	19	1433	17.16	6531	343.74	United States
Nature Reviews Drug Discovery	2.68	202	5827	15.67	7865	38.94	United Kingdom
Trends in Pharmacological Sciences	1.64	84	2588	9.56	5718	68.07	Netherlands
Drug Resistance Updates	1.52	16	530	11.79	1836	114.75	United States
DNA Repair	1.44	169	2237	4.15	10528	62.3	Netherlands
Pharmacology and Therapeutics	1.22	104	3367	9.23	20152	193.77	United States
Current Opinion in Pharmacology	1.14	117	2138	7.57	6206	53.04	Netherlands
Advanced Drug Delivery Reviews	1.1	143	4030	12.34	15219	106.43	Netherlands
10 top journals by total documents in 2009	SJR	Ouput (2009)	Citations (3years)	Citations per paper (2years)	Refs	Ref per doc	Country
Bioorganic and Medicinal Chemistry Letters	0.21	1546	10591	2.72	39742	25.71	Netherlands
Pharmaceutical Journal	0.03	1058	124	0.1	972	0.92	United Kingdom
Deutsche Apotheker Zeitung	0.02	967	11	0.02	1440	1.49	Germany
Bioorganic and Medicinal Chemistry	0.2	910	7859	2.88	34194	37.58	Netherlands
Chemosphere	0.15	905	11704	3.41	32003	35.36	Netherlands
European Journal of Pharmacology	0.27	619	6875	2.76	26762	43.23	Netherlands
British Journal of Pharmacology	0.6	616	6819	5.29	28480	46.23	United Kingdom
Medical Hypotheses	0.12	612	1835	1.55	16902	27.62	United States
Japanese Journal of Cancer and Chemotherapy	0.03	611	163	0.09	889	1.45	Japan
International Journal of Pharmaceutics	0.19	528	5930	3.33	17075	32.34	Netherlands

Table 4. Pharmacology journals: SJR, output, citations, citations per paper, references, references per paper and country of publication (Scopus), 2009

The large and unwieldy original table was abbreviated to build Table 4, which gives the values for only the journals with the 10 highest SJR and the 10 scientific journals that published the largest number of pharmacological articles in the last year of the series. Note that none of these journals appears on both lists.

Of the scientific journals with the highest SJR, two were published in the US, *Annual Review of Pharmacology and Toxicology* and *Pharmacological Review*, and one in the United Kingdom, *Nature Reviews and Drug Discovery*. These three journals had SJR scores of 3.56, 3.3 and 2.68, respectively. That means that they received large numbers of citations, but also that since they are weighted by journal prestige to calculate the indicator, those citations appeared in other high quality journals. Neither of the US journals was very productive, with only 19 papers each in 2009, compared to a much larger output by the English periodical, which published a total of 202 articles.

The scientific journals with the highest output in pharmacology were The Netherlands' *Bioorganic and Medicinal Chemistry Letters*, with 1 546 papers, followed by the UK's *Pharmaceutical Journal*, with 1 058 and Germany's *Deutsche Apotheker Zeitung*, with 967. Their SJR indices were lower than for the journals mentioned in the preceding paragraph, however, with scores of 0.21, 0.03 and 0.02, respectively. In other words, in the period calculated for the SJR index (three years), either the absolute number of citations received by this group of more productive journals was very low or the citations were published in lower quality journals.

Each country's contribution to pharmacological scientific output can be analysed from two perspectives: as specified earlier, by the contribution made by its scientists through their published papers, or by the journals edited in the country. These two factors are compared in Figure 5. Each country's scientific output is shown in red and its publishing activity in blue. Many countries, such as the United States, show similar percentages for both types of contribution, while in others the values vary widely. A case in point is The Netherlands, whose scientific output was a mere 2 % while its journals published over 20 % of the pharmacological articles.

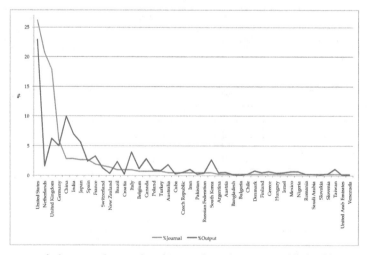

Fig. 5. Percentage of pharmacology-related journals and papers published by country (Scopus, 2009)

3.5 Scientometric indicators for pharmaceutical companies

The pharmaceutical industry, in addition to being one of the most profitable, is also one of the most globalised and fastest growing lines of business. Moreover, its large investment in research makes it an innovation-intensive activity. This innovation is the result of the direct or indirect interaction of a large number of actors: different types of companies, research institutes, financial institutions, public bodies and authorities, public and private universities, research centres, regulating bodies, governments, health systems, consumers and physicians, to name a few.

The industry comprises three categories of companies. The first covers (primarily North American and European) multinational companies that operate globally and invest huge sums in R&D, which is centralised in some cases and decentralised with laboratories in many countries and on many continents in others. The second category consists of small companies that supply their domestic markets with drugs that require no substantial R&D investment. The third includes firms that specialise in biotechnology and invest considerable sums in research despite their small size.

In 2010, biopharmaceutical companies invested an estimated 67.4 **billion** dollars in pursuit of new drugs (Figure 6). The total R&D spending by Pharmaceutical Research and Manufacturers of America (PhRMA) members, including industry majors such as AstraZeneca, Bayer, Boehringer, Ingelheim, Bristol-Myers, Squibb, Eli Lilly, Genzyme, GlaxoSmithKline, Hoffmann-La Roche, Merck, Novartis, Pfizer, and Sanofi-Aventis, as well as non-members, are shown in the figure.

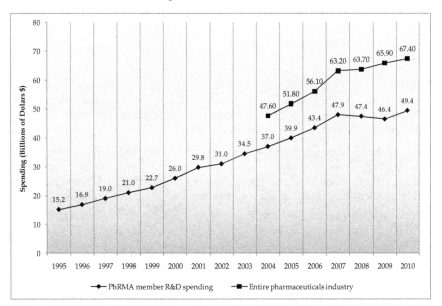

Fig. 6. Biopharmaceutical company R&D and PhRMA member R&D: 1995–2010 (Sources: Burrill and Company, analysis for PhRMA, 2005–2011 (Includes PhRMA research associates and non-members); PhRMA, PhRMA Annual Member Survey, 1996-2010)

Figure 7 shows the R&D spending by PhRMA members in and outside the United States. The total R&D investment by pharmaceutical companies has continued to rise. In 2010 PhRMA members invested 49.4 **billion** dollars, up 6 % from 2009 and 90 % since 2009.

PhRMA members spent most of their R&D budgets (76.1 %) in the United States, Western Europe (16.6 %) and Japan (1.5 %), while spreading the rest across other countries around the world (PhRMA, 2011).

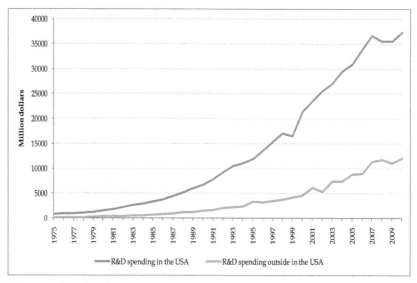

Fig. 7. R&D spending by Pharmaceutical Research and Manufacturers of America (PhRMA) members, 1975-2010 (PhRMA, 2011)

Bibliometric indicators can be constructed for the pharmaceutical industry on the grounds of the research results made public by the authors. As noted earlier, the industry has been gradually internationalising its high research and innovation potential since the mid nineteen seventies (McMillan and Hamilton, 2000).

The values of the bibliometric parameters for the pharmaceutical majors are given in Table 5. The data, which cover a seven-year period and are based on these companies' research publications, reveal a number of interesting differential characteristics. The ranking criterion followed was scientific output defined as the number of papers published in 2003-2009, initially disaggregated, although some of the companies listed had parent-subsidiary relationships.

The first significant result was the volume of scientific papers published by these companies. These elite, all of whose members published at least 125 papers in the period considered, was headed by the Pfizer headquarters site, which averaged 353 papers yearly throughout the period, followed by Merck with a yearly mean of 251.

The second statistic of interest was the citations per paper, which ranged from fairly low (7.86 for Dow Chemical Co., 8.47 for the Indian firm Dr Reddy´s and 9.26 for Sanofi-Aventis GmbH in Germany) to very high values (18.47 for Astra Zeneca in the United Kingdom and

18.21 for Hoffmann-La Roche in Switzerland). These findings suggest substantial differences in the visibility or quality of firms' scientific knowledge.

Organisation	Country	Output	Citations per paper	International collaboration	Normalised Citation	% Output in Q1
Pfizer Inc.	USA	2476	12.4	18.54	1.55	79.36
Merck & Co., Inc.	USA	1759	14.34	18.08	1.74	83.63
Eli Lilly and Company	USA	820	16.13	25.24	1.68	81.1
GlaxoSmithKline. United States	USA	788	15.17	29.7	1.77	86.68
GlaxoSmithKline. United Kigdom	GBR	781	13.76	42.77	1.74	85.66
Bristol-Myers Squibb Company	USA	677	12.97	13	1.58	87.59
Novartis	CHE	595	16.82	66.72	1.8	77.98
Abbott Laboratories United States	USA	571	14.75	12.61	1.65	88.27
Amgen	USA	497	12.27	16.9	1.59	77.46
F. Hoffmann-La Roche. Ltd.	USA	452	14.81	21.46	1.84	83.19
Pfizer Ltd	GBR	379	14.8	43.54	1.73	79.16
Bayer AG	DEU	362	10.46	36.74	1.34	64.36
Johnson & Johnson Pharmaceutical Research	USA	356	13.45	18.54	1.68	87.64
AstraZeneca R&D	SWE	294	14.64	57.82	1.8	87.07
F. Hoffmann-La Roche. Ltd.	CHE	272	18.21	55.15	1.86	83.09
Sanofi-Aventis. S.A.	FRA	224	15.64	43.75	1.55	66.52
Laboratoires SERVIER	FRA	200	17.16	37.5	1.71	91.5
Novartis Pharma SA. East Hanover	USA	192	16.2	34.9	1.89	73.96
AstraZeneca Pharmaceuticals. LP	USA	188	15.77	30.85	1.69	75
Sanofi-Aventis Deutschland GmbH	DEU	167	9.26	26.35	0.95	57.49
Schering-Plough Research Institute	USA	165	12.8	12.73	1.46	86.67
AstraZeneca	GBR	161	18.47	40.37	1.81	77.64
Novartis Institutes for Biomedical Research	USA	161	12.93	60.87	1.77	84.47
Laboratoires Pierre Fabre. S.A.	FRA	155	10.18	23.23	1.17	81.94
Novo Nordisk A/S	DNK	153	12.77	46.41	1.32	77.12
Dr. Reddy's Laboratories Ltd.	IND	150	8.47	7.33	0.88	59.33
H. Lundbeck A/S	DNK	150	18.11	45.33	1.73	91.33
GlaxoSmithKline. Italy	ITA	127	11.52	66.14	1.57	81.89
Dow Chemical Company	USA	125	7.86	34.4	0.9	66.4

Table 5. Bibliometric performance indicators for pharmaceutical firms, 2003-2009 (www.scimagoir.com)

Pharmaceuticals is generally agreed to be one of the industries whose research is most intensely internationalised, defining that to mean the proportion of the research conducted outside the headquarters country. The industry's business has become more international since the nineteen nineties as a result of the convergence of a number of processes. New industrial activities have cropped up around biotechnological research, primarily in the US;

market dynamics with a view to capitalising on research incentives has favoured the location of new laboratories in different countries; global excellence centres with research responsibilities have been created; and inter- and intra-firm networking has been intensified.

When companies were ranked in descending order of the percentage of their papers involving international collaboration, two different patterns emerged, one for European and the other for North American companies. The percentages were higher in the former than in the latter. Several explanations can be given for this difference between countries on the two sides of the Atlantic. The United States is the critical location for pharmaceutical alliances as a result of the quality of the research conducted there, but especially of the size of its research base, i.e., the number and size of universities, companies and research departments. Other factors that distinguish the European and US include the latter's easy financing and marketing terms and fairly large number of start-up incubators and venture capitalists.

The result is that companies based in the US have lower percentages of internationally co-authored papers than European companies: Abbott Laboratories 12.67 %, Schering-Plough Research Institute, 12.73 %, Bristol-Myers Squibb Company, 13 %.

Switzerland's Novartis, by contrast, co-authored 66.72 % of its papers with other countries. Its US subsidiary had a collaboration rate of 69.87 %, while the figure for the French firm Sanofi-Aventis was 43.75 %.

The final indicator analysed was normalised citation, which measures a company's impact on the scientific community as a whole and compares the quality of the research conducted by organisations of different sizes. The highest score was obtained by Swiss Novartis' North American subsidiary, with a mean citation value 89 % higher than the world-wide mean (1.89). It was followed by its parent company, which had a mean citation value 86 % higher than the world-wide mean, and the Swiss subsidiary of North America's F. Hoffman La Roche, with a score of 84 %. The lowest values were recorded for Dow Chemical's pharmaceuticals division (US) and the Dr. Reddy laboratories in India, whose citation values were below the international average.

4. Conclusions

This chapter reports on a multi-level analysis of scientific results in pharmacology. The findings confirmed that despite its scant weight in world-wide science, pharmacological scientific output is characterised by high quality and has citation per paper values higher than the mean for international scientific output as a whole.

Two regions of the world have traditionally occupied the leading positions in terms of pharmacological scientific output, North America and Western Europe. Moreover, the impact of this output is high, measured in terms of citations in other papers. When only citations outside the home region are considered, however, other regions, such as Northern Africa, prove to have higher values. The regions with the largest absolute number of citations also have the highest percentage of domestic citations. By contrast, since the regions with smaller numbers of citations in absolute terms receive fewer domestic citations, the acknowledgement coming primarily from countries outside their own region carries much heavier weight.

During the period studied, certain emerging countries such as Brazil or India joined the list of top ten producers, while China, which was already on the list, climbed almost to the summit. As might be expected, the countries in the most productive regions occupied the highest positions throughout the period analysed, but the appearance of these BRIC countries should prompt reflection on their scientific potential in the field of pharmacology.

The most productive journals, i.e., the ones that publish the largest number of pharmacological articles, do not generally earn high SJR impact values. These values are attained by journals publishing smaller numbers of papers. Consequently, journal quality and the number of papers published are inversely related. An analysis relating papers published and journals edited in each country showed that intense pharmacological publishing is not necessarily attendant upon the presence of numerous researchers working in the field (The Netherlands). US publishing in pharmacology, by contrast, is as predominant in the area as its research community.

Companies carry specific weight in pharmacology. Their investment and innovative capacity are mirrored by the scientific results attained, primarily by US and European pharmaceutical laboratories.

5. Acknowledgement

The authors wish to thank Scimago Lab for its generous assistance in compiling the data used.

6. References

Biglu, M.H. and Omidi, Y. (2010). Scientific profile of Pharmacology, Toxicology and Pharmaceutics fields in Middle East Countries: Impacts of Iranian Scientists. *International Journal of Advances in Pharmaceutical Sciences*, Vol. 1, pp. 122-127, ISSN 0976-1055

Braun, T.; Glänzel, W. and Schubert, A. Scientometric indicators: a 32-country comparative evaluation of *publishing performance and citation impact.* Singapore, Philadelphia: World Scientific, 1985, 425 p.

Congressional Budget Office. (2006). *A CBO Study: Research and Development in hte Pharmaceutical Industry.* Congress of the United States. 20/08/2011. Available from http://www.cbo.gov/ftpdocs/76xx/doc7615/10-02-DrugR-D.pdf

Fingerman, S. (2006). Web of Science and Scopus: current features and capabilities. Issues in *Science and Technology Librarianship*, Fall, ISSN 1092-1206, 20/08/2011, Available from http://www.istl.org/06-fall/electronic2.html

Gambardella, A. (1995). *Science and innovation: the US pharmaceutical industry during the 1980s.* Cambridge: Cambridge University Press. ISBN: 0521451183

González-Pereira, B.; Guerrero-Bote, V. and Moya-Anegón, F. (2009). The SJR indicator: A new indicator of journals' scientific prestige. *Arxiv Preprint* arXiv:0912.4141, 02/08/2011, Available from http://arxiv.org/ftp/arxiv/papers/0912/0912.4141.pdf

Gorraiz, J. and Schloegl, C. (2008). A bibliometric analysis of pharmacology and pharmacy journals: Scopus versus Web of Science. *Journal of Information Science*, Vol. 34, No. 5, pp. 715-725, ISSN 0165-5515

Gupta, B.M. and Kaur, H. (2009). Status of India in science and technology as reflected in its publication output in the Scopus international database, 1996-2006. *Scientometrics*, Vol. 80, No. 2, pp. 473-490, ISSN 0138-9130

Kaur, H. and Gupta, B.M. (2009). Indian Contribution in Pharmacology, Toxicology and Pharmaceutics during 1998-2007: A Scientometric Analysis. *Collnet Journal of Scientometrics and Information Management*, Vol. 3, No. 1, pp. 1-9, ISSN 0973-7766

Koening, M. (1983). Bibliometric analysis of pharmaceutical research. Research Policy, Vol. 12, No. 1, pp. 15-36, ISSN 0048-7333

LaGuardia, C. (2005). E-views and reviews: Scopus vs Web of Science. Library Journal, (January 2005), eISSN 0000-0027, 20.08.2011, Available from http://www.libraryjournal.com/article/CA491154.html

McMillan, G.S. and Hamilton, R.D. (2000). Using Bibliometrics to Measure Firm Knowledge: An Analysis of the US Pharmaceutical Industry. Technology *Analysis and Strategic Management*. Vol. 12, No. 4, pp. 465-475. ISSN 0953-7325

Noisi, J. (1999). The internationalization of industrial R&D from technology transfer to the learing organization. *Research Policy*, Vol. 28, pp. 107-117, ISSN 0048-7333

Narin, F. and Rozek, R.P. (1988). Bibliometric analysis of United States pharmaceutical industry research performance. *Research Policy*, Vol. 17, No. 3, pp. 139-154, ISSN 0048-7333

Patel, P. and Pavitt, K. (2000). National systems of innovation under strain: The internationalization of coporate R&D. In: Barrel, R.; Mason, G.; Mahony, M. (eds). *Productivity, Innovation and Economic Performance*. Cambridge: Cambridge University Press, pp. 217-235. ISBN 0521780314

Perianes-Rodríguez, A.; Rafols, I.; O'Hare, A.; Hopkins, M.M. and Nightingale, P. (2011). Benchmarking and visualizing the knowledge base of pharmaceutical firms (1995-2009). *Proceedings of the 13th ISSI Conference*. Durban: International Society for Scientometrics and Informetrics, Vol. 2, pp. 656-661, ISBN 9789081752701

Pharmaceutical Research and Manufacturers of America. *Pharmaceutical Industry Profile 2011*. Washington, DC: PhRMA, April 2011

Rafols, I.; O'Hare, A.; Perianes-Rodríguez, A.; Hopkins, M.M. and Nightingale, P. (2010). *Collaborative practices and technological trajectories in large pharmaceutical firms. Tentative Governance in Emerging Science and Technology*. Enschede: University of Twente, pp. 93-95.

Rehn, C. (2007). Bibliometric indicators: definitions and usage at Karolinska Institutet. 20/08/2011, Available from http://ki.se/content/1/c6/01/79/31/Bibliometric%20indicators%20-%20definitions_1.0.pdf

Sciverse Scopus (2011). What dos it Cover?. 2.08.2011. Available from http://www.info.sciverse.com/scopus/scopus-in-detail/facts

SJR. SCImago Research Group. *SCImago Journal and Country Rank*. 2007. 20/08/2011. Available from: http://www.scimagojr.com

5

Novel Strategies in Drug-Induced Acute Kidney Injury

Alberto Lázaro, Sonia Camaño, Blanca Humanes and Alberto Tejedor
Renal Physiopathology Laboratory, Department of Nephrology,
Hospital General Universitario Gregorio Marañón, Madrid,
Spain

1. Introduction

1.1 Renal toxicity

Renal toxicity associated with commonly prescribed drugs lengthens hospital stay, worsens prognosis, and limits the potential benefits obtained from therapy (Peracella, 2011; Servais et al., 2008).

Proximal tubule preservation is a clue in strategies aimed to prevent nephrotoxicity. The proximal tubule is a target for filtered drugs that are reabsorbed by solvent drag or pinocytosis, but also for drugs that are secreted into the luminal side.

Proximal tubules recover more than 60% of total filtered load, i.e., a single molecule of toxin that is filtered and reabsorbed will pass through the proximal tubule cell more than 50 times per day. Such a high degree of exposure implies a risk of cell damage causing a variety of clinical syndromes, from proximal acidosis and acquired Fanconi syndrome to tubular cell necrosis (Oh, 2010). This spectrum of diseases is known as acute kidney injury (AKI), which also includes cell death by apoptosis, anoikis, necrosis, or cell dysfunction (Lorz et al., 2006).

Nephrotoxicity can often be expected with certain drugs, such as vancomycin, gentamicin, foscarnet, cisplatin, cyclosporine A (CsA), and tacrolimus. Less often, the toxic effect is unexpected and not predictable, as is the case with iodinated contrast agents and paracetamol.

1.2 Cell death mediation

Intrinsic pathway–mediated apoptosis and extrinsic pathway–mediated apoptosis are both involved in toxic proximal tubule cell death (Pabla & Dong, 2008; Servais et al., 2008; Xiao et al., 2011). With most of toxins, cell death is followed by detachment and anoikis. Paracetamol is a notable exception to this behavior. Caspases activation, mitochondrial depolarization, release of cytochrome C from mitochondria, cell membrane modification, and nucleosome formation are all hallmarks of apoptosis that are regularly observed in toxin-damaged proximal tubules (Camano et al., 2010). Nitric oxide, soluble oxygen radicals, and proinflammatory cytokines are released by damaged proximal tubules, thus amplifying the lesion.

1.3 Nephrotoxicity prevention strategies

Overhydration is the most common maneuver to prevent toxic concentrations in urine and, consequently, inside the cell. However, nephrotoxicity usually requires dose adjustment or drug withdrawal, thus limiting effectiveness.

Other strategies aimed at inhibiting cell drug transport or interfering with mediation of apoptosis also tend to interfere with the therapeutic targets and, consequently, limit the effectiveness of therapy (Pabla & Dong, 2008; Servais et al., 2008).

During the last 5 years, our work on nephrotoxicity has enabled us to better understand the role of proximal tubule behavior in the adaptation of the kidney to toxic aggressions (Camano et al., 2010; Camaño-Paez et al., 2008; Neria et al., 2009; Perez et al., 2004; Tejedor et al., 2007).

Therefore, not surprisingly, the search for alternative protective strategies against toxic damage to the proximal tubule is an important area of investigation today.

1.4 Ability of cilastatin to prevent drug toxicity targeting the proximal tubule

Cilastatin is an inhibitor of brush border dehydropeptidase I (DHP-I), which is present in renal proximal tubular epithelial cells (RPTECs). It was initially designed to inhibit hydrolysis and uptake of the carbapenem antibiotic imipenem, thus enabling it to be more easily recovered from urine (Birnbaum et al., 1985; Norbby et al., 1983). However, cilastatin is also able to inhibit uptake of CsA and cisplatin by RPTECs by decreasing in a dose-dependent way the toxic effect of CsA and cisplatin on RPTECs (Camano et al., 2010; Perez et al., 2004). Clinical studies also support this protective role of cilastatin against CsA-induced nephrotoxicity (Carmellini et al., 1997, 1998; Gruss et al., 1996; Markewitz et al., 1994; Mraz et al., 1987, 1992; Tejedor et al., 2007). Experimental evidence suggests that cilastatin binding to brush border DHP-I could interact with apical cholesterol lipid rafts (Camano et al., 2010; Perez et al., 2004; Tejedor et al., 2007).

The aim of this brief report is to determine whether cilastatin is able to interfere with the direct toxic effect of several known nephrotoxic drugs on cultured RPTECs. We investigated the effect of cilastatin on the toxicity of gentamicin, vancomycin, iodinated contrast agent, amphotericin B, foscarnet, cisplatin, mannitol, chloroform, paracetamol, CsA and tacrolimus.

We describe for the first time the effects of a drug that specifically targets the renal proximal tubule brush border and seems to be able to reduce accumulation and toxicity of the main nephrotoxic drugs by inhibiting internalization of brush border–bound lipid rafts.

2. Methods

2.1 Drugs

We used commercially available parenteral formulations of gentamicin (powder, Guinama, Alboraya, Spain), vancomycin (powder, Combino Pharm, Barcelona, Spain), iodinate contrast agent (iopamidol, Laboratorios Farmacéuticos Rovi, Madrid, Spain), amphotericin B (Bristol Myers Squibb, Madrid, Spain), foscarnet (Foscavir, AstraZeneca, Madrid, Spain), cisplatin (Pharmacia, Barcelona, Spain), mannitol 20%, (Osmofundin®, Braun Medical S.A., Barcelona, Spain), chloroform (Scharlau, Barcelona, Spain), CsA (Sandimmun Neoral®,

Novartis Farmaceutica S.A., Spain), tacrolimus (Prograf®, Fujisawa S.A., Spain), and paracetamol (Perfalgan, Bristol Myers Squibb). The concentrations used were similar to the pharmacologically active recommended plasma level.

Crystalline cilastatin was provided by Merck Sharp & Dohme S.A. (Madrid, Spain). A dose of 200 µg/ml was chosen, because it is cytoprotective and falls within the reference range for clinical use (Camano et al., 2010; Perez et al., 2004).

All drug dilutions were performed with sterile culture medium and cilastatin, and the tested drugs were added simultaneously.

2.2 Primary cultures of renal proximal tubule epithelial cells

Porcine RPTECs were obtained as previously described (Camano et al., 2010; Perez et al., 2004). Briefly, the cortex was sliced and incubated for 30 minutes at 37°C with 0.6 mg/ml of collagenase A (Boehringer Mannheim, Germany) in Ham's F-12 medium. Digested tissue was then filtered through a metal mesh (250 µm), washed 3 times with Ham's F-12 medium, and centrifuged using an isotonic Percoll gradient (45% [v/v]) at $20,000g$ for 30 minutes. Proximal tubules were recovered from the deepest fraction, washed, and resuspended in supplemented DMEM/Ham's F-12 at a 1:1 ratio (with 25 mM HEPES, 3.7 mg/ml sodium bicarbonate, 2.5 mM glutamine, 1% non-essential amino acids, 100 U/ml penicillin, 100 mg/ml streptomycin, 5 x 10^{-8} M hydrocortisone, 5 mg/ml insulin-transferrin-sodium selenite media supplement, and 2% fetal bovine serum). Proximal tubules were seeded at a density of 0.66 mg/ml and incubated at 37°C in a 95% air/5% CO_2 atmosphere. Culture medium was renewed every 2 days. RPTECs were used after they had reached confluence (80%).

2.3 Cell death studies

2.3.1 Nuclear morphology

Cell nuclei were visualized following DNA staining with the fluorescent dye DAPI (Sigma-Aldrich, Missouri, USA). Briefly, cells were seeded on cover slips in a 24-well plate, fixed in 4% formaldehyde for 10 minutes, and permeabilized with 0.5% Triton X-100. They were then rinsed with PBS and incubated with DAPI (12.5 µg/ml) for 15 minutes. Excess dye was removed. Cells imaging was performed with the 40X PL-APO 1.25 NA oil objective of a Leica-SP2 confocal microscope (Leica Microsystems, Heidelberg, Germany). DAPI was excited with a 405 nm laser-diode. Emission between 420 nm and 490 nm was collected following the manufacturer's recommendations. Six fields with ~200 cells per field were examined in each condition to estimate the percentage of nuclei with an apoptosis-like appearance.

2.3.2 Nucleosomal quantification

To evaluate DNA fragmentation in the context of apoptosis, RPTECs were incubated for 48 hours under specific conditions with the nephrotoxic compounds selected. At the end of this period RPTECs were lysed and centrifuged at $200g$ for 10 minutes to remove cell debris. DNA and histones present in the soluble fraction were quantified using an enzyme-linked immunosorbent assay (*Cell Death Detection ELISAPLUS* kit, Boehringer Mannheim, Germany), as previously described (Camano et al., 2010; Perez et al., 2004).

2.3.3 Cell viability assay

The cell survival assay relies on the capacity of cells to reduce 3-(4, 5- dimethylthiazol-2-yl)-2, 5-diphenyltetrazolium bromide (MTT) (Calbiochem, California, USA) to colored formazan in metabolically active cells. RPTECs were seeded onto 96-well plates and incubated with toxins alone or in combination with cilastatin. Twenty-four hours later, 0.5 mg/ml of MTT was added, plates were incubated for 3 hours in the dark at 37°C, and 100 μL of 50% dimethylformamide in 20% SDS (pH 4.7) was added. Plates were incubated at 37°C overnight, and absorbance was measured at 595 nm. All assays were performed in triplicate.

Alternatively, MTT assays were performed in real time, following MTT reduction on single cells, with an Olympus IX70 inverted microscope fitted to a spectrofluorometer SLM AMINCO 2000. MTT was measured by reading cell absorbance at 570 nm.

2.4 Cell viability: Quantification of colony-forming units

RPTECs were treated for 24 hours with CsA, tacrolimus or paracetamol in the presence or absence of cilastatin (200 μg/ml). Adherent cells were washed in saline serum, harvested with trypsin-EDTA, seeded in Petri dishes (100 mm), and cultured for 7 days in drug-free complete medium. Surviving adherent cells were fixed for 5 minutes with 5% paraformaldehyde/PBS and stained with 0.5% crystal violet/20% methanol for 2 minutes. Excess dye was rinsed with PBS. Finally, the intracellular dye was eluted with 50% ethanol/50% sodium citrate 0.1 M (pH 4.2) and quantified by spectrometry at 595 nm.

2.5 Cellular drug transport and accumulation

RPTECs incubated for 24 hours with increasing concentrations of CsA, tacrolimus or paracetamol in the presence or absence of cilastatin (200 μg/ml), were scraped and lysed in 400 μL of lysis buffer at 70°C (2.22% [w/v] SDS; 19.33 % [v/v] glycerol [87% v/v]; 790 mM Tris HCl pH 6.8 in dH$_2$O, phenylmethylsulfonyl fluoride, and protease inhibitors). Cell lysates were heated at 100°C for 5 minutes, homogenized in ice, and centrifuged at 12,000g for 5 minutes at 4°C. The supernatant was analyzed for total protein content and the presence of nephrotoxins. The concentrations of CsA, tacrolimus and paracetamol were measured using fluorescence polarization immunoassay technology on a TDX Chemistry Analyzer (Abbot Laboratories, USA) in accordance with the instructions provided by the manufacturer. The calibrators and controls supplied with each kit were applied, and the results were expressed as ng drug/μg protein.

2.6 Localization of lipids rafts by immunofluorescence

To study the interaction of cilastatin with cholesterol lipid rafts, we used FITC-conjugated cholera toxin B (Molecular Probes, Oregon, USA), as its internalization is mediated by lipid rafts.

RPTECs cultured on glass coverslips were preincubated with culture medium alone or cilastatin 200 μg/ml for 15 minutes. The cells were then incubated with 10 μg/ml FITC-labelled cholera toxin B for 1 and 2.5 hours. Cells were washed with PBS and fixed in 4%

formaldehyde in PBS for 10 minutes before being rinsed with PBS. The nuclei were counterstained with DAPI. After washing, cells were mounted in fluorescent mounting medium (Dako North America, Inc., Carpinteria, California). Images of the distribution of cholera toxin immunolocalization across membranes were obtained with the 20X PL-APO 0.7-numerical aperture objective of a Leica-SP2 confocal microscope (Leica Microsystems).

2.7 Dehydropeptidase I and IV activity assays

RPTECs were incubated overnight with Gly-Phe-p-nitroanilide (DHP-I substrate; Sigma-Aldrich) 1mM in PBS for DHP-I activity determination or with Gly-Pro-p-nitroanilide (DHP-IV substrate; Sigma-Aldrich) 1 mM for DHP-IV activity determination. Both activities were measured in the presence or absence of cilastatin (200 µg/ml). P-Nitroanilide was quantified in aliquots from supernatants by measuring at 410 nm absorbance.

2.8 Statistical analysis

Quantitative variables were expressed as the mean ± standard error of the mean (SEM). Differences were considered statistically significant for bilateral alpha values less than 0.05. Factorial ANOVA was used when more than 1 factor was considered. When a single factor presented more than 2 levels and the model showed significant differences between factors, a post-hoc analysis (least significant difference) was performed. When results are shown, they represent a minimum of at least 3 repeats. When possible, a quantification technique (e.g. dye recovery) was used to illustrate reproducibility. When figures illustrated an effect, paracetamol was chosen as the example.

3. Results

3.1 Cilastatin as a broad nephroprotective drug: reduction of toxin-induced proximal tubular cell death

After 48 hours of exposure to the drugs tested, apoptosis of RPTECs measured as nucleosomal DNA fragmentation and migration from nuclei to cytosol was quantified and compared with apoptosis under the same conditions, although in the presence of cilastatin (Fig. 1). RPTECs exposed to toxins present different increases in the number of nucleosomes recovered from cytosol. Cilastatin significantly partially or totally prevented these changes in most of the selected drugs (Fig. 1).

When the magnitude of cilastatin protection was plotted against the magnitude of basal cell death under every treatment tested, a clear linear trend was observed (r=0.839, p<0.0005). None of the drugs tested differed significantly from this trend (Fig. 2).

We made a detailed study of the effect of 3 of these drugs: CsA, tacrolimus and paracetamol. A more selective qualitative estimation of apoptotic cell death was also obtained in adherent cells treated with CsA, tacrolimus, and paracetamol and stained with DAPI (Fig. 3). Incubation with toxins led to cell shrinkage with significant nuclear condensation, fragmentation, and formation of apoptosis-like bodies (see arrows). Cilastatin was able to reduce nuclear damage in all cases. Apoptosis-like nuclei are quantified in Fig. 3B, C, and D.

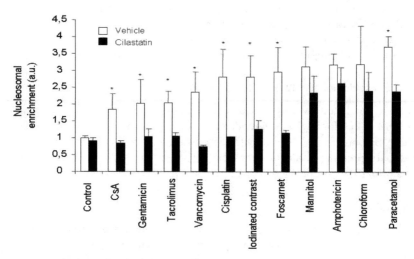

Fig. 1. Effect of cilastatin on nephrotoxin-induced apoptosis. Renal proximal tubular epithelial cells were exposed to CsA (1 µg/ml), gentamicin (20 mg/ml), tacrolimus (50 ng/ml), vancomycin (600 µg/ml), cisplatin (10 µM), iodinated contrast (1 mg/ml), foscarnet (1 mM), mannitol (100 mosm/l), amphotericin B (10 µg/ml), chloroform (100 µg/ml), and paracetamol (300 µg/ml) with and without cilastatin (200 µg/ml) for 48 hours. Oligonucleosomal DNA fragmentation was detected by ELISA. Data are represented as the mean ± SEM of at least 3 separate experiments. ANOVA model: p<0.0001. *p<0.05 vs. same data with cilastatin.

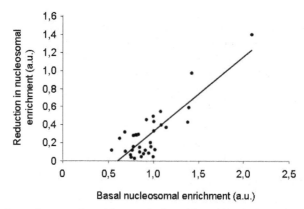

Fig. 2. Reduction in nucleosomal enrichment induced by cilastatin over basal nucleosomal enrichment induced by each toxin. Individual experimental data are provided. There is a common trend for all the data, suggesting a common behavior, with cilastatin protection being proportional to basal damage. Linear regression of "cilastatin-induced reduction" vs. "basal nucleosomal enrichment", slope=0.82, r=0.839, adjusted r^2=0.695, p<0.0005.

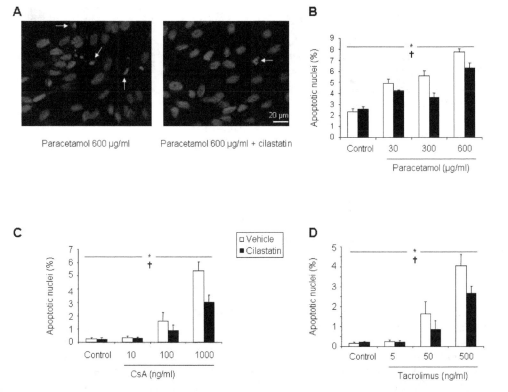

Fig. 3. Effects of cilastatin on the nuclear morphology of renal proximal tubular epithelial cells (RPTECs) during treatment with toxins. RPTECs were cultured in the presence of paracetamol (30, 300 and 600 μg/ml), cyclosporine (CsA, 10, 100, and 1000 ng/ml) and tacrolimus (5, 50, and 500 ng/ml) with or without cilastatin (200 μg/ml) for 24 hours. A, Example of nuclear staining with DAPI to determine whether an apoptotic-like nuclear morphology was present. Arrows point to fragmented, apoptotic nuclei. B, C and D, Quantitative approach to staining for paracetamol, CsA and tacrolimus, respectively. Data are represented as the mean ± SEM of at least 3 separate experiments. ANOVA models p<0.0001. * cilastatin effect, p<0.05; †dose effect, p<0.05.

We quantified the functional impact of CsA, tacrolimus and paracetamol treatments on cell survival by measuring the percentage of adherent cells still able to reduce MTT to formazan after exposure to increasing doses of toxins. After 24 hours of incubation with toxins, the amount of surviving cells able to reduce MTT decreases progressively as the concentrations of CsA, tacrolimus, and paracetamol increase. However, in the presence of cilastatin, all surviving cells keep their capacity to reduce MTT (Fig. 4). Cilastatin is able to counteract both the structural and functional damage induced by toxins.

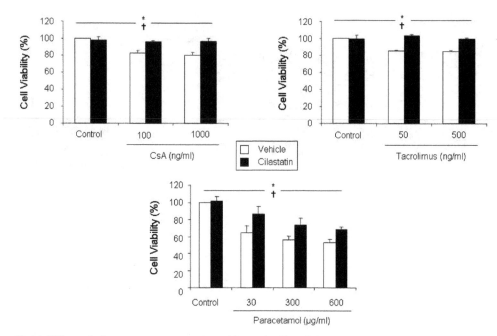

Fig. 4. Effect of cilastatin on toxin-induced loss of cell viability determined by the ability to reduce MTT (see Methods). Renal proximal tubular epithelial cells were exposed to toxins and toxins + cilastatin (200 µg/ml) for 24 hours. Results are expressed as the percentage of the value obtained relative to control (without toxins and cilastatin) of at least 3 separate experiments. ANOVA: for CsA, *dose effect, p≤0.05; †cilastatin effect, p<0.05; for tacrolimus, *dose effect, p<0.05; †cilastatin effect, p≤0.04; for paracetamol, *dose effect, p≤0.05; †cilastatin effect, p≤0.05.

3.2 Cilastatin prevents toxin-induced mitochondrial damage

The effect of cilastatin on mitochondria may be observed very early after CsA, tacrolimus, or paracetamol is added to cell culture plates. In Fig. 5, an inverted IX-80 microscope was fitted with a black chamber, a photomultiplier, and a spectrofluorimeter (SML Aminco) to obtain absorbance readings at specific wavelengths on single (or small groups of) cells in culture. This set-up allows real time follow-up of colorimetric in vivo reactions.

Recording the first seconds after MTT addition shows the initial kinetics of MTT reduction and formazan precipitation, thus offering a first approach to the activity of the mitochondrial chain in intact cells. Although not suitable for detailed kinetic studies, this method allows a quick check of mitochondrial oxidative activity.

RPTECs exposed to toxins showed a quick and deep depression in the reduction of MTT activity compared with controls (Fig. 5). Coincubation with cilastatin partially recovers this effect, although the effect was less visible for paracetamol. Differences are observed even during the first 5 minutes of drug additions.

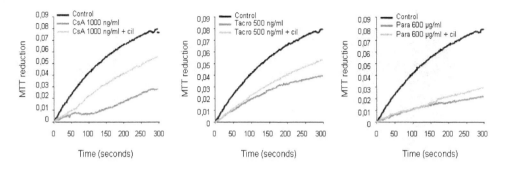

Fig. 5. Effect of cilastatin on toxin-induced mitochondrial damage. Changes in the mitochondrial oxidative capacity of RPTECs were assessed by MTT reduction at 570 nm. The graphs show formation of formazan as detected in isolated cells in real time with no treatment (control) and CsA (cyclosporin, 1000 ng/ml), tacro (tacrolimus, 500 ng/ml) and para (paracetamol, 600 μg/ml) with or without 200 μg/ml cilastatin, after the incubation times on the X-axis.

3.3 Cilastatin improves long-term recovery and viability of RPTECs after exposure to CsA, tacrolimus, and paracetamol

To know the long-term viability of surviving RPTECs after 24 hours of exposure to CsA, tacrolimus, or paracetamol, we tested the ability of those cells to proliferate into new cell colonies. Colony-forming units (CFUs) were quantified as specified in Methods. The CFUs count decreased after 24 hours of treatment with CsA, tacrolimus, and paracetamol, and this decrease was clearly dose-dependent (Fig. 6). If the cells were exposed to toxins in the presence of cilastatin, the number of CFUs was significantly greater after 7 days of recovery for every CsA, tacrolimus, and paracetamol concentration studied. The intracellular dye was extracted, and absorbance was quantified al 595 nm (Fig. 6B, C and D).

3.4 Cilastatin reduces intracellular accumulation of CsA, tacrolimus, and paracetamol

In many cases, nephrotoxicity is largely dependent on the intracellular concentration of drug reached. As cilastatin is a ligand of the brush border membrane, we investigated whether it affected toxin uptake by RPTECs. To test this hypothesis, we measured the intracellular content of CsA, tacrolimus, and paracetamol by TDX analysis, as described in Methods. Cellular CsA, tacrolimus and paracetamol content increased progressively in a dose-dependent manner when RPTECs were incubated for 24 hours in the presence of different concentrations of toxins (Fig. 7). Coincubation with cilastatin consistently reduced accumulation of CsA, tacrolimus and paracetamol in the cells for every concentration studied (Fig. 7). These results confirm that adding cilastatin to primary cultures of proximal cells decreases cellular toxin accumulation. This effect may be involved in the reduced impact of CsA, tacrolimus, and paracetamol on damage to and survival and death of RPTECs.

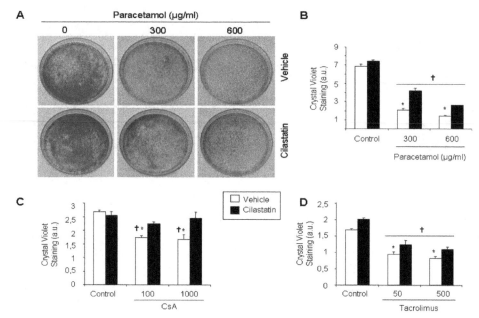

Fig. 6. Cilastatin preserves long-term recovery of toxin-treated RPTECs. A, RPTECs were incubated with paracetamol, CsA (cyclosporin), or tacrolimus in the presence or absence of 200 µg/ml cilastatin for 24 hours. The number of colony-forming units was determined by staining with crystal violet after 7 days (the figure shows the experiment with paracetamol). B, C, and D, Quantification of crystal violet staining for paracetamol, CsA and tacrolimus, respectively. Data are expressed as mean ± SEM; of 3 separate experiments. ANOVA model, p<0.0001. †p<0.05 vs. control; *p≤0.05 vs. same data with cilastatin.

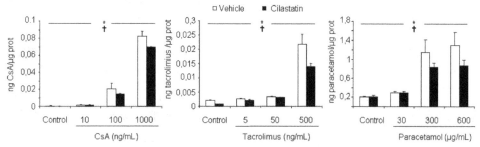

Fig. 7. Effects of cilastatin on accumulation of toxins by RPTECs. Intracellular accumulation was measured in the lysates of RPTECs treated with nephrotoxins for 24 hours, in the presence or absence of cilastatin (200 µg/ml), using a specific fluorescence polarization immunoassay (TDX). Cilastatin was shown to prevent entry of all nephrotoxins into RPTECs. Values were expressed as means ± SEM of drug concentrations (n=4 different experiments). ANOVA model, p<0.0001; *, cilastatin effect p<0.05; †, dose effect p<0.05.

3.5 Effect of cilastatin on lipid rafts distribution

According to these results, which suggest that cilastatin interferes with intracellular administration of the nephrotoxins tested, cilastatin appears to be able to inhibit an intracellular nephrotoxin accumulation pathway as a result of its binding to renal DHP-I. We explored the possibility that cilastatin, through its interaction with DHP-I and when anchored to cholesterol lipid rafts by a glycosyl-phosphate-inositol (GPI) group (Adachi et al., 1990; Parkin et al., 2001), could block transport through lipid rafts or interfere with the cholesterol lipid raft–dependent endocytic pathway. The expression and cell membrane localization of cholera toxin, which specifically binds to its ganglioside GM1 receptor present in cholesterol lipid rafts, were assessed using confocal microscopy in RPTECs treated for very short periods. In Fig. 8, cholera toxin is identified on the cell surface after 15 minutes incubation, but it disappeared from the membrane after 1 hour (top) and accumulated in a perinuclear position. In the presence of 200 µg/ml cilastatin and after 1 hour of treatment, cholera toxin was still attached to the membrane, suggesting interference with the cholera toxin internalization site. No significant changes in FITC-cholera toxin staining patterns were observed at 2.5 hours in the presence of cilastatin.

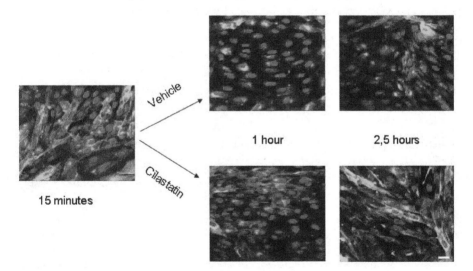

Fig. 8. Blockade of circulation of cholesterol rafts by cilastatin. This picture shows the change in cholera toxin fluorescence internalization over time in control cells and cells incubated in the presence of cilastatin (200 µg/ml). Bar, 20 µm.

4. Conclusion

We report that cilastatin, a powerful and specific inhibitor of DPH-I, is able to reduce both intracellular accumulation and induction of apoptosis by antibiotic, cytotoxic, anti-inflammatory, antiretroviral, anesthetic, and immunosuppressive drugs. These findings expand our previous results with cisplatin (Camano et al., 2010) and CsA (Perez et al., 2004; Tejedor et al., 2007).

Cilastatin inhibits the activity of DPH-I, but not of DPH-4, in the brush border of renal RPTECs (Fig. 9).

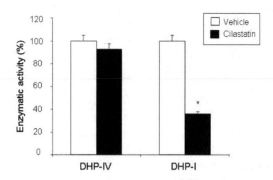

Fig. 9. Effect of cilastatin on the activity of dehydropeptidase I and IV. Activities were determined by the hydrolysis of specific substrates. Results are expressed as a percentage of enzyme activity compared to untreated controls (100% activity) and as the mean ± SEM of 3 experiments. ANOVA model, p<0.0001. * p<0.01 vs. the same data without cilastatin.

Although this inhibition is probably irrelevant in the degree of nephroprotection observed — none of the nephrotoxins studied have a chemical structure that could potentially be affected by dipeptidase activity — binding to DPH-I may partially explain this protection.

DPH-I is anchored to brush border lipid rafts (Pang et al., 2004; Parkin et al., 2001). Binding of FITC-labelled B-cholera toxin to lipid rafts leads to their rapid internalization. However, internalization does not occur in the presence of cilastatin.

This mechanism is probably behind the reduction observed in the intracellular concentration of the different drugs analyzed.

We previously showed that cilastatin modifies brush border membrane fluidity by interfering with membrane-bound cholesterol (Perez et al., 2004).

The drugs tested in Fig. 1 have many different chemical structures, and their mechanisms of cell permeation are not well established in some cases. However, for all those drugs, intracellular concentrations were measured and cilastatin always reduced intracellular accumulation. By inhibiting lipid raft–dependent vesicle circulation, cilastatin seems able to reduce luminal entry of drugs, even if they are not substrates for DPH-I activity.

This interference with drug entry may explain the almost instantaneous protection observed in the real-time experiments of MTT reduction. MTT reduction relies on mitochondrial oxidative chain integrity. When single cell oxidative capacity is recorded in real time, addition of the toxin inhibits MTT reduction activity relative to the single control cell, and this is evident from the first seconds. Cilastatin partially protects against this effect. The quick time course of the effect strongly suggests that a mechanism of cilastatin inhibits drug intake by the cell.

However, other mechanisms may be implicated in the broad renal protection observed. We recently published that, when exposed to toxic concentrations of cisplatin, RPTECs increase expression of Fas and Fas L. Fas targets brush border lipid rafts (Dimanche-Boitrel et al., 2005), binds its ligand, and triggers the extrinsic pathway of apoptosis. Internalization of Fas/Fas L seems a necessary step (Camano et al., 2010).

Cilastatin reduced cisplatin-induced cell apoptosis but not cell necrosis (Camano et al., 2010). When the extrinsic apoptosis pathway was checked, the initial step blocked by cilastatin was Fas L/Fas internalization (Camano et al., 2010).

Cilastatin reduces apoptosis (nuclear damage, nucleosome formation, MTT reduction capacity) and ameliorates surviving cell recovery. Both reductions in drug intake by proximal cells and blockade of lipid raft internalization are probably involved in these protective actions (Fig. 10).

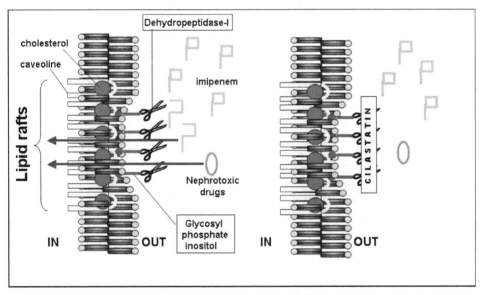

Fig. 10. Diagram of the possible protective mechanism of cilastatin. Cilastatin is a dehydropeptidase-I inhibitor used in human clinical practice combined with imipenem. Dehydropeptidase inhibition affects the structure of lipid rafts by preventing hydrolysis of the lactam ring and inhibits the absorption of imipenem and other nephrotoxic drugs, thus reducing their renal toxicity.

Protection by cilastatin depends on its interaction with DPH-I, an enzyme that is found almost exclusively in proximal tubules. Therefore, cilastatin-induced nephroprotection is specific for tissue and cell type, but not for the drug tested.

More research is necessary to confirm the mechanism of protection, the ability to protect in animal models of acute renal failure, and the absence of an effect on the pharmacological targets of tested drugs. Nevertheless, cilastatin offers a new protective strategy, as it is a tissue-specific designed drug, with unexpected tissue-specific antiapoptotic actions.

5. Acknowledgments

This work was partially supported by the Fondo de Investigaciones Sanitarias [Grants FIS-PI05/2259, FIS-PI 08/1481], Comunidad de Madrid [Grant BIO-S-0283/2006], and Fundacion Mutua Madrileña. AL holds a "Sara Borrell" post-doctoral research contract from the ISCIII.

The authors are grateful to Dr. Rafael Samaniego for help with confocal microscopy, Dr. Miguel L.F. Ruano for technical assistance with the TDX assays, and Merck Sharp & Dohme for providing cilastatin.

6. References

Adachi, H.; Tawaragi, Y.; Inuzuka, C.; Kubota, I.; Tsujimoto, M.; Nishihara, T. & Nakazato, H. (1990). Primary structure of human microsomal dipeptidase deduced from molecular cloning. *The Journal of Biological Chemistry*, Vol.265, No.7, (March 1990), pp. 3392-5, ISSN 0021-9258

Birnbaum, J.; Kahan, F.M.; Kropp, H. & MacDonald, .JS. (1985). Carbapenems, a new class of beta-lactam antibiotics. Discovery and development of imipenem/cilastatin. *The American Journal of Medicine*, Vol.78, No.6A, (June 1985), pp. 3-21, ISSN 0002-9343

Camano, S.; Lazaro, A.; Moreno-Gordaliza, E.; Torres, A.M.; de Lucas, C.; Humanes, B.; Lazaro, J.A.; Gomez-Gomez, M.; Bosca, L. & Tejedor, A. (2010). Cilastatin attenuates cisplatin-induced proximal tubular cell damage. *The Journal of Pharmacology and Experimental Therapeutics*, Vol.334, No.2, (April 2010), pp. 419-29, ISSN 0022-3565

Camaño-Páez, S.; Lázaro-Fernández, A.; Callejas-Martínez, R.; Lázaro-Manero, J.A.; Castilla-Barba, M.; Martín-Vasallo, P.; Martínez-Escandel, A: & Tejedor-Jorge A. (2008). Study on the role of the tubule in renal vasoconstriction induced by cyclosporine. *Actas Urológicas Españolas*, Vol.32, No.1, (January 2008), pp. 128-39, ISSN 0210-4806

Carmellini. M.; Frosini, F.; Filipponi, F.; Boggi, U. & Mosca, F. (1997). Effect of cilastatin on cyclosporine-induced acute nephrotoxicity in kidney transplant recipients. *Transplantation*, Vol.64, No.1, (July 1997), pp. 164-6, ISSN 0041-1337

Carmellini, M.; Matteucci, E.; Boggi, U.; Cecconi, S.; Giampietro, O. & Mosca, F. (1998). Imipenem/cilastatin reduces cyclosporin-induced tubular damage in kidney transplant recipients. *Transplantation Proceedings*, Vol.30, No.5, (August 1998), pp. 2034-5, ISSN 0041-1345

Dimanche-Boitrel, M.T.; Meurette, O.; Rebillard, A. & Lacour, S. (2005) Role of early plasma membrane events in chemotherapy-induced cell death. *Drug Resistance Update: reviews and commentaries in antimicrobial and anticancer chemotherapy*, Vol.8, No.1-2, (April 2005), pp. 5-14, ISSN 1368-7646

Gruss. E.; Tomas, J.F.; Bernis, C.; Rodriguez, F.; Traver, J.A. & Fernandez-Ranada, J.M. (1996). Nephroprotective effect of cilastatin in allogeneic bone marrow transplantation. Results from a retrospective analysis. *Bone Marrow Transplantation*, Vol.18, No.4, (October 1996), pp. 761-5, ISSN 0268-3369

Lorz, C.; Benito-Martin, A.; Justo, P.; Sanz, A.B.; Sanchez-Niño, M.D.; Santamaria, B.; Egido, J. & Ortiz, A. (2006). Modulation of renal tubular cell survival: where is the evidence?. *Current Medicinal Chemistry*, Vol.13, No.4, pp. 449-54, ISSN 0929-8673

Markewitz, A.; Hammer, C.; Pfeiffer, M.; Zahn, S.; Drechsel, J.; Reichenspurner, H. & Reichart, B. (1994). Reduction of cyclosporine-induced nephrotoxicity by cilastatin following clinical heart transplantation. *Transplantation*, Vol.57, No.6, (March 1994), pp. 865-70, ISSN 0041-1337

Mraz, W.; Modic, P.K. & Hammer, C. (1992). Impact of imipenem/cilastatin on cyclosporine metabolism and excretion. *Transplantation Proceedings*, Vol.24, No.5, (October 1992), pp. 1704-8, ISSN 0041-1345.

Mraz. W.; Sido, B.; Knedel, M. & Hammer, C. (1987). Concomitant immunosuppressive and antibiotic therapy--reduction of cyclosporine A blood levels due to treatment with imipenem/cilastatin. *Transplantation Proceedings*, Vol.19, No.5, (October 1987), pp. 4017-20, ISSN 0041-1345

Neria, F.; Castilla, M.A.; Sanchez, R.F.; Gonzalez-Pacheco, F.R.; Deudero, J.J.; Calabia, O.; Tejedor, A.; Manzarbeitia, F.; Ortiz, A. & Caramelo, C. (2009). Inhibition of JAK2 protects renal endothelial and epithelial cells from oxidative stress and cyclosporin A toxicity. *Kidney International*, Vol.75, No.2, (September 2008), pp. 227-34, ISSN 0085-2538

Norrby, S.R.; Alestig, K.; Björnegård, B.; Burman, L.A.; Ferber, F.; Huber, J.L.; Jones, K.H.; Kahan, F.M.; Kahan, J.; Kropp, H.; Meisinger, M.A. & Sundelof, J.G. (1983). Urinary recovery of N-formimidoyl thienamycin (MK0787) as affected by coadministration of N-formimidoyl thienamycin dehydropeptidase inhibitors. *Antimicrobial Agents and Chemotherapy*, Vol.23, No.2, (February 1983), pp. 300-7, ISSN 0066-4804

Oh, M.S. (2010). Unconventional views on certain aspects of toxin-induced metabolic acidosis. *Electrolyte & Blood Pressure*, Vol.8, No.1, (June 2010), pp.32-7, ISSN 17385997

Pabla, N. & Dong, Z. (2008) Cisplatin nephrotoxicity: mechanisms and renoprotective strategies. *Kidney International*, Vol.73, No.9, (May 2008), pp. 994-1007, ISSN 0085-2538

Pang, S.; Urquhart, P. & Hooper, N.M. (2004). N-glycans, not the GPI anchor, mediate the apical targeting of a naturally glycosylated, GPI-anchored protein in polarised epithelial cells. *Journal of Cell Science*, Vol.117, No.Pt21, (October 2004), pp. 5079-86, ISSN 0021-9533

Parkin, E.T.; Turner, A.J. & Hooper, N.M. (2001). Differential effects of glycosphingolipids on the detergent-insolubility of the glycosylphosphatidylinositol-anchored membrane dipeptidase. *The Biochemical Journal*, Vol.358, No.Pt1, (August 2005), pp. 209-16, ISSN 0264-6021

Perazella, M.A. (2009). Renal vulnerability to drug toxicity. *Clinical Journal of the American Society of Nephrology*, Vol.4, No.7, (July 2009), pp. 1275-83, ISSN 1555-9041

Perez, M.; Castilla, M.; Torres, A.M.; Lázaro, J.A.; Sarmiento, E. & Tejedor, A. (2004) Inhibition of brush border dipeptidase with cilastatin reduces toxic accumulation of cyclosporin A in kidney proximal tubule epithelial cells. *Nephrology, dialysis, transplantation*, Vol.19, No.10, (July 2004), pp. 2445-55, ISSN 0931-0509

Servais, H.; Ortiz, A.; Devuyst, O.; Denamur, S.; Tulkens, P.M. & Mingeot-Leclercq, M.P. (2008). Renal cell apoptosis induced by nephrotoxic drugs: cellular and molecular mechanisms and potential approaches to modulation. *Apoptosis*, Vol. 13, No.1, (January 2008), pp. 11-32, ISSN 1360-8185

Tejedor, A.; Torres, A.M.; Castilla, M.; Lazaro, J.A.; de Lucas, C. & Caramelo, C. (2007). Cilastatin protection against cyclosporin A-induced nephrotoxicity: clinical evidence. *Current Medical Research Opinion*, Vol.19, No.10, (March 2007), pp. 505-13, ISSN 0300-7995

Xiao, Z.; Li, C.; Shan, J.; Luo, L.; Feng, L.; Lu, J.; Li, S.; Long, D. & Li, Y. (2011). Mechanisms of renal cell apoptosis induced by cyclosporine A: a systematic review of in vitro studies. *American Journal of Nephrology*, Vol.33, No.69, (May 2011), pp. 558-66, ISSN 0250-8095

6

Mephedrone-Related Fatalities in the United Kingdom: Contextual, Clinical and Practical Issues

John M. Corkery, Fabrizio Schifano and A. Hamid Ghodse
University of Hertfordshire & St George's, University of London
United Kingdom

1. Introduction

The misuse of mephedrone (4-methylmethcathinone) has been increasing greatly in Western countries over the last two years or so, especially in the club and dance scenes. This period has also been marked by claims that the substance has been implicated in a rising number of deaths in the USA and Western Europe, especially the United Kingdom (UK).

This chapter explores the context(s) and evolution of mephedrone use in the UK, and the circumstances in which these fatalities occurred. Particular attention is paid to the settings in which these incidents took place, their symptomatology and physical characteristics; intervention/treatment opportunities; and toxicological and pathological findings. These results are related to the known pharmacological facts regarding mephedrone, its possible interactions with alcohol and other psychoactive drugs, and suggested clinical interventions and treatment(s).

The relationship between mephedrone, other methcathinones, and other emerging novel psychoactive substances, as well as established stimulants is also examined. These developments are important as novel substances used for recreational use become more globally accessible through the use of the Internet.

2. Recreational use

Mephedrone (4-methylmethcathinone; 'Plant Food', 'Meow Meow', 'Miaow', 'Drone', 'Meph', 'Bubbles', 'Spice E', 'Charge', 'M-Cat', 'Rush', 'Ronzio', 'Fiskrens' and 'MMC Hammer') (Schifano et al, 2011) is the most popular of the cathinone derivatives, which also include butylone, flephedrone, MDPV, methedrone, methylone, pentylone, and other compounds (ACMD, 2010; Morris, 2010). It has been readily available for purchase both online and in head shops as a 'legal high', and more recently as a 'research chemical'; its circulation has been promoted by aggressive web-based marketing (Deluca et al., 2009). Mephedrone elicits stimulant and empathogenic effects similar to amphetamine, methylamphetamine, cocaine and MDMA (Winstock et al., 2010). However, as we write, relatively few formal related papers and experimental/clinical data have been published (Dargan et al., 2010; Winstock et al., 2010; Winstock et al., 2011).

The synthesis of mephedrone was first described over 80 years ago (Saem de Burnaga Sanchez, 1929). However, the first Internet reference to it occurred reportedly in May 2003 (Power, 2009), but both its availability for purchase online (Camilleri et al., 2010; Roussel et al., 2009) and its related popularity only started in 2007 (Deluca et al., 2009). Data collected by the European Monitoring Centre for Drugs and Drug Addiction (EMCDDA) indicate that during the first quarter of 2010, there were detections in some 20 EU Member States, with most of them reporting small- to medium-sized seizures (Europol-EMCDDA, 2010). During the second quarter of 2009, the UK Forensic Science Service received submissions of three times as many samples of mephedrone for analysis than it had in the previous 12-month period (ACMD, 2010; Ghodse et al., 2010). Since mephedrone appeared comparatively recently on the market, it does not feature in most drug use household surveys, and it is uncertain how many people present with a history of mephedrone misuse. Most available data originate from self-reported surveys and small focus group research.

The main settings for mephedrone use appear to be nightclubs, parties and people's homes (Newcombe, 2009). A survey of readers of the dance magazine 'Mixmag' found that 41.7% of respondents had ever tried mephedrone and 33.2% had used it during the previous month (Winstock et al., 2011). Dargan et al. (2010) assessed both the prevalence and frequency of use of mephedrone by students in Tayside (Scotland) in February 2010. Some 20.3% reported previous use of mephedrone; 23.4% reported using only using mephedrone on one occasion previously and 4.4% reported daily use. A total of 48.8% of users had sourced mephedrone from street-level dealers and 10.7% from the Internet. Heightened awareness and interest in mephedrone was reflected by a rise in the number of both telephone inquiries and visits to both the TOXBASE and FRANK web sites (ACMD, 2010; James et al., 2010). The 2011 sweep of the British Crime Survey, which covers households in England and Wales, found that 4.4% of adults aged 16 to 24 years had used mephedrone in the last year, compared to only 0.6% of those aged 25 to 59 years (Smith & Flatley, 2011). The rate for the younger age-group is similar to that for cocaine. The majority of respondents who had taken mephedrone in the last year had also taken another drug. It is, therefore, likely that it is existing users of drugs that are taking mephedrone rather than new users drawn to drug taking.

The emergence of mephedrone on the UK recreational drug scene may be linked to decreasing purity in the UK of both MDMA (ecstasy) and cocaine (Mulchandani et al., 2010; Fleming, 2010; Measham et al., 2010; NTA, 2010). As a consequence, drug users may have switched to mephedrone, as it was seen as cheaper and more powerful than the currently available 'traditional' stimulants (Deluca et al., 2009). Its availability over the Internet and its status as a 'legal high' (and therefore presumed not to be harmful) may have boosted its appeal (Daly, 2010; Ramsey et al., 2010).

3. Legal status

Mephedrone is not scheduled under the 1971 United Nations Convention on Psychotropic Substances. In Australia, New Zealand, and the USA mephedrone is considered as an analogue of other illegal substances already and can be controlled by laws similar to the Federal Analog Act. In March 2010, the EMCDDA and Europol submitted a joint report on mephedrone to the Council of the European Union, the European Commission and the European Medicines Agency (EMA), presenting the case for a formal risk assessment of the drug (Europol-EMCDDA, 2010). The risk assessment report, which was submitted to the European Commission and the Council of the European Union on 26 May 2010, examined the health and social risks of the drug, as well as information on international trafficking and the involvement of organised crime. Furthermore, the report considers the potential implications for placing the drug under control in the EU. On the basis of this report – and on the initiative of the European Commission – on 2 December 2010, the Council decided that mephedrone is to be subject to control measures (EMCDDA, 2011).

In the UK, where mephedrone had been attracting great attention from both the mass media and the Government, the Advisory Council on the Misuse of Drugs (ACMD) submitted a report to the Home Office on the cathinone derivatives, recommending their inclusion in the Misuse of Drugs Act 1971 as a Class B drug (ACMD, 2010). The Home Office announced on 30 March 2010 that this recommendation would be enforced from 16 April 2010 (Home Office, 2010).

4. Chemistry

Mephedrone is a semi-synthetic compound belonging to the chemical class of cathinone derivatives (or substituted cathinones). Cathinone is a natural amphetamine-like alkaloid found in the fresh leaves and stems of the African shrub Khat (Catha edulis) (Kalix, 1992). The systematic name of mephedrone is 2-(methylamino)-1-(p-tolyl)propan-1-one(2S)-2-(methylamino)-1-(4-methylphenyl)propan-1-one, in accordance with the International Union of Pure and Applied Chemistry. The structure of mephedrone differs from cathinone by methylation of the amino group and the benzene ring present (Gustaffsson and Escher, 2009; Osorio-Olivares et al., 2003). The cathinones are beta-keto derivatives of phenethylamines, and hence analogues of amphetamines (Chemspider, 2010). Since they are mainly synthetic in origin, beta-keto amphetamines are also known as 'bk designer drugs'. It is relatively easy to produce mephedrone in nonprofessional laboratories via bromination of 4-methylpropiophenone followed by reaction with methylamine or by oxidation of 4-methylephedrine (Archer, 2009; Europol-EMCDDA, 2010).

Although mainly sold in powder and crystal forms, mephedrone may be commercially available in tablets and included within vegetable-based capsules. It has been reported that mephedrone is sometimes sold in some countries as either ecstasy or 'synthetic' cocaine (Deluca et al., 2009; Schifano et al., 2011). Furthermore, it may be found mixed with adulterants, such as caffeine, paracetamol and even cocaine, amphetamine and ketamine (Camilleri et al., 2010), as well as with other methcathinones (as revealed by information supplied to the National Programme on Substance Abuse Deaths by coroners – see below).

5. Pharmacology

Given the affiliation of cathinone derivatives to beta-keto amphetamines, mephedrone would be expected to act as a Central Nervous System stimulant. In vitro studies on the effects of the cathinone derivatives methcathinone and methylone confirm that the main mechanism of action is very similar to that of amphetamine, being characterised by a predominant action on plasma membrane catecholamine transporters (Cozzi et al., 1999). The presence of the ring substituent on the phenethylamine core modifies the pharmacological properties by giving the compound some MDMA-like effects (Europol-EMCDDA, 2010). Cathinones' potencies are mostly lower than those of amphetamines as beta-keto amphetamines show a reduced ability to cross the blood–brain barrier due to the presence of the beta group (Nagai et al., 2007; Gygi et al., 1996).

N-demethylation to the primary amine, reduction of the keto moiety to the respective alcohol, and oxidation of the tolyl moiety to the corresponding alcohols and carboxylic acid is the major metabolic pathway for mephedrone, followed by N-dealkylation.

6. Routes of administration, dosage, use in combination with other drugs, effects

The most common routes for recreational use include insufflation (snorting) and oral ingestion. Because of its solubility in water, mephedrone is reportedly used by rectal administration or injected intravenously. Other typical methods of intake include oral ingestion as capsules or tablets; swallowing mephedrone powder wrapped up in cigarette paper (bombing); or mixed with water. Insufflation is likely to be the most common modality as, when snorted, mephedrone elicits its effects within a few minutes, with the peak being reached in less than 30 min followed by a rapid comedown. According to online users, the mephedrone dosage for snorting may range between 25 and 75 mg, with a lower threshold at 5-15 mg and levels in excess of 90 mg considered a high dosage (Sumnall and Wooding, 2009). Dosing is more frequent when taken intranasally; this route is allegedly associated with greater abuse liability than the oral route (Winstock et al., 2010, 2011). On average, the most common oral dosages are higher than the snorting ones (Sumnall & Wooding, 2009), in the range 150 to 250 mg.

Time of onset may be from 45 min to 2 h and may vary in association with the amount of food in the stomach. Because of this, users suggest taking mephedrone on an empty stomach. Psychoactive effects may last longer (up to 2-4 h) with oral ingestion; side-effects might be milder and the need to re-dose less urgent. Some users employ both insufflation and oral ingestion in combination to obtain faster onset and long-lasting effects (Deluca et al., 2009). Users report that rectal administration is characterised by faster onset of the effects and requires lower doses, e.g. 100 mg on average than oral ingestion (Deluca et al., 2009). Although not typically advised, because this may increase the drug's addictive liability levels (Deluca et al., 2009), mephedrone may also be injected either intramuscularly (Wood et al., 2010a) or intravenously, at one half or two-thirds of the oral dose (Deluca et al., 2009). According to online user fora, mephedrone may be taken in combination with a number of stimulants, sedatives and psychedelics (Deluca et al., 2009; Schifano et al., 2011).

As mephedrone has the capacity to induce tolerance on repeated dosing, an increasing number of user reports have stated a quick progression to either regular drug use and/or uncontrolled bingeing behaviour (known as 'fiending'), with 1-4 g of mephedrone consumed in a session to prolong the duration of its effects (Deluca et al., 2009; Europol-EMCDDA, 2010; Dargan et al., 2010). A recent survey carried out by a drug-related web site has unveiled an average monthly use of 11.16 g for each mephedrone consumer (Drugs-forum, 2010). Although withdrawal symptoms are not commonly reported, users often display strong cravings for mephedrone (Newcombe, 2009).

The effects of mephedrone have been compared by users variously to those of cocaine, amphetamine and MDMA. Self-reported subjective effects may include (Winstock et al., 2011; Deluca et al., 2009): intense stimulation and alertness, euphoria; empathy/feelings of closeness, sociability and talkativeness; intensification of sensory experiences; moderate sexual arousal; and perceptual distortions (reported with higher dosages only).

7. Adverse effects

Dargan et al. (2010) report that some 56% of those who had used mephedrone may complain of at least one unwanted effect associated with mephedrone use. These may include (ACMD, 2010; Deluca et al., 2009; James et al., 2010; Wood et al., 2009, 2010b): loss of appetite, nausea, vomiting and stomach discomfort; tremors, headache (very common), dizziness/light-headedness, seizures, nystagmus, pupil dilation, blurred vision, numbness of tactile sensitivity (reported at higher dosages); anxiety, confusion, dysphoria, aggression, depression, long-lasting hallucinations, paranoid delusions, short-term psychosis, short-term mania, insomnia and nightmares, impaired short-term memory, poor concentration, tachycardia, elevated blood pressure, respiratory difficulties, chest pain. Possibly due to vasoconstriction, users have anecdotally described cold/blue fingers. Of particular interest are recent reports of clinical significance: severe refractory left ventricular failure (Chhabra et al., 2010); and acute myocarditis (Nicholson et al., 2010). Further unwanted effects may include: difficulties in urination, possible nephrotoxicity, anorgasmia; changes in body temperature regulation, with hot flushes and sweating; immunological toxicity (vasculitis, infections and ulcerations); posterior reversible encephalopathy syndrome (Omer & Doherty, 2010); and finally serotonin syndrome (Garrett & Sweeney, 2011).

Most of the above untoward effects seem to be similar to those already documented for amphetamine, methylamphetamine and MDMA (Schifano et al., 2010), implicitly supporting a sympathomimetic activity of mephedrone. Conversely, symptoms of depression and anhedonia could be tentatively associated to a putative depletion of serotonin and dopamine as a consequence of drug use (ACMD, 2010), similarly to what may occur with other stimulants (Schifano, 1996). It is impossible to determine a 'safe' dose for mephedrone since negative side-effects may present in association with any dosage taken. Furthermore, similar dosages may have dramatically different consequences in different individuals (Dickson et al., 2010).

8. Fatalities

During the last few months of 2009 and the first few months of 2010, the UK media were constantly reporting fatalities allegedly related to mephedrone consumption, but only a proportion of them had by that time been formally confirmed. A report on a mephedrone-related fatality first appeared in Sweden, referring to an 18-year-old female death which occurred in December 2008. No other drugs, apart from mephedrone, were identified by the toxicological screenings (Gustaffson & Escher, 2009). Previously, a Danish teenager found in possession of mephedrone died in May 2008, although toxicology reports were inconclusive (Campbell, 2009). The first mephedrone-related death in the USA involved the combined use of mephedrone and heroin (Dickson et al., 2010). More recently, the first cases from the Netherlands (Lusthof et al., 2011) and the Republic of Ireland (EMCDDA, 2011:85) have been reported.

Given the potentially large numbers of consumers involved in the use of mephedrone across both the EU and the UK (EMCDDA, 2011), the main aims of this study were to report and analyse information relating to the socio-demographics and clinical circumstances of all recorded mepherone-related deaths for the whole of the UK, both when the index drug was taken on its own and when in combination with other drugs. The rationale for doing this is to make accessible a corpus of material which will help inform treatments and interventions so as to reduce deaths associated with the use of this drug and other methcathinones.

9. Methodology for identifying potential mephedrone-related fatalities

In the UK and Islands all sudden, unexpected or violent deaths - as well as deaths in custody - are formally investigated by Coroners (or their equivalent in the Islands), or Procurators Fiscal in the case of Scotland. Most drug-related deaths are subject to these processes, typically by way of a coronial inquest (Corkery, 2002).

Since its establishment in 1997, the National Programme on Substance Abuse Deaths (np-SAD) has been regularly receiving coroners' information on drug-related deaths amongst both addicts and non-addicts in the UK, the Channel Islands and the Isle of Man. The average annual response rate from coroners in England and Wales to np-SAD has been between 89% and 95% (Ghodse et al., 2010). Since 2004, information has also been received from the Scottish Crime &Drug Enforcement Agency and the General Register Office for Northern Ireland. To date, details of some 25,000 deaths have been received. The information reported here on deaths associated with mephedrone consumption are based on all relevant cases recorded in the Special Mortality Register of the np-SAD based at St George's Hospital Medical School, University of London.

To be recorded in the np-SAD database as a drug-related death, at least one of the following criteria must be met: (a) presence of one or more psychoactive substances directly implicated in death; (b) history of dependence or abuse of drugs; and (c) presence of controlled drugs at post-mortem. Full details of the np-SAD data collection form and its surveillance work can be found in the Programme's annual report (Ghodse et al., 2010). Ethical approval is not required in the UK for studies whose subjects are deceased. However, confidentiality arrangements are in place with each of the respective data providers.

A range of documents are contained in coronial inquest files, although the variety differs from case to case. Typically, the coroner has access to: statements from witnesses, family and friends; General Practitioner records (if the deceased is registered with one); reports from ambulance, police or other emergency services; hospital Emergency Department and clinical ward reports; psychiatric and substance abuse team reports; as well as post mortem and toxicology reports. Internet searches of toxicological as well as newspaper and other media websites revealed information on further cases. The media reports available for some cases were used to supplement the information provided on the np-SAD data collection form, especially where access to the full coronial files was not possible.

In addition to its routine surveillance activities, the Programme also provides real-time information on the emergence of novel substances or new ways of taking existing substances to the UK Early Warning System and the Advisory Council on the Misuse of

Drugs (ACMD). This information comes both from notifications of deaths and from 'alerts' or other information provided by the various agencies and networks, national and international, with which the Programme maintains contacts. Regular searches of media reports are also undertaken.

Through these channels (including coroners, forensic toxicologists – principally the London Toxicology Group, Drug & Alcohol Action Teams, and the Scottish Crime & Drug Enforcement Agency) the Programme became aware of the emerging issue of the use of methcathinones, especially mephedrone, and similar substances (including chemicals), and of their potential adverse health consequences. It was decided to take a pro-active approach to monitor the situation especially in respect of the potential role of these new substances in causing or contributing to death. For those cases not formally reported to the Programme, contact was made with the relevant coroners to request the submission of an np-SD form so as to obtain the appropriate information. Information on these cases was added to the database when forms were received by the Programme team.

The np-SAD database was searched using the terms 'mephedrone' and '4-methylmethcathinone' to identify potentially relevant cases. The database fields searched were those holding data on: drugs present at post-mortem; drugs implicated; cause(s) of death; accident details; and 'other relevant information'. The data presented here relate to all concluded cases for which forms had been submitted to the Programme by 31 August 2011. Details of some of these cases have previously been published (Torrance & Cooper, 2010; Wood et al., 2010b; Maskell et al., 2011; EMCDDA, 2011:78-85).

Analyses were performed using IBM® SPSS® Statistics, version 18 for Windows™. Demographic details, risk factors, and categorical data were expressed as frequencies and percentages within groups; ages were compared using Levene's Test for Equality of Variances (two-tailed). The results for statistical tests were regarded as significant at or below the 5% probability level.

10. Results

A total of 125 alleged or suspected mephedrone-associated fatalities have been identified by the np-SAD team (Fig. 1). However, in 25 cases (20.0%) mephedrone was not found at post mortem and for 13 cases (10.4%) the toxicology results are still pending. For those 87 cases (69.6%) where mephedrone was identified at post mortem, inquests have been concluded in 60 cases. These were considered as confirmed fatalities meeting the above inclusion criteria, and on which the present analysis will focus.

10.1 Demographics

The mean age of the sample was 28.7 years (SD 11.3), range 14-64 years old. The mean age for males was 28.9 years compared to 28.0 years for females; this difference was not statistically significant (t = 0.27 (two-tailed for equality of means) p = 0.79 (95% CI = -5.87 to +7.72). Where known, most victims were described as 'White' (Table 1). Where place of birth was given, 39 were born in the UK and Islands and 8 overseas. Many were in employment (n = 25), but one-quarter (n = 16) were unemployed, and 11 were students.

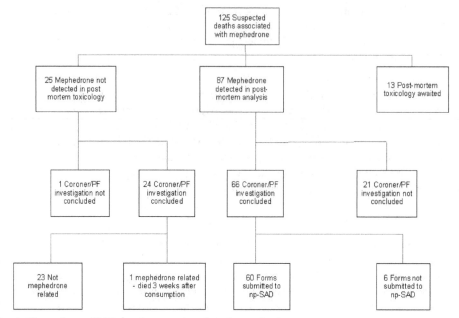

Fig. 1. Flow-chart of UK deaths associated with mephedrone

Demographic variable	Characteristics

Age (years):
    male (n=45)
 	
    female (n=15)
 	
    all (n=60)
	mean = 28.9, median = 24.9, minimum = 17.1, maximum = 63.8, range = 46.8, SD = 11.1.
	mean = 28.0, median = 24.9, minimum = 14.8, maximum = 55.1, range = 40.3, SD = 12.2.
	mean = 28.7, median = 24.9, minimum = 14.8, maximum = 63.8, range = 49.0, SD = 11.3.

Age-group (years)	< 15 = 1; 15-24 = 30; 25-34 = 16; 35-44 = 6; 45-54 = 5; 55-64 = 2; >64 = 0.
Ethnicity	White = 50; Black = 0; Asian = 1; Other (Filipina) = 1; Not known = 8.
Country of birth	England = 32, Wales = 2, Scotland = 1, Northern Ireland = 2, Guernsey = 2; overseas = 8; unknown/unavailable = 13.
Employment status	non-manual = 9; manual = 14; unemployed = 16; self-employed = 2; invalidity/sickness = 1; student = 11; housewife = 0; unknown = 7.
Living arrangements	alone = 11; with parents = 20; with partner = 14; with partner and children = 2; with friends = 4; no fixed abode = 2; self & children = 1; Other = 1; unknown = 5.
Addict status	non-addict = 10; addict/drug abuser = 27; unknown = 23.

Table 1. Socio-demographics of 60 UK deaths associated with mephedrone reported to np-SAD

Just over half (33) died in their home or that of a friend and 12 in hospital (Table 2). The verdict/conclusion returned by the coroners or procurators fiscal in 35 instances was accidental death or misadventure; (non-dependent) abuse of drugs in 5 cases, suicide in 10 cases, homicide in one case, natural causes in one case, and an open verdict in 8 cases. Forty-four of these deaths occurred in England; nine in Scotland, four in Northern Ireland, two on Guernsey, and one in Wales.

Twenty-seven were known to be as 'addicts' (either dependent on or misusing drugs), and 10 were not addicts; for 23 cases the information was not known. Only 11 of the deceased were known to have been prescribed psychoactive drugs: these included diazepam, antidepressants, antipsychotics, antiepileptics, methadone, and opioid analgesics, often in combination.

Demographic variable	Characteristics
Place of death	at home = 28; friend's home = 5; hospital = 12; open space/woodland/river = 7; other = 7; unknown = 1.
Country of death	England = 44; Wales = 1; Scotland = 9; Northern Ireland = 4; Guernsey = 2; Jersey = 0; Isle of Man = 0.
Day of week of death (this is not necessarily day of consumption)	Sunday = 13; Monday = 12; Tuesday = 10; Wednesday = 8; Thursday = 2; Friday = 5; Saturday = 10.
Month of death	Sep 2009 = 1; Oct 2009 = 1; Nov 2009 = 1; Dec 2009 = 5; Jan 2010 = 7; Feb 2010 = 7; Mar 2010 = 9; Apr 2010 = 6; May 2010 = 3; Jun 2010 = 1; Jul 2010 = 7; Aug 2010 = 2; Sep 2010 = 0; Oct 2010 = 2; Nov 2010 = 2; Dec 2010 = 0; Jan 2011 = 0; Feb 2011 = 2; Mar 2011 = 0; Apr 2011 = 2; May 2011 = 2; Jun 2011 = 0; Jul 2011 = 0; Aug 2011 = 0.
Verdict (legal conclusion)	accident/misadventure = 35; (non-dependent) abuse of drugs = 5; open/undetermined = 8; suicide = 10; killed unlawfully = 1; other = 1.
Manner of death (intentionality)	natural = 1; accidental = 41; suicidal = 11; homicidal = 1; undetermined = 6.

Table 2. Circumstances of 60 deaths associated with mephedrone reported to np-SAD

The first known death in the UK occurred in September 2009. The number steadily rose to 7 both in January and February 2010, peaked at 9 in March, falling to 6 in April, and declining in the next couple of months to one in June. However, there was a further peak of 7 cases in July, followed by two deaths in August and another 2 in both October and November. There then followed a period of a few months without any reported fatalities, but the most recent deaths occurred in April and May 2011 (Fig. 2). There were twice as many deaths on Saturdays, Sundays, Mondays and Tuesdays (n = 45, average 11.2 per day) compared to the other days of the week (n = 15; average of 5.0 per day). It should be noted that the day of death was not necessarily the day that mephedrone was consumed, as in a few cases death occurred several days later in hospital – in one case three weeks after the event.

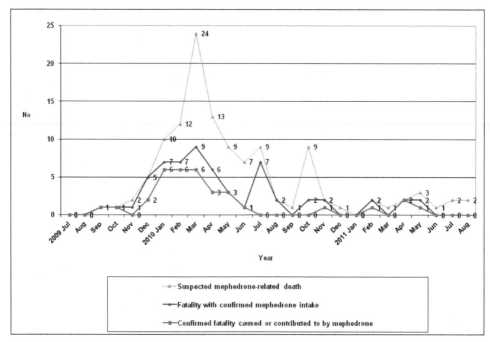

Fig. 2. Evolution of suspected deaths (n = 125) and cases with confirmed positive toxicology for mephedrone submitted to np-SAD as at 31 August 2011 (n = 60)

10.2 Events leading to death

As might be expected given the typical purpose of using mephedrone to experience its psychoactive effects, many deaths occurred following recreational consumption of the drug (Table 3), often in the deceased's or another's home. However, some deaths (road traffic collisions, drowning, hypothermia, etc.) occurred as the result of accidents through impaired judgement due to mephedrone use. In two cases, the deceased had been engaged in sexual activity.

There was a significant number (n = 18) of deaths involving violent means, and especially hanging (13 cases). In several of these cases, mephedrone was considered by the pathologist/coroner/Procurator Fiscal to have played a role although it was not being specifically mentioned in the cause of death field. Mephedrone withdrawal was considered a contributory factor in one suicide by hanging. There were also three fatal road traffic accidents following consumption of mephedrone (and other drugs), and one homicide when the deceased was killed for his supply of mephedrone (about 500 g).

10.3 Cause(s) of death

The effects ('adverse', poisoning, intoxication, toxicity) of mephedrone, including other substances, were recorded in the cause of death for 24 cases (Table 4). Consumption of mephedrone led to a seizure in one case, and cardiac arrest in another. In a further case, cardiac arrest was caused by multiple drug toxicity (including mephedrone) and/or excited delirium. In two cases the ingestion of mephedrone with other drugs led to hypoxic brain injury (one with cerebral oedema). Health issues were present in a number of cases. These, along with mephedrone (and other substances) contributed to death; for example, cardiovascular conditions - 4, bronchopneumonia - 3.

Found unresponsive/dead after taking mephedrone (and other substance) – 14
Found hanging after paranoiac/suicidal behaviour - 6
Found hanging following depression relationship broke up – 1
Found hanging following row with girlfriend over his drug misuse - 1
Self-suspension when intoxicated with alcohol and cocaine – 1
Found hanging after no apparent untoward behaviour – 1
Found dead after cutting own throat – 1
Suicide by gun-shot following consumption of mephedrone, other methcathinone(s) and cocaine – 1
Had consumed mephedrone and other substances, jumped from bridge where relative had previously committed suicide – 1
Committed suicide by drug overdose, including mephedrone – 2
Following family argument, took fatal levels of amitriptyline and methadone, consumed mephedrone – 1
Reported missing after argument with partner, found dead next day on running track with suicide note, had consumed prescribed medications and mephedrone - 1
Had taken mephedrone, but was stabbed and his large supply of mephedrone was stolen, bled to death – 1
Took drugs (including mephedrone and cocaine), started behaving bizarrely, aggressively and abusively; police tried unsuccessfully to calm him down and had to arrest him; collapsed whilst under restraint and suffered cardiac arrest - 1
Attended party, collapsed with cardiac arrest, died in hospital – 1
Attended party, collapsed with breathing difficulties, died in hospital – 1
Attended party, took mephedrone 'bomb', collapsed with very high temperature which prevented blood from clotting, causing abdominal haemorrhages, never regained consciousness - 1
Took mephedrone and other substances, collapsed with chest pains – 2
Took mephedrone and other methcathinones, together with cocaine, which caused fatal heart attack – 1
Took cocaine and mephedrone at party, collapsed and died following day - 1
Had consumed mephedrone but died from heroin and alcohol toxicity – 1
Found dead after consuming Datura, dihydrocodeine, alcohol and mephedrone - 1
Had consumed mephedrone and other stimulants, attempted to swim across river but drowned - 1
Had taken mephedrone and other drugs, driving vehicle involved in fatal road traffic accident – 3
Following consumption of alcohol and mephedrone, felt sick, collapsed, died in hospital – 1

Took alcohol and mephedrone, collapsed and unrouseable, died in hospital - 1
Collapsed after taking mephedrone, died in hospital 3 weeks later from acute liver failure – 1
Attended party where took mephedrone and heroin, collapsed died in hospital 3 weeks later – 1
Died in hospital after taking mephedrone – 1
Indulged in sexual activity, self-injected mephedrone, had seizure and collapsed – 1
Had taken large amounts of methcathinones, engaged in auto-erotic asphyxiation with plastic bag over head, but accidentally suffocated - 1
Consumed amphetamine & mephedrone, vomited, felt cold & sleepy; taken to hospital where, despite treatment, suffered liver problems & multi-organ failure – 1
Found unresponsive in bed, death certified at scene; had been feeling unwell, on medication for chronic abdominal & back pain – 1
Admitted to Emergency Department previous day with drug overdose, had been partying but later found hanging – 1
Aspirated blood following mixed drug (including mephedrone) intoxication - 1
Had consumed GHB and mephedrone; found dead beside bed at home by a friend – 1
Not known – 2

Table 3. Events leading to death

1a Hanging – 10
1a Hanging; 2 Mephedrone withdrawal – 1
1a Hanging; 2 alcohol and mephedrone use – 1
1a Hanging; 2 using mephedrone - 1
1a Shotgun wound to head; 2 Use of mephedrone, methylone and cocaine – 1
1a Blood loss following fatal stabbing to thigh [inflicted by third party] – 1
1a Exsanguination; 1b Neck laceration cutting left jugular vein [self-inflicted] – 1
1a Multiple injuries; 1b Blunt force trauma; 1c Vehicular collision (driver) – 1
1a Ruptured inferior vena cava with haemorrhage in abdominal cavity & cervical spine fracture; 1b Road traffic accident; 2 Cirrhosis of liver & misuse of drugs – 1
1a Multiple injuries [road traffic accident] – 1
1a Multiple injuries [fall from height] – 1
1a Drowning; 2 Multiple drug overdose – 1
1a Hypothermia; 1b Drug overdose [quetiapine, lorazepam, venlafaxine, mephedrone] - 1
1a Adverse effects of mephedrone - 1
1a Poisoning by mephedrone – 1
1a Mephedrone toxicity - 1
1a Mephedrone poisoning; 2 Coronary artery disease – 1
1a Adverse effects of mephedrone; 2 Atherosclerotic coronary artery disease; myocardial fibrosis – 1
1a Mephedrone intoxication – 2
1a Cardiac arrest following ingestion of mephedrone – 1

1a Seizure; 1b Effect of mephedrone – 1
1a Cardiac arrest, cause unascertained between multiple drug toxicity [mephedrone, MDPV, fluoromethcathinone] and/or Excited Delirium – 1
1a Aspiration of blood; 1b Mixed drug intoxication [inc. mephedrone] - 1
1a Adverse effects of methadone and mephedrone – 1
1a Overdosage of mephedrone (meow meow) compounded by cocaine; 2 Cocaine abuse - 1
1a Mixed MDMA and mephedrone toxicity – 1
1a Combined toxic effects of amphetamine and mephedrone – 1
1a Patchy bronchopneumonia & pulmonary oedema; 1b Cardiac ischaemia, contributed to by mephedrone, citalopram and diazepam - 1
1a Ischaemic heart disease; 1b Illicit use of cathinones - 1
1a Toxic effects of drugs [inc. mephedrone] – 1
1a Fatal drug intoxication [inc. mephedrone] – 1
1a Mixed drug toxicity [inc. mephedrone] – 1
1a Hypoxic brain injury; 1b Mixed drug overdose [inc. mephedrone] - 1
1a Hypoxic brain injury; 1b Cerebral oedema; 1c Ingestion of psychoactive drug [inc. mephedrone] – 1
1a Toxic effects of alcohol and cocaine – 1
1a Heroin and alcohol toxicity - 1
1a GHB intoxication – 2
1a Acute alcohol poisoning – 1
1a Morphine (heroin) toxicity - 1
1a Morphine toxicity (on balance of probability) – 1
1a BZP and TFMPP toxicity – 1
1a Illicit methadone misuse – 1
1a Combined effects of alcohol and GBL intoxication – 1
1a Combined toxic effects of alcohol, dihydrocodeine and atropine/hyoscine (from Datura Stramonium) together with postural asphyxia - 1
1a Systemic sepsis, resulting in cardiac arrest; 1b Bronchopneumonia; 1c Beta haemolytic Streptococcal Group A infection – 1
1a Medication toxicity; 2 Acute & chronic debilitating back pain, early stage bronchopneumonia - 1
1a Combined methadone and alcohol overdose – 1
1a Amitriptyline/Methadone overdose - 1
1a Asphyxia [plastic bag suffocation] – 1
(Where cause of death sections of the death certificate specifically mentioned mephedrone or where it was included in verdict. Mephedrone was implicated on its own in 18 cases, with other substances in 18 cases. In many of the hanging causes, mephedrone was considered to have played a contributory role although not recorded in the cause of death.)

Table 4. Cause of deaths associated with mephedrone reported to np-SAD

10.4 Drugs implicated

Mephedrone was specifically mentioned as being present at post-mortem in 59 cases. The drug was formally included in the cause of death in 18 cases and implicitly (e.g. polydrug toxicity given in the cause of death without specifying particular drugs, but mephedrone was found in post-mortem analysis or mentioned by the pathologist as contributing to death) in 10 further cases. In a further case, the drug was not mentioned either as being present at post-mortem (death occurred 3 weeks after mephedrone consumption) or in the cause of death although stated by witnesses to have been consumed.

Where details of the drugs present at post-mortem (or ante-mortem) were given, mephedrone alone was used on eight occasions, solely with alcohol in four cases, and in combination with further substances in 18 cases (Table 5). In 15 cases mephedrone was ingested with stimulants, and with diazepam in 13 cases. It is noteworthy that other newly emerging psychoactive substances were also here identified, including: GBL/GHB, ketamine, and piperazines, as well as other methcathinones (n = 8), especially MDPV. Prescribed medications were also present: opioids including methadone; hypnotics/sedatives; antidepressants; antipsychotics; and antiepileptics.

(Mephedrone was present in 59 cases, including 2 ante-mortem. It had been consumed in all cases in the period leading up the incident causing death.)

Mephedrone sole mention – 8
Mephedrone with alcohol – 4
Mephedrone and alcohol and other drugs - 18
Mephedrone with cannabis – 4
Mephedrone with stimulants – 15
Mephedrone with diazepam - 13
Mephedrone with opiates – 12
Mephedrone with piperazines – 7
Mephedrone with GBL/GHB – 5
Mephedrone with ketamine – 2
Mephedrone with other methcathinones – 8
Mephedrone with antidepressants – 5
Mephedrone with antipsychotics - 2
Mephedrone with antiepileptics - 1
Mephedrone with hypnotics/sedatives (exc. Diazepam) – 3

Table 5. Summary of drug combinations and positive toxicological findings for deaths associated with mephedrone reported to np-SAD

10.5 Toxicology

Full details of mephedrone levels are given in Table 6; actual levels were quantified in 36 cases (Table 6). Overall: (n = 36) mean = 1.586mg/l, range = <0.01 – 22.0mg/l; mono-mephedrone cases (n = 10) mean = 1.996mg/l range = <0.01 – 12.15mg/l; combined mephedrone cases (n = 26): mean = 1.429mg/l; range = 0.03 – 22.0mg/l. These figures exclude one combined mephedrone case with a level of >2000mg/l.

Case No.	Mephedrone present	Mephedrone levels	Second drug present	Third drug present	Fourth drug present	Fifth drug present	Sixth drug present
1	Yes	bl 0.04mg/l	methadone	diazepam	olanzapine	chlorpromazine	
2	Yes	bl <0.01mg/l ur +					
3	Yes	bl 0.76mg/l	alcohol	GBL	diazepam & metabolites		
4	Yes	bl 1.3mg/l ur +					
5	Yes	bl 0.07mg/l, 0.15mg/l ur 16mg/l	alcohol	diazepam			
6	Yes	bl 0.41mg/l, 0.42mg/l	diazepam	citalopram			
7	Yes	bl +	alcohol	cocaine & metabolite	lignocaine		
8	Yes	bl 16ug/l	alcohol				
9	Yes	bl detected	alcohol	cocaine	cocaethylene	levamisole	lignocaine
10	Yes	bl 2.1ug/ml	alcohol				
11	Yes	bl 0.21ug/ml ur +	GBL	TFMPP	ketamine	methylamphetamine	diazepam
12	Yes	bl 2.24mg/l, ur +	TFMPP	alcohol			
13	Yes	bl 1.0mg/l	MDMA				
14	Yes	bl 0.32mg/l					
15	Yes	bl 0.88mg/l, ur +, stomach +	paracetamol				
16	Yes	bl 22mg/l	alcohol	amphetamine	diazepam		
17	Yes	bl 0.04mg/l, 0.19mg/l, ur 64.8mg/l, stomach 2.65mg/l					
18	Yes	bl 0.108mg/l, 0.08mg/l	alcohol	diazepam			
19	Yes	bl 3.3mg/l, stomach +, hair 4.2ng/mg, 4.7ng/mg					
20	Yes	bl > 2.0mg/ml	amphetamine	BZP	TFMPP	chlorpheniramine	
21	Yes	bl 9.01ug/ml, ur 0.01ug/ml, stomach +	morphine	cannabis			

Case No.	Mephedrone present	Mephedrone levels	Second drug present	Third drug present	Fourth drug present	Fifth drug present	Sixth drug present
22	No	-	morphine				
23	Yes	AM serum 0.042mg/l, ur +					
24	Yes	bl 12.15mg/l, ur +					
25	Yes	ur +	cocaine	methylone			
26	Yes	ur +	alcohol	pyrovalerone	BZP	FTMPP	
27	Yes	bl 0.31ug/ml	cannabis				
28	Yes	bl trace	morphine	quetiapine			
29	Yes	bl 0.07mg/l	alcohol				
30	Yes	bl +	alcohol	BZP	TFMPP	paracetamol	citalopram
31	Yes	bl +	alcohol	paracetamol	citalopram	zopiclone	
32	Yes	AM bl +					
33	Yes	bl 0.08ug/ml	methylone	MDPV	GBL		
34	Yes	bl +	methadone	alcohol	cocaine		
35	Yes	bl + recent use	alcohol	benzocaine			
36	Yes	bl + recent use	alcohol	benzocaine			
37	Yes	bl 0.03ug/ml	cannabis				
38	Yes	bl + ur +	diazepam				
39	Yes	bl low level	diazepam	cannabis			
40	Yes	bl +	amphetamine				
41	Yes	ur +	alcohol	cocaine & metabolites			
42	Yes	bl 6.2mg/l	diazepam & metabolites	gabapentin	oxycodone		
43	Yes	bl +	alcohol	cannabis	diazepam		
44	Yes	bl 0.05mg/l	GHB	alcohol	amphetamine	cocaine & metabolites	methadone
45	Yes	bl 0.033ug/ml, bile 0.05ug/ml, ur 0.24ug/ml					
46	Yes	bl 1.7mg/l	BZP	TFMPP	codeine	diazepam	
47	Yes	bl <0.05mg/l, ur 11.67mg/l	alcohol	venlafaxine	quetiapine	halperidol	lorazepam
48	Yes	bl 0.51mg/l	alcohol				
49	Yes	bl <0.3125, ur +	alcohol	MDPV	cocaine	levamisole	quinine

Case No.	Mephedrone present	Mephedrone levels	Second drug present	Third drug present	Fourth drug present	Fifth drug present	Sixth drug present
50	Yes	bl 0.17mg/l	MDPV	MDMA	MDA	cocaine	diazepam
51	Yes	ur +	methylam-phetamine	amphetamine	GHB	ketamine	
52	Yes	n/k	alcohol	morphine	cocaine	fluoxetine	
53	Yes	bl 0.04mg/l, ur +	alcohol	dihydroco-deine	atropine	hyoscine butylbromide	diazepam
54	Yes	bl <0.005mg/l	morphine	nitrazepam	buprenor-phine	mirtazapine	
55	Yes	bl 0.21mg/l	cocaine	levamisole	alcohol		
56	Yes	n/k	methadone	amitriptyline	nitrazepam		
57	Yes	ur <0.005mg/l	flephedrone	MDPV	ibuprofen	unidentified compounds	
58	Yes	n/k	MDPV	MDPBP	pentylone	cocaine metabolites	
59	Yes	bl 0.05mg/l, ur 0.05mg/l	MDPV	fluoromethcat hinone	diazepam		
60	Yes	bl 1.94mg/l	BZP	TFMPP	diazepam		

Table 6. Combinations of post mortem drugs in deaths associated with mephedrone (levels) reported to np-SAD

11. Discussion

The existence of the Special Mortality Register maintained by the National Programme on Substance Abuse Deaths fulfills several major roles: it provides a unique UK-wide historic repository of unparalleled detailed information on drug-related deaths and deaths of drug addicts since 1997; the provision of a nation-wide surveillance capability for monitoring substance-related deaths; and the provision of information on the epidemiology of such events.

This paper contributes to the knowledge-base on mephedrone by providing supplementary/complementary information on the epidemiology of its use in the UK through the provision of centralised collation of post mortem toxicological results. Furthermore, this report has provided an analysis of the only UK-wide, mephedrone-specific mortality dataset. Although not all cases have yet been fully investigated, to the best of our knowledge this is the most comprehensive and detailed study of deaths associated with mephedrone in the literature.

11.1 User profile

One in five of 'mephedrone fatalities' turned out here not to be actually related to mephedrone, since the drug was actually not identified at post mortem. This might be understood in the context of the high levels of both media attention and public concerns surrounding the unprecedented rapidity of the appearance of mephedrone in the UK recreational drug market (Davey et al., 2010). However, some of these cases turned out to involve other methcathinones such as MDPV.

Typical mephedrone victims in this study were young (78% under 35 years of age); male (75%); White (96% where ethnicity was known); either in full time employment, unemployed or students; and with a previous history of drug misuse (73% where known). With an average age of 29 years and nearly four-fifths under the age of 35, the age profile of this dataset is much younger than cases typically reported to np-SAD (Ghodse et al., 2010).

Mephedrone misuse in the UK is likely to have started as early as 2007 (Davey et al., 2010), and the first mephedrone-related fatality recorded on the np-SAD database occurred in September 2009. Although further studies are needed to confirm present observations, it seems from the information presented here that reports of mephedrone fatalities dropped in the months following the announcement by the Home Office on 30 March 2010 that the chemical, together with other related substances, was going to become a Controlled Drug. However, there was a further peak in July 2010, as well as additional deaths occurring in February, April and May 2011. This suggests that mephedrone, as well as other illegal methcathinones, are still being consumed in the UK.

The excess number (doubling) of observed mephedrone-associated fatalities between Saturdays and Tuesdays, compared to other days of the week, might be explained by its more frequent intake over the weekend, confirming once again its recreational drug profile.

An issue of particular concern and, to the best of our knowledge, something previously unreported is that 16 victims (about 1 in 3 cases of the current sample) either hanged themselves (13 cases), or used particularly violent means to terminate their own lives. In 10 cases, the coroner gave a verdict of suicide and in 8 further cases an open verdict was returned. In most of these cases, mephedrone was considered to have played a contributory role. Although a full psychiatric history is not typically made available to np-SAD, it is worth emphasizing that, out of the whole sample, antipsychotics were here identified at post mortem in 2 cases and antidepressants in 5 cases. Therefore, it can be postulated that mephedrone (either on its own, or in a polydrug misuse combination) has the potential to cause and/or exacerbate psychosis and/or depression, thus facilitating the occurrence of bizarre behaviour/self harm with particularly violent means. In one instance, the possibility of Excited Delirium was recorded. Although the present report comments on only 60 cases, the suicide rates in our other UK studies of stimulant-related fatalities were quantitatively less significant, being in the range of 3-6%: amphetamine-type drugs (Schifano et al., 2010); MDMA/ecstasy (Schifano et al., 2010; Schifano et al., 2003b); cocaine (Schifano & Corkery, 2008). The rate for khat-related fatalities was about 31% (sample size = 13) (Corkery et al., 2010).

Contributory clinical (e.g. sepsis; bronchopneumonia; pre-existing atherosclerotic cardiovascular conditions) and environmental (e.g. involvement in traffic accidents, drowning, hypothermia) factors were here identified at post mortem in respectively 5 and 5 mephedrone fatalities. These observations are overall consistent with the existing literature on stimulant misuse and may reflect the sympathomimetic actions of mephedrone and the accident-proneness or risk-taking behaviour of stimulant, including mephedrone, misusers (Schifano et al., 2011).

Mean mephedrone blood levels at post mortem were of either about 1.43mg/l (in polydrug cases) or 2.00mg/l (mono-intoxication fatalities), which is broadly in line with previous, small scale, anecdotal observations (Dickson et al., 2010; Lusthof et al., 2011).

11.2 Mephedrone use with other substances

Although mephedrone was here identified on its own in the cause of death in only one-third of cases (n = 18, 30%), this finding confirms some of the concerns recently expressed regarding the acute toxicity potential of the drug itself (James et al., 2011; Maskell et al., 2011; Schifano et al., 2011; Torrance & Cooper, 2010; Wood et al., 2010; Regan et al., 2010). It could be argued that the fact there are such a relatively large number of deaths in a comparatively short period (two years) underlines the need to inform consumers of its potential to cause death on its own.

Conversely, most mephedrone victims died of polydrug, and especially alcohol, consumption. Anecdotally, it appears that alcohol is taken in association with stimulants to get a stronger/better 'high'. Similarly, other stimulants such as MDMA/ecstasy, whilst in the presence of alcohol, show more significant physiopathological effects (Pacifici et al., 2002; Schifano et al., 2003a). In 15 cases mephedrone was ingested with stimulants. Cocaine, amphetamines, other methcathinones and/or ecstasy tablets may be taken to maintain arousal and a state of alertness, since the stimulant desired effects of mephedrone fade away in a few hours (Schifano et al., 2011). However, co-ingestion of two stimulants could increase, in a synergic way, both the dopaminergic and serotonergic stimulation, and this is likely to increase mephedrone toxicity effects and harm potential (Schifano et al., 2011). In other cases, arguably to modulate its stimulant effects, mephedrone was associated in this study with opiates (12 cases) and/or diazepam (13 cases). This is likely to be consistent with the observation made here that, where known, about 3 out of 4 victims had a history of drug misuse. It is noteworthy that other newly emerging psychoactive substances (including: GBL/GHB, ketamine, piperazines, as well as other methcathinones) were also found in several cases in conjunction with mephedrone; this is in line with the literature (Deluca et al., 2009; Schifano et al., 2011). In all of these polydrug abuse cases, the precise role of mephedrone in causing fatality was due to simultaneous drug use and remains unclear. Conversely, the use of stimulants might afford some protective effects to those who overdosed with sedatives.

11.3 Treatment and prevention of fatalities

The patterns of drug use evidenced by post mortem toxicology results are similar to those reported by surveys and online users' fora; polysubstance use is common, especially the co-ingestion of alcohol, stimulants and other 'legal highs'. The pathologies (including psychopathologies) exhibited in many of these cases exhibit close similarities to those previous noted for amphetamine, cocaine, MDMA and khat. The implication of these findings is that similar advice to that already given for adverse events caused by other stimulants should be provided to clinicians, the emergency services and first-aiders. It is suggested that the treatment for more life-threatening conditions might be broadly similar to that for amphetamine poisoning. Individuals with less severe symptoms should be assessed and managed as for any psychoactive drug user; they may simply need reassurance, support and observation. People with underlying cardiac, neurological and psychiatric conditions, especially those on medication, are likely to be at greatest risk of serious adverse events (Winstock et al., 2010).

Although our knowledge of mephedrone's potential neurotoxicity or long-term consequences of its use is still very limited, it is sensible to offer the following advice: avoiding regular use to avoid developing tolerance; not using the drug in combination with other stimulants or large amounts of alcohol and other depressants; not injecting the drug; remaining well hydrated when using the drug; and avoiding becoming overheated. Brief motivational interventions and appropriately adapted psychosocial intervention may be employed to treat mephedrone addiction (Winstock et al., 2010).

11.4 Limitations

A number of limitations need to be borne in mind in respect of this study: (a) not all suspected cases may have been identified; (b) remaining 'positive' cases are awaiting further inquiries or inquest; (c) the fact that mephedrone may have been involved in death cannot be confirmed until the relevant Coroner or Procurator Fiscal has concluded her/his inquest or other formal inquiry; (d) the presence of mephedrone in post mortem toxicology does not necessarily imply that it caused or contributed to a death; (e) not all completed cases have been formally notified to the Programme for recording. Hence, the number of identified cases reported here is likely to be an underestimation.

It is thought unlikely that the changes in fatality rates over time observed here are related to parallel changes in coroner methods, which would in turn affect surveillance. Data collection methods have remained unchanged. However, greater awareness of the phenomenon, improved case identification methods, and the devopment of new approaches in forensic toxicology and the range of substances now routinely screened for may have led to more potential cases being notified and registered.

Further limitations of the present report may include: lack of analytical attention to the role of the possible triggering environmental factors (i.e. overcrowding; hot settings etc); lack of total geographical coverage of coroner's jurisdictions; possible incomplete information relating to the prescription of psychoactive medications; and lack of information for some fatalities on the concentration of mephedrone detected in body fluids, so that some victims might have had only traces of the substance. Finally, since mortality rates (e.g. number of deaths out of number of mephedrone intake occasions) were not here calculated, it may be difficult to determine the true extent of risks associated with mephedrone consumption. However, in at least one case death occurred on the first use of mephedrone (albeit in combination with amphetamine).

12. Conclusions

This chapter has highlighted the dangers associated with mephedrone consumption, especially with regard to recreational use. This study represents the most detailed analysis to date of the largest number of mephedrone-related fatalities world-wide. It is hoped that it will thereby make a major contribution to the evidence-base being built up on this drug, and therefore, to reducing drug-related deaths.

Although identified on its own in only a minority of cases, present data confirm concerns regarding the acute toxicity potential of the drug. It is of concern that about 1 in 3 cases of the current sample used particularly violent means to terminate their own lives.

The number of mephedrone intake occasions was not calculated here, and so it may be difficult to determine the true extent of risks associated with mephedrone consumption. It may be possible to compare the lethality of mephedrone with other substances building on methods developed by King and Corkery (2010).

Further studies of a similar nature should be conducted in other countries, to see if the clinical and toxicity patterns associated with mephedrone use described here are confirmed. Notwithstanding the possible biases outlined above, the number of cases reported here may however suggest a significant level of caution when ingesting mephedrone for recreational purposes.

The limited information yet available on mephedrone underlines the need for basic pre-clinical and in-vitro research (and the necessary funding to carry it out) on the pharmacology, metabolism, etc. of methcathinones so as to provide evidence-based interventions and treatments.

13. Acknowledgements

The authors wish to thank coroners and their staff in England & Wales, Northern Ireland, and the Islands; Procurators Fiscal in Scotland; and the Scottish Crime & Drug Enforcement Agency for their assistance in providing data to the National Programme on Substance Abuse Deaths. Thanks are also due to colleagues in UK forensic toxicology agencies for assistance in identifying and confirming suspected deaths in which mephedrone consumption was positive. The np-SAD regularly received support from the Department of Health in the time frame 2004-2010.

This publication arises as well from the activities of the ReDNet Research Project, for which FS has received funding from the European Commission, in the framework of the Public Health Programme (2009 12 16).

14. Conflicts of interest

No conflicts of interest are declared here which may have influenced the interpretation of present data. Please note the following: JC has been the UK Focal Point expert on Drug-Related Deaths for the European Monitoring Centre for Drugs and Drugs Addiction since 2000; FS is a full member of the UK Advisory Council on the Misuse of Drugs (ACMD); JC and FS are members of the ACMD Working Group on Novel Psychoactive Substances, the UK Early Warning System. All authors are members of the International Centre for Drug Policy (ICDP). AHG is current President of the International Narcotics Control Board (INCB). The views expressed here reflect only those of authors and not necessarily those of the Department of Health, Home Office, the ACMD, the ICDP, the EMCDDA, or the INCB.

15. References

ACMD. (2010). *ACMD letter to Home Secretary - Mephedrone (and related cathinones)*. 13 January. Advisory Council on the Misuse of Drugs, London, Available from: http://www.homeoffice.gov.uk/publications/alcohol-drugs/drugs/acmd1/acmdmephedrone?view=Binary

Archer, R.P. (2009). Fluoromethcathinone, a new substance of abuse, *Forensic Science International*, Vol.185:10–20.

Camilleri, A., Johnston, M.R., Brennan, M., Davis, S. & Caldicott, D.G. (2010). Chemical analysis of four capsules containing the controlled substance analogues 4-

methylmethcathinone, 2-fluoromethamphetamine, alpha-phthalimidopropiophenone and N-ethylcathinone, *Forensic Science International*, Vol.197:59–66.

Campbell, D. (2009). Online sales of legal alternatives to class A drugs raise safety fears. *The Guardian*, 12.03.09, Available from:
http://www.guardian.co.uk/society/2009/mar/12/online-legal-drugs-stimulants

Chhabra, J.S., Nandalan, S. & Saad, R. (2010). Mephedrone poisoning – a case of severe refractory left ventricular failure, Poster Presentation 33, *The State of the Art Meeting*, London, 13-14 December 2010, pp. 74-75.

Chemspider. (2010). Mephedrone, Available from:
http://www.chemspider.com/Chemical-Structure.21485694.html

Corkery, J.M. (2002). Drug-related mortality in the United Kingdom, in Ghodse, H., Oyefeso, A., Corkery, J. & Baldacchino, A. (eds.), *Drug-related Mortality: Perspectives across Europe*, European Collaborating Centres for Addiction Studies, London, Monograph Series No. 2, pp. 155-184.

Corkery, J.M., Schifano, F., Oyefeso, A., Ghodse, A.H., Tonia, T., Naidoo, V. & Button, J. (2011). 'Bundle of fun' or 'bunch of problems'? Case series of khat-related deaths in the UK, *Drugs Education, Prevention and Policy*, Vol.18(6):408-425.

Cozzi, N.V., Sievert, M.K., Shulgin, A.T., Jacobill, P. & Ruoho, A.E. (1999). Inhibition of plasma membrane monoamine transporters by betaketoamphetamines, *European Journal of Pharmacology*, Vol. 381:63–69.

Daly, M. (2010). Teenage kicks, *Druglink*, Vol.25(No.1) (Jan/Feb):8-10, Available at:
http://www.drugscope.org.uk/OneStopCMS/Core/CrawlerResourceServer.aspx
?resource=359F1F2D-3D94-4061-AB88-
25AFFF1C801C&mode=link&guid=677eca484c614bf995ba90f8f81449d7

Dargan, P.I., Albert, S. & Wood, D.M. (2010). Mephedrone use and associated adverse effects in school and college/university students before the UK legislation change, *Quarterly Journal of Medicine*, Vol.103(No.11):875-9.

Davey, Z., Corazza, O., Schifano, F., Deluca, P. & the Psychonaut Web Mapping Group. (2010). Mass-information: Mephedrone, myths, and the new generation of legal highs, *Drugs and Alcohol Today*, Vol.10:24-28.

Deluca, P., Schifano, F., Davey, Z., Corazza, O., Di Furia, L. & the Psychonaut Web Mapping Research Group. (2009). *Mephedrone Report*, Institute of Psychiatry, King's College London, London (UK), Available from: http://www.psychonautproject.eu

Dickson, A.J., Vorce, S.P., Levine, B. & Past, M.R. (2010). Multiple-Drug Toxicity Caused by the Coadministration of 4-Methylmethcathinone (Mephedrone) and Heroin, *Journal of Analytical Toxicology*, Vol.34:162-168.

Drugsforum. (2010). Mephedrone (4-methylmethcathinone, 4-MMC) Experiences, www.drugs-forum.com, Available at:
http://www.drugs-forum.com/forum/showthread.php?t=43273

EMCDDA. (2011). *Report on the risk assessment of mephedrone in the framework of the Council Decision on new psychoactive substances*, May 2011, European Monitoring Centre for Drugs and Drug Addiction, Lisbon, Available from:
http://www.emcdda.europa.eu/html.cfm/index116639EN.html

Europol-EMCDDA. (2010). *Europol–EMCDDA Joint Report on a new psychoactive substance: 4-methylmethcathinone (mephedrone)*, March 2010, European Monitoring Centre for Drugs and Drug Addictions, Lisbon, Available from:

http://www.emcdda.europa.eu/html.cfm/index132196EN.html

Feyissa, A.M. & Kelly, J.P. (2008). A review of the neuropharmacological properties of khat, *Progress in Neuro-Psychopharmacology and Biological Psychiatry*, Vol.32:1147-1166.

Fleming, N. (2010). Miaow-miaow on trial: truth or trumped-up charges?, *New Scientist*, 29 March, Available at: http://www.newscientist.com/article/dn18712-miaowmiaow-on-trial-truth-or-trumpedup-charges.html

Garret, G. & Sweeney, M. (2010). The serotonin syndrome as a result of mephedrone toxicity, *BMJ Case Reports*, Doi:10.1136/bcr.04.2010.2925.

Gibbons, S. & Zloh, M. (2010). An analysis of the 'legal high' mephedrone, *Bioorganic & Medicinal Chemistry Letters*, Vol.20:4135–4139

Ghodse, A.H., Corkery, J., Oyefeso, A., Schifano, F., Ahmed, K. & Naidoo, V. (2010). *Drug-related deaths in the UK. Annual Report 2010*. International Centre for Drug Policy, St George's, University of London (UK). Available from: http://www.sgul.ac.uk/research/projects/icdp/pdf/np-SAD%2011th%20annual%20report%20Final.pdf

Gustaffsson, D. & Escher, C. (2009). Mefedron. Internetdrog som tycks ha kommit för att stanna [Mephedrone-Internet drug that seems to have come to stay], *Läkartidningen*, Vol.106:2769-2771.

Gygi, M.P., Gibb, J.W. & Hanson, G.R. (1996). Methcathinone: an initial study of its effects on monoaminergic systems, *Journal of Pharmacology and Experimental Therapeutics*, Vol.276:1066–1072.

Home Office. (2010). A change to the Misuse of Drugs Act 1971: Control of mephedrone and other cathinone derivatives, Home Office Circular 010/2010, 14 April 2010, Home Office, London, Available at: http://www.homeoffice.gov.uk/about-us/corporate-publications-strategy/home-office-circulars/circulars-2010/010-2010/

James, D., Adams, R.D., Spears, R., Cooper, G., Lupton, D.J., Thompson, J.P. & Thomas, S.H.; on behalf of the National Poisons Information Service. (2011). Clinical characteristics of mephedrone toxicity reported to the UK National Poisons Information Service, *Emergency Medical Journal*, Aug, Vol.28(No.8):686-689.

Kalix, P. (1990). Pharmacological properties of the stimulant khat, *Pharmacology and Therapeutics*, Vol.48:397-416.

Kalix, P. (1992). Cathinone, a natural amphetamine, *Pharmacology & Toxicology*, Vol.70:77–86.

King, L.A. & Corkery, J.M. (2010). An index of fatal toxicity for drugs of misuse, *Human Psychopharmacology*, Vol.25(No.2):162-166.

Lee, W.S., Chan, M.F., Tam, W.M. & Hung, M.Y. (2007). The application of capillary electrophoresis for enantiomeric separation of N,Ndimethylamphetamine and its related analogs: intelligence study on N,N-dimethylamphetamine samples in crystalline and tablet forms, *Forensic Science International*, Vol.165:71–77.

Lusthof, K.J., Oosting, R., Maes, A., Verschraagen, M., Dijkhuizen, A. & Sprong, A.G.A. (2011). A case of extreme agitation and death after the use of mephedrone in The Netherlands, *Forensic Science International*, Vol. 206:e93–e95

Mackay, K., Taylor, M. & Bajaj, N. (2011). The adverse consequences of mephedrone use: a case series, *The Psychiatrist*, Vol.35: 203-205.

Maskell, P.D., De Paoli, G., Seneviratne, C. & Pounder, D.F. (2011). Mephedrone (4-Methylmethcathinone)-related deaths, *Journal of Analytical Toxicology*, Vol. 35:188-191.

Measham, F., Moore, K., Newcombe, R. & Welch, Z. (2010). Tweaking, bombing, dabbing and stockpiling: the emergence of mephedrone and the perversity of prohibition, *Drugs and Alcohol Today*, Vol.10:14-21.

Morris, K. (2010). UK places generic ban on mephedrone drug family, *The Lancet*, Vol.9723:1333-1334.

Mulchandani, R., Hand, T. & Panesar, L.K. (2010). *Seizures of drugs in England and Wales, 2009/10*, Home Office Statistical Bulletin 17/10, 28 October 2010, Home Office Research Development and Statistics Directorate, London, Available from: http://webarchive.nationalarchives.gov.uk/20110218135832/rds.homeoffice.gov.u k/rds/pdfs10/hosb1710.pdf

Nagai, F., Nonaka, R. & Kamimura, K.S.H. (2007). The effects of nonmedically used drugs on monoamine neurotransmission in rat brain, *European Journal of Pharmacology*, Vol.559:132-137.

National Treatment Agency. (2010). *Drug treatment in 2009-2010*, National Treatment Agency, London, Available from: http://www.nta.nhs.uk/uploads/nta_annualreport_0910.pdf

Newcombe, R. (2009). *Mephedrone: the use of mephedrone (M-cat, meow) in Middlesbrough*, Lifeline Publications, Manchester

Nicholson, P.J., Quinn, M.J. & Dodd, J.D. (2010). Headshop heartache: acute mephedrone 'meow' myocarditis, *Heart*, Vol.96:2051-2052.

Odenwald, M., Neuner, F., Schauer, M., Elbert, T., Catani, C., Lingenfelder, B., Hinkel, H., Häfner, H. & Rockstroh, B. (2005). Khat use as risk factor for psychotic disorders: a cross-sectional and case-control study in Somalia, *BMC Medicine*, Vol.12:3-5.

Odenwald, M., Hinkel, H., Schauer, E., Schauer, M., Elbert, T., Neuner, F. & Rockstroh, B. (2009). Use of khat and posttraumatic stress disorder as risk factors for psychotic symptoms: a study of Somali combatants, *Social Science & Medicine*, Vol.69:1040-1048

Omer, T.A. & Doherty, C. (2011). Posterior reversible encephalopathy syndrome (PRES) complicating the 'legal high' mephedrone, *BMJ Case Reports*, Doi:10.1136/bcr.02.2011.3904

Osorio-Olivares, M., Caroli Rezende, S., Sepulveda-Boza, B.K., Cassels, R.F. et al. (2003). A two-step method for the preparation of homochiral cathinones, *Tetrahedron: Asymmetry*, Vol.14:1473-1477.

Pacifici, R., Zuccaro, P., Farre, M., Pichini, S., Di Carlo, S., Roset, P.N., Palmi, I., Ortuno, J., Menoyo, E., Segura, J. & de la Torre, R. (2002). Cell-mediated immune response in MDMA users after repeated dose administration: studies in controlled versus noncontrolled settings, *Annals of the New York Academy of Sciences*, Vol.965:421-433.

Power, M. (2009). Mephedrone: the future of drug dealing, *Druglink*, Vol.24.(No.2) (Mar/Apr):6,7,9. Available from: http://www.drugscope.org.uk/Resources/Drugscope/Documents/PDF/Good%2 0Practice/Druglink_March_09_mephedrone.pdf

Ramsey, J., Dargan, P.I., Smyllie, S., Davies, S., Button, J., Holt, D.W. & Wood, D.M. (2010). Buying 'legal' recreational drugs does not mean that you are not breaking the law, *Quarterly Journal of Medicine*, Vol.103:777–783.

Roussel, O., Perrin, M., Herard, P., Chevance, M. Arpino, P. (2009). La 4-méthyléphédrone sera-t-elle une "Ecstasy" du XXIème siècle?, *Annales de toxicologie analytique*, Vol. 21:169–177.

Regan, L., Mitchelson, M. & Macdonald, C. (2010). Mephedrone toxicity in a Scottish emergency department, *Emergency Medicine Journal*, Dec 23. [Epub ahead of print]

Saem de Burnaga Sanchez, J. (1929). Sur un homologue de l'ephedrine, *Bulletin de la Société Chimique de France*, Vol.45:284–286.

Schifano, F. (1996). Cocaine misuse and dependence, *Current Opinion in Psychiatry*, Vol.9:225–230

Schifano, F., Corkery, J., Naidoo, V., Oyefeso, A. & Ghodse, A.H. (2010). Comparison between amphetamine/ methylamphetamine and ecstasy (MDMA, MDEA, MDA, 4-MTA) mortality data in the UK (1997-2007), *Neuropsychobiology*, Vol.61:122-130.

Schifano, F., Oyefeso, A., Corkery, J., Cobain, K., Jambert-Gray, R., Martinotti, G. & Ghodse, A.H. (2003a). Death rates from ecstasy (MDMA, MDA) and polydrug use in England and Wales 1996-2002, *Human Psychopharmacology Clinical and Experimental*, Vol. 18:519-524.

Schifano, F., Oyefeso, A., Webb, L., Pollard, M., Corkery, J. & Ghodse, A.H. (2003b). Review of deaths related to taking ecstasy, England and Wales, 1997-2000, *British Medical Journal*, Vol. 326:80-81.

Schifano, F. & Corkery, J. (2008). Cocaine/crack cocaine consumption, treatment demand, seizures, related offences, prices, average purity levels and deaths in the UK (1990-2004), *Journal of Psychopharmacology*, Vol. 22:71-79.

Schifano, F., Albanese, A., Fergus, S., Stair, J.L., Deluca, P., Corazza, O., Davey, Z., Corkery, J., Siemann, H., Scherbaum, N., Farre', M., Torrens, M., Demetrovics, Z., Ghodse, A.H., Psychonaut Web Mapping & ReDNet Research Groups. (2011). Mephedrone (4-methylmethcathinone; 'meow meow'): chemical, pharmacological and clinical issues, *Psychopharmacology (Berlin)*, Vol. 214:593-602.

Smith, K. & Flatley, J. (Eds.). (2011). *Drug Misuse Declared: Findings from the 2010/11 British Crime Survey England and Wales*, Home Office Statistical Bulletin 12/11, 28 July 2011, Home Office Research, Development and Statistics Directorate, London, Available from: http://www.homeoffice.gov.uk/publications/science-research-statistics/research-statistics/crime-research/hosb1211/hosb1211?view=Binary

Sumnall, H. & Wooding, O. (2009). *Mephedrone: an update on current knowledge*. Centre for Public Health, Liverpool John Moores University, Liverpool, Available from: http://www.cph.org.uk/showPublication.aspx?pubid=614

Torrance, H. & Cooper, G. (2010) The detection of mephedrone (4-methylmethcathinone) in 4 fatalities in Scotland, *Forensic Sciences International*, Vol.202(No.1-3):e62-3.

Winstock, A.R., Marsden, J. & Mitcheson, L. (2010). What should be done about mephedrone? *British Medical Journal*, Vol.340:c1605.

Winstock, A., Mitcheson, L., Deluca, P., Davey, Z., Corazza, O. & Schifano, F. (2011). Mephedrone; new kid for the chop, *Addiction*, Vol.106(No.1):154-61.

Wood, D.M., Davies, S., Puchnarewicz, M., Button, J., Archer, R., Ovaska, H., Ramsey, J., Lee, T., Holt, D.W. & Dargan, P.I. (2010a). Recreational use of mephedrone (4-

methylmethcathinone, 4-MMC) with associated sympathomimetic toxicity, *Journal of Medical Toxicology*, Vol.6:327–330.

Wood, D.M., Davies, S., Puchnarewicz, M., Button, J., Archer, R. et al. (2009). Recreational use of 4-methylmethcathinone (4-MMC) presenting with sympathomimetic toxicity and confirmed by toxicological screening, *Clinical Toxicology*, Vol.47:7331.

Wood, D.M., Greene, S.L. & Dargan, P.I. (2010b). Clinical pattern of toxicity associated with the novel synthetic cathinone mephedrone, *Emergency Medical Journal*, doi:10.1136/emj.2010.092288

7

Chemical and Physical Enhancers for Transdermal Drug Delivery

José Juan Escobar-Chávez[1,*], Isabel Marlen Rodríguez-Cruz[2]
and Clara Luisa Domínguez-Delgado[2]
*[1]Unidad de Investigación Multidisciplinaria,
Laboratorio 12: Materiales Nanoestructurados y Sistemas Transdérmicos,
Facultad de Estudios Superiores Cuautitlán-Universidad
Nacional Autónoma de México, Carretera Cuautitlán–Teoloyucan,
San Sebastián Xhala, Cuautitlán Izcalli, Estado de México,
[2]Departamento de Ingeniería y Tecnología,
Sección de Tecnología Farmacéutica,
Facultad de Estudios Superiores Cuautitlán-Universidad
Nacional Autónoma de México,
Cuautitlán Izcalli, Estado de México,
México*

1. Introduction

The application of preparations to the skin for medical purposes is as old as the history of medicine itself, with references to the use of ointments and salves found in the records of Babylonian and Egyptian medicine.(López-Castellano & Merino, 2010) The historical development of permeation research is well described by Hadgraft & Lane, 2005. Over time, the skin has become an important route for drug delivery in which topical, regional or systemic effects are desired (Domínguez-Delgado, et al., 2010). Nevertheless, skin constitutes an excellent barrier and presents difficulties for the transdermal delivery of therapeutic agents, since few drugs possess the characteristics required to permeate across the stratum corneum in sufficient quantities to reach a therapeutic concentration in the blood. In order to enhance drug transdermal absorption different methodologies have been investigated developed and patented (Rizwan et al., 2009). To date many chemical and physical approaches have been applied to increase the efficacy of the material transfer across the intact skin. These are termed 'Novel' due to recent development with satisfactory results in the field of drug delivery (Patel et al., 2010). Improvement in physical permeation-enhancement technologies has led to renewed interest in transdermal drug delivery. Some of these novel advanced transdermal permeation enhancement technologies include: iontophoresis, electroporation, ultrasound, microneedles to open up the skin and the use of transdermal nanocarriers (Díaz-Torres, 2010; Escobar-Chávez & Merino, 2010a).

---

* Corresponding Author

2. Chemical enhancers

Chemical percutaneous enhancers have long been used to increase the range of drugs that can be effectively delivered through the skin (López-Castellano & Merino, 2010). To date, a plethora of chemicals have been evaluated as enhancers, but their inclusion in topical or transdermal formulations is limited due to fact that the underlying mechanisms of action of these agents remain unclear. Although different chemicals are employed by the industry as percutaneous enhancers, some of which have several desirable properties, to date none has proved to be ideal. An ideal chemical penetration enhancer should have the following attributes (Barry, 1983; López- Castellano & Merino, 2010): a) It should be non-toxic, non-irritating and non-allergenic, b) It should work rapidly, and its activity and duration of effect should be both predictable and reproducible, c) It should exert no pharmacological activity within the body, d) It should work unidirectionally, e) When removed, the skin's barrier properties should return both rapidly and fully, f) It should be compatible with both excipients and drugs, and g) It should be cosmetically acceptable and, ideally, odourless and colourless.

2.1 Percutaneous penetration routes of drugs

There are three major potential routes of percutaneous penetration: appendageal, transcellular (through the stratum corneum), and intercellular (through the stratum corneum) (Figure 1). There is a weight of evidence that suggests that passage through the intact stratum corneum constititus the predominant route by which most molecules penetrate the skin, as the appendageal route is characterized by a limited available fractional

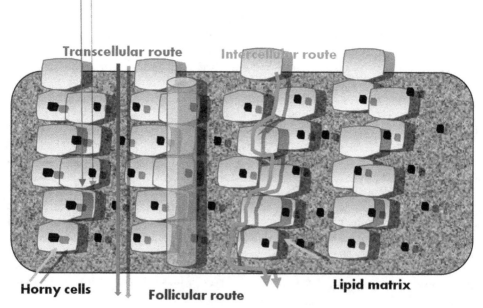

Fig. 1. Processes of percutaneous absorption

area of 0.1%. In this way, diffusion through the skin is controlled by the particular characteristics of the stratum corneum. In order to obtain a sufficient drug flux and, in turn, the therapeutical objectives in question, an alternative is to use chemical percutaneous enhancers. These substances alter some of the properties of the stratum corneum. (López-Castellano & Merino, 2010)

2.2 Direct effects on the skin due to the use of transdermal penetration enhancers

The lipid–protein-partititioning theory sets out the mechanisms by which enhancers alter skin lipids, proteins and/or partitioning behaviour (Barry, 1991): i) They act on the stratum corneum intracellular keratin by denaturing it or modifying its conformation, causing subsequent swelling and increased hydration; ii) They affect the desmosomes that maintain cohesion among corneocytes; iii) They modify the intercellular lipid domains to reduce the barrier-like resistance of the bilayer lipids. Disruption to the lipid bilayers can be homogeneous when the enhancer is distributed evenly within the complex bilayer lipids, but the accelerant is more likely to be heterogeneously concentrated within the domains of the bilayer lipids and iv) They alter the solvent nature of the stratum corneum, thus aiding the partitioning of the drug or a co-solvent into the tissue.(López-Castellano & Merino, 2010)

2.3 Indirect effects on the skin due to the use of transdermal penetration enhancers

Chemical enhancers can produce: a) Modification of the thermodynamic activity of the vehicle. The permeation of a good solvent from the formulation, such as ethanol, can increase the thermodynamic activity of a drug; b) It has been suggested that, by permeating through the membrane, a solvent can 'drag' the permeant with it, though this concept is somewhat controversial and requires confirmation; c) Solubilising the permeant within the donor, especially when solubility is very low, as in the case of aqueous donor solutions, can reduce depletion effects and prolong drug permeation.(López-Castellano & Merino, 2010)

2.4 Classification of percutaneous chemical enhancers

The classification of percutaneous enhancers is frequently based on the chemical class to which the compounds belong. Table 1 shows the principal classes of percutaneous enhancers.

CHEMICAL CLASS	COMPOUNDS
Water	Water
Sulfoxides and similar chemicals	Dimethyl sulfoxide, Dodecyl methyl sulfoxide
Ureas	Urea
Alcohols	Ethanol, Caprylic alcohol, Propylene glycol
Pyrrolidones and derivatives	N-methyl-2-pyrrolidone, 2-pyrrolidone
Azone and derivatives	Azone® (1-dodecylazacycloheptan-2-one)
Dioxolane derivatives	SEPA®
Surfactants (Anionic, Cationic, Nonionic, Zwitterionic)	Sodium lauryl sulfate, Cetyltrimethyl amonium bromide, Sorbitan monolaurate, Polisorbate 80, Dodecyl dimethyl ammoniopropane sulfate
Terpenes	Menthol, Limonene
Fatty acids	Oleic acid, Undecanoic acid

Table 1. Principal classes of percutaneous enhancers.

2.5 Determination of permeation enhancement

The great majority of studies of the effects of enhancers on skin permeability have been carried out by means of *in vitro* diffusion experiments in which various kinds of diffusion cells have been used. The most well-known of these cells are the Franz diffusion systems. These cells have two receptor compartments - donor and receptor (donor positioned above receptor) – between which the skin is placed. In general, the skin is pretreated with a solution of the chemical enhancer to be evaluated. The transdermal flux (J) of drugs can be estimated from the slope of the linear region (steady-state portion) of the accumulated amount of drug in the receptor compartment versus time plot. Permeation enhancing activity, expressed as enhancement ratio of flux (ER_{flux}), is determined as the ratio between the flux value obtained with the chemical enhancer and that obtained with the control. A number of variables can strongly influence the permeation enhancement of drugs. The most important are the skin used in the experiments, temperature, humidity, enhancer concentration, vehicle employed and degree of saturation of the drug in the donor and receptor compartments. (López-Castellano & Merino, 2010)

2.6 Uses in topical/transdermal formulations

Some examples of drugs delivered throughout the skin using chemical enhancer are shown in Table 2.

Drug	Chemical enhancer
Sodium salicylate (Hadgraft et al., 1985; Smith & Irwin, 2000); *Sodium naproxen* (Escobar-Chavez et al., 2005); *Ibuprofen* (Philips & Michniak,1995; Shen et al., 2007); *Nonivamide acetate* (Fang et al., 1997); *Meloxicam* (Zhang et al., 2009); *Flurbiprofen* (Ma et al., 2010); *Naloxone* (Xu et al., 2007); *Furosemide* (Agyralides et al., 2004); *Methotrexate* (Allan, 1995); *Sumatriptan succinate* (Balaguer-Fernandez et al., 2010).	Azone®
Sodium naproxen (Escobar-Chavez et al., 2005); *Sodium diclofenac* (Escribano et al., 2003); *Lidocaine* (Cazares-Delgadillo et al., 2005); *Testosterone* (Hathout et al., 2010); *Mometasone furoate* (Senyiğit et al., 2009); *Ketorolac* (Amrish et al., 2009).	Transcutol ®
Haloperidol (Vaddi et al., 2009); *Indomethacin* (Ogiso et al., 1995); *Leuprolide* (Lu et al., 1992).	Urea
Tizanidine hydrochloride (Mutalik et al., 2009); *Minoxidil* (Mura et al., 2009); *Metopimazine* (Bounoure et al., 2008); *Nortriptyline hydrochloride* (Merino et al., 2008; Escobar-Chavez et al., 2011).	Alcohols
Lidocaine (Lee et al., 2006); *Bupranolol* (Babu et al., 2008); *Propanolol* (Amnuaikit et al., 2005); *Acyclovir* (Montenegro et al., 2003).	Pyrrolidones
Tizanidine hydrochloride (Mutalik et al., 2009); *Daphnetin* (Wen et al., 2009); *Nitrendipin* (Mittal et al., 2008).	Fatty acids
Diclofenac (Kigasawa et al., 2009); *Nortiptyline hydrochloride* (Merino et al., 2008); *Verapamil hydrochloride* (Güngör et al., 2008); *Minoxidil* (Mura et al., 2009)	Terpenes
Retinol (Mélot et al., 2009); *Morphine* (Monti et al., 2001); *Arginine vasopressin* (Nair&Pachangula, 2003); *Insulin* (Pillai & Pachangula, 2003); *Enoxacin* (Fang et al., 1998).	Surfactants

Table 2. Examples of drugs delivered throughout the skin using chemical penetration enhancers.

3. Sonophoresis

Absorption of ultrasonic energy leads to tissue heating, and this has been used with therapeutic intent in many conditions. More recently it has been realized that benefit may also be obtained from the non-thermal effects that occur as ULTS travels through tissue. ULTS therapies can broadly be divided into "high" power and "low" power therapies where high power applications include high intensity focused ULTS and lithotripsy, and low power encompasses sonophoresis, sonoporation, gene therapy and bone healing. There are three distinct sets of ULTS conditions based on frequency range and applications: 1) High frequency (3-10 MHz) or diagnostic ULTS, 2) Medium frequency (0.7-3 MHz) or therapeutic ULTS, and 3) Low frequency (18 to 100 KHz) or power ULTS.

3.1 The ultrasound

The term ultrasonic refers to sound waves whose frequency is >20 KHz. The intensity (I, expressed in W/cm^2), or concentration of power within a specific area in an ULTS beam, is proportional to the square of the amplitude, p, which is the maximum increase or decrease in the pressure relative to ambient conditions in the absence of the sound wave. The complete relationship is: $I = p^2/2\rho c$, where ρ is the density of the medium and c is the speed of the sound (in human soft tissue, this velocity is 1540 m/s). The intensity is progressively lost when a sound wave passes through the body or is deviated from its initial direction, a phenomenon referred to as attenuation. In homogeneous tissue, the attenuation occurs as a result of absorption, in which case the sound energy is transformed into heat and scattered. The sound waves are produced in response to an electrical impulse in the piezoelectric crystal, allowing the conversion of electrical into mechanical or vibrational energy; this transformation requires a molecular medium (solid, liquid, or gas) to be effective. The ULTS beam is composed of two fields, the "near field," in the region closest to the transducer face, and the "far field," corresponding to the conical diverging portion of the beam (Figure 2). The parameters controlling this configuration of the ULTS beam are principally the frequency and the size of transducer.

3.2 Mechanisms of action

3.2.1 Cavitation effects

Cavitation is the formation of gaseous cavities in a medium upon ULTS exposure. The primary cause of cavitation is ULTS-induced pressure variation in the medium. Cavitation involves both the rapid growth and collapse of a bubble (inertial cavitation), or the slow oscillatory motion of a bubble in an ULTS field (stable cavitation). Collapse of cavitation bubbles releases a shock wave that can cause structural alteration in the surrounding tissue (Clarke et al., 2004) ULTS can generate violent microstreams, which increase the bioavailability of the drugs (Tachibana & Tachibana, 1999). Tissues contain air pockets that are trapped in the fibrous structures that act as nuclei for cavitation upon ultrasound exposure. The cavitational effects vary inversely with ULTS frequency and directly with ULTS intensity. Cavitation might be important when low-frequency ULTS is used, gassy fluids are exposed or when small gas-filled spaces are exposed. Cavitation occurs due to the nucleation of small gaseous cavities during the negative pressure cycles of ULTS, followed by the growth of these bubbles throughout subsequent pressure cycles (Tang et al., 2001).

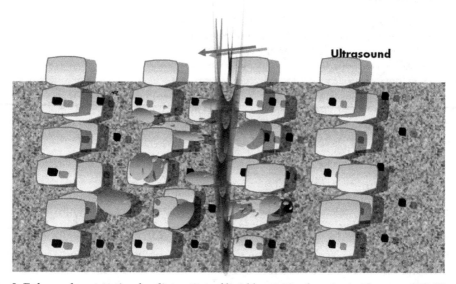

Fig. 2. Enhanced permeation by disruption of lipid barrier and cavitation by use of ULTS.

3.2.2 Thermal effects

Absorption of ULTS increases temperature of the medium. Materials that possess higher ULTS absorption coefficients, such as bone, experience severe thermal effects compared with muscle tissue, which has a lower absorption coefficient (Lubbers et al., 2003). The increase in the temperature of the medium upon ULTS exposure at a given frequency varies directly with the ULTS intensity and exposure time. The absorption coefficient of a medium increases directly with ULTS frequency resulting in temperature increase.

3.2.3 Convective transport

Fluid velocities are generated in porous medium exposed to ultrasound due to interference of the incident and reflected ULTS waves in the diffusion cell and oscillations of the cavitation bubbles. Fluid velocities generated in this way may affect transdermal transport by inducing convective transport of the permeant across the skin, especially through hair follicles and sweat ducts.

3.2.4 Mechanical effects

ULTS is a longitudinal pressure wave inducing sinusoidal pressure variations in the skin, which, in turn, induce sinusoidal density variation. At frequencies greater than 1 MHz, the density variations occur so rapidly that a small gaseous nucleus cannot grow and cavitational effects cease. But other effects due to density variations, such as generation of cyclic stresses because of density changes that ultimately lead to fatigue of the medium, may continue to occur. Lipid bilayers, being self-assembled structures, can easily be disordered by these stresses, which result in an increase in the bilayer permeability. This increase is, however, non-significant and hence mechanical effects do not play an important role in therapeutic sonophoresis. Thus cavitation induced lipid bilayer disordering is found to be the most important cause for ultrasonic enhancement of transdermal transport.

3.3 Advantages and disadvantages of sonophoresis

Sonophoresis is capable of expanding the range of compounds that can be delivered transdermally. In addition to the benefits of avoiding the hepatic first-pass effect, and higher patient compliance, the additional advantages and disadvantages that the sonophoretic technique offers can be summarized as follows in Table 3.

Advantages	Disadvantages
Enhanced drug penetration (of selected drugs) over passive transport.	Can be time-consuming to administer.
Allows strict control of transdermal penetration rates. Permits rapid termination of drug delivery through termination of ULTS. Skin remains intact, therefore low risk of introducing infection. Less anxiety provoking or painful than injection	Minor tingling, irritation, and burning have been reported (these effects can often be minimized or eradicated with proper ULTS adjustment (Maloney et al., 1992). SC must be intact for effective drug penetration.
In many cases, greater patient satisfaction.	
Not immunologically sensitizing.	
Less risk of systemic absorption than injection.	

Table 3. Advantages and disadvantages of using sonophoresis as a physical penetration enhancer.

3.4 Applications of ultrasound

Table 4 summarizes the research on sonophoresis uses in the transdermal administration of drugs.

Anesthetics		
Research	Outcome	References
Topical skin penetration of lidocaine	Increase in the concentration of lidocaine transmitted into rabbit subdermal tissues when topical application was followed by use of ULTS	Wells et al., 1977.
Double blind, vehicle-controlled, crossover trial in healthy volunteers for lidocaine cream	No increase in absorption of lidocaine cream by using ULTS	McEnlay et al., 1985.
Trial in healthy volunteers for lidocaine oil	Other variables include differences in ULTS frequencies and drug concentrations.	Novak et al., 1964.

Skin lidocaine penetration	250 kHz induced the highest penetration of lidocaine.	Griffin & Touchstone, 1972.
Anesthetic effect of lidocaine in legs of hairless mice	ULTS in conjunction with a topical aqueous lidocaine solution was rapidly effective in inducing an anesthetic effect in the legs of hairless mice	Tachibana et al., 1993
Sonophoresis of topical benzocaine and dibucaine	No detectable increase in the rate of anesthetic penetration	Williams et al., 1990.
Administration of lidocaine hydrochloride trandermally on healthy volunteers applying 0.5 MHz ULTS.	0.5 MHz ULTS in sonophoresis for conduction anesthesia using lidocaine hydrochloride for a nerve block, it is more effective than the 1 Mhz that is widely used in clinical situations	Kim et al., 2007.
Permeation of procaine hydrochloride through cell monolayers applying therapeutical ULTS.	Extent and velocity of the permeation of procaine hydrochloride through MDCK monolayer can be controlled by sonophoresis	Hehn et al., 1996.
Analgesic and anti-inflammatory drugs		
Effect of intensity, mode, and duration of ULTS application on the transport of three non steroidal anti-inflammatory drugs (NSAIDs) across cellulose membrane and hairless rabbit-skin	Demonstrated the synergistic effect of temperature and ULTS operation parameters on drug transport of NSAIDs	Meshali et al., 2008.
Effect of an ULTS (1 MHz) on transdermal absorption of indomethacin from an ointment in rats	Intensity and duration of application play an important role in the transdermal sonophoretic delivery; intensity of 0.75 W/cm² for 10 min was most effective for delivering indomethacin	Miyazaki et al., 1992.
Study of the influence of ultrasound on percutaneous absorption of ketorolac tromethamine *in vitro* across hairless rat skin	A significant increase in permeation of ketorolac through rat skin was observed with the applied sonication at 3 W/cm² when compared with permeation at 1 and 2 W/cm².	Tiwari et al., 2004.
To determine if a ketorolac tromethamine (KT) gel solution could be administered *in vivo* via phonophoretic transdermal delivery using pulsed ULTS by examining its anti-inflammatory effects in a rat carrageenan inflammation model.	The transdermal application of KT gel using sonophoresis had significant anti-hyperalgesic and anti-inflammatory effects. These findings suggest that the transdermal administration of a KT gel using sonophoresis with pulsed ULTS might be useful for treating acute inflammation and pain.	Yang et al., 2008.
Application of ultraphonophoresis of 5% ibuprofen nurofen gel to affected joints of 20 patients.	Analgesic efficacy of transcutaneous 5% gel nurofen in osteoarthrosis.	Serikov et al., 2007.

Examination of therapeutic effects of sonophoresis with ketoprofen in gel form in patients with enthesopathy of the elbow.	Positive effects of sonophoresis using a pharmacologically active gel with ketoprofen were shown to be highly significant in assessments, objective (clinical examination) and subjective (interview). The pain symptoms in the elbow resolved in most of the patients.	Cabak et al., 2005.
Quantitative study of sodium diclofenac (Voltaren Emulgel, Novartis) phonophoresis in humans	Previously applied therapeutic ULTS irradiation enhances the percutaneous penetration of the topical diclofenac gel, although the mechanism remains unclear	Rosim et al., 2005.
Investigation of *in vitro* penetration and the *in vivo* transport of flufenamic acid in dependence of ULTS.	Using this *in vitro* model it is possible to compare the transdermal delivery of commercial flufenamic ointment in volunteers.	Hippius et al., 1998.
Antibiotics		
Effect of ULTS on the delivery of topically applied amphotericin B ointment in guinea pigs.	Amphotericin B content in the skin and subcutaneous fatty tissues was much higher when the drug was delivered in the presence of ULTS.	Rornanenko & Araviiskii, 1991.
Administration of tetracycline in healthy rabbits using electrophoresis and sonophoresis	It was found that the tissue levels of tetracycline administered with the modified methods of electro and sonophoresis increased with an increase in the current density or ULTS intensity, the procedure time and antibiotic concentration.	Ragelis et al., 1981.
Immunosuppressives		
Investigated the topical transport of Cyclosporin A using low-frequency US throughout rat skin	The enhanced skin accumulation of Cyclosporin A by the combination of low-frequency ULTS and chemical enhancers could help significantly to optimize the targeting of the drug without of a concomitant increase of the systemic side effects.	Liu et al., 2006.
Evaluation of the efficacy of low frequency sonophoresis (LFS) at 25KHz produced by a sonicator apparatus for treatment of alopecia areata, melasma and solar lentigo.	The study showed that LFS, a not aggressive technique, enhanced penetration of topic agents obtaining effects at the level of the epidermis, dermis and appendages (intradermal delivery), giving better results in the treatment of some cosmetic skin disorders.	Santoianni et al., 2004.

Anticancer drugs		
Application of a method using ULTS and nano/microbubbles to cancer gene therapy using prodrug activation therapy.	Dramatic reductions of the tumor size by a factor of four.	Aoi et al., 2007.
Investigation of competitive transport across skin of 5-fluorouracil into coupling gel under the influence of ULTS, heat-alone and Azone® enhancement.	Ultrasonication produced a decrease in percutaneous drug penetration. This effect was due to the diffusive loss of the hydrophilic substance 5-fluorouracil from the skin surface.	Meidan et al., 1999.
Insulin		
To determine if the 3x1 rectangular cymbal array perform significantly better than the 3x3 circular array for glucose reduction in hyperglycemic rabbits.	Using the rectangular cymbal array, the glucose decreased faster and to a level of -200.8±5.9 mg/dL after 90 min.	Luis et al., 2007.
To demonstrate ultrasonic transdermal delivery of insulin *in vivo* using rabbits with a novel, low-profile two-by-two ULTS array.	For the ULTS-insulin group, the glucose level was found to decrease to -132.6 ± 35.7 mg/dL from the initial baseline in 60 min	Lee et al., 2004.
The purpose of this study was to demonstrate the feasibility of ULTS-mediated transdermal delivery of insulin *in vivo* using rats with a novel, low profile two-by-two US array based on the "cymbal" transducer.	For the 60-min ULTS exposure group, the glucose level was found to decrease from the baseline to -267.5 ± 61.9 mg/dL in 1 h. Moreover, to study the effects of ULTS exposure time on insulin delivery, the 20-min group had essentially the same result as the 60-min exposure at a similar intensity.	Smith et al., 2003.
Corticosteroids		
Determination of the effect of ULTS on the transcutaneous absorption of dexamethasone.	A sonophoretic effect occurred with dexamethasone when its application saturated the skin.	Saliba et al., 2007.
To determine if ULTS enhances the diffusion of transdermally applied corticosteroids.	The effects of sonophoresed dexamethasone can be measured in terms of reduced collagen deposition as far down as the subcutaneous tissue but not in the submuscular or subtendinous tissue	Byl et al., 1993.
Comparison of effectiveness of 0.4% Dexamethasone sodium phosphate (DEX-P) sonophoresis (PH) with 0.4% DEX-P iontophoresis (ION) therapy in the management of patients with knee joint osteoarthritis	Significant improvement in total WOMAC scores was observed in 15 (60%) and 16 (64%) patients in the PH and ION groups respectively, indicating no significant difference in the improvement rate.	Akinbo et al., 2007.

Designing a sonophoretic drug delivery system to enhance the triamcinolone acetonide (TA) permeability.	The highest permeation of TA was observed under the ULTS treatment conditions of low frequency, high intensity, and in continuous mode.	Yang et al., 2006.
Cardiotonics		
The sonophoresis of digoxin *in vitro* through human and hairless mouse skin.	There was no enhancement of digoxin absorption across human skin by ULTS.	Machet et al., 1996.
Vasodilators		
Skin penetration enhancement effect of ULTS on methyl nicotinate in 10 healthy human volunteers.	ULTS treatment applied prior to methyl nicotinate led to enhanced percutaneous absorption of the drug	McEnlay et al., 1993.
Hormones		
Effect of permeation enhancers and application of low frequency (LUS) and high frequency ultrasound (HUS) on testosterone (TS) transdermal permeation after application of testosterone solid lipid microparticles (SLM).	Skin exposure to HUS or LUS before application of 1% dodecylamine for 30 min had no superior enhancement effect over application of either LUS or HUS alone. Application of drug loaded SLM offered skin protection against the irritation effect produced by TS and 1% DA.	El-Kamel et al., 2008.
Cicatrizants		
The effectiveness of sonophoresis on the delivery of high molecular weight (MW) hyaluronan (HA) into synovial membrane using an animal model of osteoarthritis (OA).	Synovial fluid analysis revealed increased absorption and fluorescence microscopy showed deeper penetration of both HA1000 and HA3000.	Park et al., 2005.
Calcein		
The skin permeation clearance of model hydrophilic solutes, calcein (MW 623) and-labeled dextrans [MW 4400 (FD-4) and MW 38000 (FD-40)], across the skin under the influence of ULTS.	Good correlations were observed between the $3H_2O$ flux and solute clearances and, unexpectedly, the slope values obtained from linear regression of the plots were consistent for all solutes examined.	Morimoto et al., 2005.
Oligonucleotids		
Assessment of the potential of low frequency ULTS (20 kHz, 2.4 W/cm²) in delivering therapeutically significant quantities of anti-sense oligonucleotides into skin.	Microscopic evaluations using revealed heterogeneous penetration into the skin. Heterogeneous penetration led to the formation of localized transport pathways, which occupied about 5% of the total exposed skin area.	Tezel et al., 2004.
Stimulants		
The effect of low-frequency sonophoresis on fentanyl and caffeine permeation through human and hairless rat skin.	Discontinuous ULTS mode was found to be more effective in increasing transdermal penetration of fentanyl while transdermal transport of caffeine was enhanced by both continuous and pulsed mode.	Boucaud et al., 2001.

Calcium		
Manipulation of the Ca^{2+} content of the upper epidermis by sonophoresis across hairless mouse SC.	Sonophoresis at 15 MHz did not alter barrier function.	Menon et al., 1994.
Panax notoginseng		
Effect of a therapeutic US coupled with a Panax notoginseng gel for medial collateral ligament repair in rats.	This study reveals a positive ultrasonic effect of Panax notoginseng extract for improving the strength of ligament repair.	Ng et al., 2008.
Other applications *i)To study the mechanisms of penetration due to US throughout the skin*		
To demonstrate the calcein permeability through the localized transport regions (LTRs) from the exposure to the ULTS/ Sodium lauryl sulphate (SLS) system.	LTRs and the non-LTRs exhibit significant decreases in skin electrical resistivity relative to untreated skin, suggesting the existence of two levels of significant skin structural perturbation due to ULTS exposure in the presence of SLS.	Kushner IV et al., 2004.
To shed light on the mechanism(s) by which low-frequency ULTS (20 KHz) enhances the permeability of the skin.	Significant fractions (30%) of the intercellular lipids of SC were removed during the application of low frequency sonophoresis.	Alvarez-Roman et al., 2003.
Investigation of short time sonication effects of human skin at variable intensities and on the dynamics of fluorescein transport across the skin.	A short application of ULTS enhanced the transport of fluorescein across human skin by a factor in the range of 2–9 for full thickness skin samples and by a factor in the range of 2–28 000 for heat-stripped SC samples	Cancel et al., 2004.
Use of quantum dots as a tracer and confocal microscopy and transmission electron microscopy (TEM) as visualization methods, on low frequency sonophoresis.	ULTS significantly increased the frequency of occurrence of the otherwise scattered and separated lacunar spaces in the SC. A significant increase in lacunar dimensions was observed when 1% w/v sodium lauryl sulfate was added to the coupling medium.	Paliwal et al., 2006.
ii)Kelloids		
ULTS therapy with a water-based gel alone	"Complete flattening" of keloids in two young men when 1 MHz at 0.8 W/cm 2 was applied for approximately 4 minutes.	Walker, 1983.
iii) Tumours		
Optimization of ULTS parameters for *in vivo* bleomycin delivery	An effective antitumor effect was demonstrated in solid tumors of both murine and human cell lines.	Larkin et al., 2008.

Investigation of high-intensity focused ULTS (HIFU) exposure of (111) In-MX-B3.	The HIFU exposure shortened the peak tumor uptake time (24 vs. 48 h for the control) and increased the peak tumor uptake value (38 vs. 25 %ID/g for the control). The HIFU effect on enhancing tumor uptake was greater at earlier times up to 24 h.	Khaibullina et al., 2008.
Supurative wounds		
Treatment of suppurative wounds with ULTS.	sonophoresis of ethylenediaminetetra acetic acid with the quinoxaline antibiotic dioxidine was effective in accelerating wound purification an delimination of necrotic issues	Levenets et al., 1989.
Treatment of suppurative wounds with ULTS.	Sonophoresis of a 1% papain solution together with dimethyl sulfoxide was an effective method for treating purulent wounds and inflammatory infiltrates.	Matinian et al., 1990.

Table 4. Research on uses of sonophoresis to administer different drugs through the skin

4. Iontophoresis

Transdermal iontophoresis consists of the application of a low density current and low voltage (typically 0.5 A/cm²) via an electrical circuit constituted by two drug reservoirs (anode and cathode) deposited on skin surface. During application of the current, the drug is repelled by the corresponding electrode and pushed through the stratum corneum. A substance can pass through the skin by electromigration, electroosmosis or passive diffusion. The latter of the three mechanisms is a result of changes caused by the electric field to the permeability of the skin, and its effects are negligible compared with those of the other two mechanisms. When ions are repelled by the electrode of the same charge and attracted by the electrode of the opposite charge is electromigration. When neutral substances are transported with the solvent flow is electroosmosis, which at physiological pH favours the movement from the anode to the skin.

The advantages and disadvantages that the iontophoretic technique offers are summarized in Table 5.

4.1 Mechanisms of action

Skin is a complex membrane and controls the movement of molecules across it in the presence of an electric field. Skin has an isoelectric point (pI) of 4–4.5. Above this pH, the carboxylic acid groups are ionized. Therefore, at higher pH values, the skin behaves as a permselective membrane which especially attracts cations that have been repelled by the anode, thus favouring the passage of molecules by electromigration (Merino et al., 1999). The movement of small sized cations (mainly Na^+) generates a solvent flow that promotes the passage of non-charged molecules through the skin. This process is identified as electroosmosis (Delgado-Charro and Guy, 1994). Electrical mobility decreases with molecular weight, and, as a consequence, the electroosmotic contribution becomes increasingly important for larger molecules (Guy et al., 2000). The dependence of iontophoretic flux on the intensity of the current applied has been clearly demonstrated by Faraday's law (Sage et al., 1992): where Ja is the flux (in moles per unit time), ta is the transport number, Za is the valence of ion a, I is the current applied (Amperes), and F is Faraday's constant (Coulombs/mol). The transport number, ta, is the fraction of the total current transported by a specific ion, and is a measure of its efficiency as a charge carrier: ta=Ia / I. It follows that knowledge of a compound's transport number allows the feasibility of its iontophoretic delivery or extraction to be predicted. The sum of the transport numbers of all the ions present during iontophoresis equals 1 ($\Sigma ti=1$), illustrating the competitive nature of electrotransport.

Advantages	Disadvantages
Enhance penetration of ionized and unionized molecules. Moreover, improving the delivery of polar molecules as well as high molecular weight compounds (e. g. peptides and oligonucleotides). Enabling continuous or pulsatile delivery of drug (depending on the current applied). Permitting easier termination of drug delivery. Offering better control over the amount of drug delivered since the amount of compound delivered depends on applied current, duration of applied current, and area of skin exposed to the current. Restoration of the skin barrier functions without producing severe skin irritation. Ability to be used for systemic delivery or local (topical) delivery of drugs. Reducing considerably the inter and intraindividual variability, since the rate of drug delivery is more dependent on applied current than on stratum corneum characteristics.	Can be time-consuming to administer. The actual current density in the follicle maybe high enough to damage growing hair. SC must be intact for effective drug penetration.

Table 5. Advantages and disadvantages of using iontophoresis as a physical penetration enhancer.

4.2 Types of iontophresis

4.2.1 Direct iontophoresis

Direct iontophoresis can be anodal if the drug is neutral or positively charged and cathodal if the drug is negatively charged. Although cations have better properties for iontophoresis, anions can also increase their transdermal drug flux with respect to passive diffusion.

4.2.2 Reverse iontophoresis

Reverse iontophoresis across the skin is a potentially useful alternative for non-invasive clinical and therapeutic drug monitoring. During current application, reverse iontophoresis allows the movement of neutral and positively charged entities into the cathode while negatively charged entities move into the anode. The main problem with this is that skin contains some of the entities to be analyzed, which implies that there is a period of time within which it is necessary to withdraw skin reserves and after which it is possible to correlate extracted levels of the analytes with levels in the blood (Leboulanger et al., 2004).

4.3 Applications of iontophoresis

The most extended uses of iontophoresis are the treatment of palmoplantar hyperhidrosis and the diagnosis of cystic fibrosis. However, iontophoresis is also used for the topical delivery of others drugs such as lidocaine, acyclovir and dexamethasone. The only system commercially available at present is the fentanyl iontophoretic transdermal system. It is indicated for the shortterm management of acute postoperative pain in adult patients requiring opioid analgesia during hospitalization. Currently, the iontophoretic delivery of apomorphine for the treatment of idiopathic Parkinson's disease is being evaluated in human subjects. Peptide drugs including various series of amino acid derivatives and tripeptides, thyrotropin release hormones, LHRH and analogues, vasopressin and calcitonin can also be administered by means of this technique. One peptide that has focused the attention of researchers in the field of iontophoresis is insulin.

5. Electroporation

Electroporation is the phenomenon in which cell membrane permeability to ions and macromolecules is increased by exposing the cell to short high electric field pulses. The increase in permeability is attributed to the electric field induced "breakdown" of the cell membrane and the formation of nano- scale defects or "pores" in the membrane – and hence electro-"poration". Electroporation can be of two types - reversible and irreversible. In irreversible electroporation the electric field is such that the membrane permeabilization leads to cell death. This may be caused by either permanent permeabilization of the membrane and cell lysis (necrosis) or by temporary permeabilization of a magnitude which can cause a severe disruption of the cell homeostasis that can finally results in cell death, either necrotic or apoptotic. In reversible electroporation the electric pulse causes only a temporary increase in permeability and the cell survives. The reversible electroporation mode has numerous applications in biotechnology and medicine both, *in vitro* and *in vivo*. Irreversible electroporation has applications in the food industry, for sterilization and in medicine for tissue ablation (Ball et al., 2010).

5.1 Mechanisms of transdermal electroporation

The theory postulates two paths for electroporation induced transdermal transport, through pores formed in the multiple lipid bilayers connecting corneocytes and through appendage cells. Small lipid-soluble molecules can partition into the SC, and then diffuse across the lipid bilayer membranes, but water soluble molecules, particularly charged molecules, cannot penetrate significantly by this route. High voltage pulsing (> 50V) creates aqueous pathways ("pore") through stratum corneum (SC) lipid bilayer membranes, and short pathway segments are formed across 5--6 lipid bilayer membranes which connect adjacent corneocyte interiors forming transcellular straight-through pathways. Moderate voltage (= 5 to 50V) pulses appear to electroporate cell linings of the appendages. Temperature is considered to play a role in the permeabilization.

5.2 Advantages and disadvantages of electroporation for transdermal drug delivery

The advantages and disadvantages that the electroporation technique offers are summarized in Table 6.

Advantages	Disadvantages
Enhanced drug penetration (of selected drugs) over passive transport. Allows strict control of transdermal penetration rates. Versatility: electroporation is effective nearly with all cells and species types (Sung et al., 2003). Efficiency: a large majority of cells take in the target DNA or molecule (Huang et al., 2005). Permits rapid termination of drug delivery through termination of electroporation. The procedure may be performed with intact tissue (Heller et al., 1996). Less anxiety provoking or painful than injection. In many cases, greater patient satisfaction.	Cell damage: If the pulses are of the wrong length or intensity, some pores may become too large or fail to close after membrane discharge causing cell damage or rupture (Murthy et al., 2004). The transport of material into and out of the cell during the time of electropermeability is relatively nonspecific (Murthy et al., 2004).
Not immunologically sensitizing.	

Table 6. Advantages and disadvantages of using electroporation as a physical penetration enhancer.

5.3 Applications of electroporation

The field of skin electroporation is made of two aspects. The first deal with electroporation in a conventional sense in relation to the cells of the skin and the second is unique and relates to transdermal effects. The concept of transdermal electroporation may be traced to fundamental research on the breakdown of flat lipid bilayer membranes. Prausnitz et al., (1993) addresses the fact that transdermal transport normally occurs primarily through the intracellular lipids organized in bilayers. Small molecular weight lipophilic drugs can be effectively delivered by passive transdermal delivery. However, the stratum corneum does not permit passage of polar/hydrophilic molecules and macromolecules. The paper suggests that microsecond to millisecond electroporation type pulsed electric fields applied across the skin produce, in a manner similar to that found in studies on flat lipid bilayers, trans bilayer aqueous pores. It reports that electroporation produces transient structural changes in the skin resulting in an up to four orders of magnitude increase in transdermal mass transfer flux of polar molecules in human skin *in vitro* and animal skin *in vivo*.

6. Microneedles

The use of microneedles is another method for bypassing the stratum corneum barrier, which have been introduced as a form of transdermal drug delivery. They can penetrate the upper layer of the skin without reaching the dermis, to be an efficient method to deliver drugs transdermally in an almost painless method. The drug diffuses across the rest of the epidermis into the dermis where it is absorbed into the blood circulation. Nowadays different types of microneedles have been designed by other researchers as well, varying in their materials of fabrication, shapes, dimensions, modes of application, etc. (Chabri et al., 2009).

6.1 Microneedle types and their methods of transdermal delivery

Microneedles are available as both solid and hollow microneedles made of various materials (Figure 3). Till date, five methods of transdermal delivery mediated by microneedles have been attempted (Gill & Prausnitz, 2007): *Poke with patch approach*: It can be inserted into the skin to pierce the stratum corneum and create micro conduits through which drug can enter into the lower layers of the epidermis (Henry et al., 1998). *Coat and poke approach:* It involves coating the drug to be delivered around the surface of the microneedle. By inserting the microneedles through the skin, the drug coating dissolves off in the skin fluid and the dissolved drug diffuses through the skin into the blood microcirculation. The coating methods are used to roll coating, spray coating and dip coating (Gill & Prausnitz, 2006). *Dip and scrape:* The dip and scrape method involves placing the array in contact with the drug solution and then scraping multiple times across the skin to create microabbrassions (Mikszta et al., 2002). *Dissolving microneedles:* It is referred to microneedles made from a biodegradable polymeric material with the drugs encapsulated inside them. In this method, the drug is released in a controlled manner as the microneedle dissolves off when inserted into the skin (Lee W. J et al., 2007). *Injection through hollow microneedles:* This occurs where the microneedles are designed with holes at the centre or with side openings through which drugs are microinjected into the lower layers of the skin and then diffuses across the viable skin until it reaches the blood vessels in the dermis (Griss & Stemme, 2003).

Solid microneedles: These are easier to fabricate, have better mechanical strength and sharper tips as compared to hollow microneedles (Rhoxed et al., 2008a). Solid silicon microneedles have been widely used for the transdermal drug delivery studies (Donnelly et al., 2009; Haq et al., 2009). However, silicon is expensive, not biocompatible and brittle. Therefore it breaks easily during the penetration across skin (Chen et al., 2008). Polymer has been used as an alternative material because it is a cheaper and stronger material which could reduce tissue damage (Fernandez et al., 2009). Polymer increases the bluntness of the microneedle tip due to the low modulus and yield strength of polymer. Polymer microneedles have a main limitation with its mechanical properties which could cause needle failure during the penetration across skin (Park et al., 2007). Bevelled tip microneedles have been fabricated using biodegradable polymers (Park, 2004). Metal is the third material used to manufacture microneedles. It is mechanically strong and relatively cheap to produce.

Hollow microneedles: The purpose of this type of microneedles is to deliver drugs through the bore at the needle tip. This reduces the sharpness of needle tip which affect the penetration of this needle into skin. These issues have been resolved recently including openings at the side in the microneedles rather than at the bottom (Roxhed et al., 2008). These microneedles have their tip closed initially; however they can be opened on insertion into the skin where the tip dissolves in the high saline solution in the interstitial fluid. The tips can also be opened as a result of applied pressure. It has been proposed the use of rotary drilling and mechanical vibration as methods to enhance insertion of hollow microneedles and the fluid infusion flow rate (Wang et al., 2006).

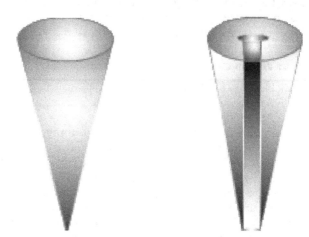

Fig. 3. Two dimensional view of hollow and solid microneedle.

6.2 Microneedles manufacturing

The methods that have been adopted for microneedle fabrication include wet etching, deep reactive ion etching (DRIE) (Teo et al., 2005), microinjection moulding (Sammoura et al., 2007), isotropic etching, isotropic etching in combination with deep etching and wet etching respectively, dry etching, isotropic and anisotropic, photolithography, thin film deposition (Moon & Lee, 2003), laser cutting (Martanto et al., 2004), and inclined LIGA process (Perennes et al., 2006). Studies have shown that factors such as microneedle geometry, coating depth on solid microneedle and skin thickness affect the drug delivery efficiency using microneedles (Al-Qallaf et al., 2009a; 2009b). To ensure that both the insertion and delivery occur at the right location, they should be sharp enough and at least 100µm in length (Stoeber & Liepmann, 2000).

6.3 Microneedles applications

Vaccination against virus: Researchers have recently presented microneedle patches as a better alternative for immunization. The vaccine can be coated unto microneedle array and presented as a simple patch which can allow patients to immunize themselves without the necessity for intense medical training (Stoeber & Liepmann, 2005). *Cutaneous fluid extraction and glucose monitoring:* A prototype of a disposable microneedle based glucose monitoring devices has been designed in which, the fluid extraction chamber attached to the microneedle can be connected to a sensing device which measures and indicates the glucose concentration in the body (Zimmermann et al., 2003). *Acne treatment:* The treatment is limited by the low rate of penetration of drugs through the stratum corneum. So, experiments have been carried out by applying the TheraJectMAT™ dissolving microneedles containing API in a GRAS matrix to the surface of human skin with acne (Kwon, 2006). *Delivery of nanoparticles:* It was showed that the delivery of particles of 1µm in diameter is enhanced when the skin is pre-treated with microneedles by adopting the poke with patch approach. Therefore, it seems to us that the delivery of micro and nano-particles is important in order to facilitate controlled/ delayed delivery after the drug is inserted into the skin (McAllister et al., 2003). *Insulin delivery:* Microneedles have been shown to deliver insulin with a significant biological effect as the blood glucose concentration was reduced by substantial amount using microneedles.

7. Nanocarriers

Nanocarriers are so small to be detected by immune system and they can deliver the drug in the target organ using lower drug doses in order to reduce side effects. Nanocarriers can be administrated into the organisms by all the routes; one of them is the dermal route. The nanocarriers most used and investigated for topic/transdermal drug delivery in the pharmaceutical field are liposomes, dendrimers, nanoparticles and nanoemulsions (Table 7).

Nanocarrier	Size	Preparation Methods	Characteristics	References
Nanoparticles	10-1000 nm	In situ polymerization, emulsification-evaporation, emulsification-diffusion, emulsification-diffusion by solvent displacement	Solid or hollow particles wich have entraped, binded or encapsulated drugs.	Domínguez-Delgado et al., 2011; oppimath et al., 2001
Solid lipid nanoparticles	50-1000 nm	High-pressure homogenization.	Similar to polymeric nanoparticles but made of solid lipids.	Almeida & Souto, 2007
Inorganic nanoparticles	<50nm	Sol-gel technique	Nanometric particles, made up of inorganic compounds such as silica, titania and alumina.	García-González, 2009
Liposomes	25 nm-100 μm	Sonication, extrusion, mozafari method	Vesicles composed of one or more concentric lipid bilayers, separated by water or aqueous buffer compartments.	El Maghraby et al., 2008
Dendrimers	3-10 nm	Polymerization	Macromolecular high branched structures.	Menjoge et al., 2010
Quantum dots	2-10nm	Colloidal assembly, viral assembly, electrochemical assembly.	Made up of organic surfactants, precursors and solvents.	Rzigalinski & Strobl, 2009
Lipid globules	1-100 nm	Emulsification espontaneous systems.	Multicomponent fluid made of water, a hydrophobic liquid, and one or several surfactants resulting in a stable system.	Dan et al., 2010

Nanocarrier	Size	Preparation Methods	Characteristics	References
Lipid microcylinders	<1 μm	Self emulsification	Self organizing system in which surfactants crystallize into tightly packed bilayers that spontaneously form cylinders	Dodla & Bellamkonda, 2008
Lipid microbubbles	<2 μm	Sonication	Gas filled microspheres stabilized by phospholipids, polymers or low density proteins.	Tartis et al., 2008
Lipospheres	0.2-100 μm	Melt method, multiple microemulsion, cosolvent method	Solid lipid core stabilized by a monolayer of phospholipids molecules embedded in the particle surface.	Fang et al., 2007
Ethosomes	<400 nm	Cold method, hot method	Non invasive delivery carriers that enable drugs to reach the deep skin layers and/or the systemic circulation.	Elsayed et al., 2006
Aquasomes	60-300 nm	Self-assembling of hydroxyapatite by co-precipitation method	The particle core is composed of noncrystalline calcium phosphate or ceramic diamond, and it is covered by a polyhydroxyl oligomeric film.	Rojas-Oviedo et al., 2007
Pharmacosomes	<200 nm	Hand-shaking method, Ether-injection method	Pure drug vesicles formed by amphiphilic drugs	Jin et al., 2006
Colloidosomes	200 nm – 1.5 μm	Self-assembly of colloidal particles at the interface of emulsion droplets	Hollow capsules with elastic shells.	Rossier-Miranda et al., 2009
Niosomes	10-1000 nm	Self-assembly of nonionic surfactant	Bilayered structures made of non-ionic surfactant vesicles.	Hong et al., 2009
Nanoemulsions	20-200 nm	High-pressure, homogenization, microfluidization, phase inversion Temperature.	Submicron emulsions o/w or w/o	Elnaggar et al., 2009

Table 7. Examples of Nanocarriers used for transdermal drug delivery

7.1 Liposomes

Liposomes are hollow lipid bilayer structures that can transport hydrophilic drugs inside the core and hydrophobic drugs between the bilayer (Bangham, 1993). They are structures made of cholesterol and phospholipids. They can have different properties depending on the excipients included and the process of their elaboration. The nature of liposomes makes them one of the best alternatives for drug delivery because they are non-toxic and remain inside the bloodstream for a long time. Liposomes can be surface-charged as neutral, negative or positive, depending on the functional groups and pH medium. Liposomes can encapsulate both lipophilic and hydrophilic drugs in a stable manner, depending on the polymer added to the surface (Rodriguez-Justo & Morae et al., 2011). There are small unilamellar vesicles (25 nm to 100nm), medium-sized unilamellar vesicles (100 nm and 500nm), large unilamellar vesicles, giant unilamellar vesicles, oligolamellar vesicles, large multilamellar vesicles and multivesicular vesicles (500 nm to microns). The thickness of the membrane measures approximately 5 to 6 nm. These shapes and sizes depend of the preparation technique, the lipids used and process variables. Depending on these parameters, the behavior both *in vivo* and *in vitro* can change and opsonization processes, leakage profiles, disposition in the body and shelf life are different due to the type of liposome (Rodriguez-Justo & Morae et al., 2011).

Liposomes preparation techniques follow three basic steps with particular features depending on safety, potential scale up and simplicity: 1) Lipid must be hydrated, 2) Liposomes have to be sized and 3) Nonencapsulated drug has to be removed. The degree of transdermal drug penetration is affected by the lamellarity, lipid composition, charge on the liposomal surface, mode of application and the total lipid concentrations (Cevc & Blume, 1992). Some examples of drugs delivered throughout the skin by using liposomes are melatonin (Dubey et al., 2007b), indinavir (Dubey et al., 2010), amphotericin B (Manosroi et al., 2004), methotrexate (Dubey et al., 2007a), ketoprofen (Maestrelli et al., 2005), estradiol (Essa et al., 2004), clindamicyn hydrochloride and lignocaine (Sharma et al., 1994).

7.2 Dendrimers

Dendrimers are monodisperse populations that are structurally and chemically uniform. They allow conjugation with numerous functional groups due to the nature of their branches. The amount of branches increases exponentially and dendrimers growth is typically about 1 nm per generation (Svenson & Tomalia, 2005). The dendrimers classification is based on the number of generations. After the creation of a core, the stepwise synthesis is called first generation; after that, every stepwise addition of monomers creates the next generation. This approach allows an iterative synthesis, providing the ability to control both molecular weight and architecture.

The kind of polymer chosen to construct the dendrimer by polimerization is very important with regard to the final architecture and features. In addition, the use of branched monomers has the peculiarity of providing tailored loci for site-specific molecular recognition and encapsulation. Notably, 3D and fractal architecture, as well as the peripheral functional groups, provide dendrimers with important characteristic physical and chemical properties. In comparison with linear polymers, dendritic structures have "dendritic voids" that give these molecules important and useful features. These spaces inside dendrimers can mimic the molecular recognition performed by natural proteins. Furthermore, dendrimers have a high surface-charge density due to ionizable groups that help them to attach drugs by electrostatic forces, regardless of the stoichimetry. This dendrimer-drug association provides drugs with better solubility, increasing their transport through biological membranes and sometimes increasing drug stability. The number of molecules that can be incorporated into dendrimers is related to the number of surface functional groups; therefore, later-generation dendrimers are more easily incorporated into dendritic structure. However, not all the functional groups are available for interaction due to steric volume, molecule rotation or stereochemistry effects. Dendrimers can have positive and negative charges, which allows them to complex different types of drugs (Kabanov et al., 1998). The main problems with this kind of transdermal carrier are poor biodegradation and inherent cytotoxicity (Parekh, 2007). In order to reduce their toxicity, dendrimers have been linked to peptides and which are formed from amino acids linked via peptide-amide bonds to the branches of dendrimers in the core or on the surface. When they are bio-transformed, dendrimer-peptide systems produce amino-acid derivatives. Finally, the synthesis of these structures is less expensive and purification does not present any difficulty (Niederhafner et al., 2005). Due to their form and size, these molecules can carry drugs, imaging agents, etc. Dendrimers interact with lipids present in membranes, and they show better permeation in cell cultures and intestinal membranes (Cheng et al., 2008). Dendrimers also act like solubility enhancers, increasing the permeation of lipophilic drugs; nevertheless, they are not good carriers for and hydrophilic drugs.

7.3 Nanoparticles

Nanoparticles are smaller than 1,000 nm. Nowadays, it is possible to insert many types of materials such as drugs, proteins, peptides, DNA, etc. into the nanoparticles. They are constructed from materials designed to resist pH, temperature, enzymatic attack, or other problems (Huang L. et al., 2010; Wei et al., 2010). The nanoparticle technology can be divided into three stages: first generation (involves those nanoparticles that had only one component in their structure and these delivery systems are able to transport drugs in the blood until they reach the target), second generation (implies nanoparticles made of one main component and additional substances and these complexes are able to cross barriers and reach difficult targets such as the brain) and third generation is represented by nanoparticles that can be made of nanoparticles with one main component combined with a second component to reach a specific target (Cui et al., 2005; Herffernan & Murthy, 2005). Moreover, nanoparticles can be classified as nanospheres or nanocapsules (Figure 4). Nanospheres are solid-core structures and nanocapsules are hollow-core structures (Yoo et al., 2005). Nanoparticles can be composed of polymers, lipids, polysaccharides and proteins (Goswami et al., 2010; Li et al., 2009). Nanoparticles preparation techniques are based on their physicochemical properties. They are made by emulsification-diffusion by solvent displacement, emulsification-polymerization, in situ-polymerization, gelation, nanoprecipitation, solvent evaporation/extraction, inverse salting out, dispersion polymerization and other derived from these one.

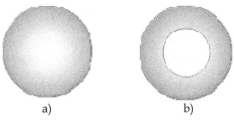

a)   b)

Fig. 4. a) Nanospheres and b) nanocapsules.

7.4 Nanoemulsions

Nanoemulsion are isotropic dispersed systems of two non miscible liquids, normally consisting of an oily system dispersed in an aqueous system (o/w nanoemulsion), or an aqueous system dispersed in an oily system but forming droplets or other oily phases of nanometric sizes (100 nm). They can be stable (methastable) for long times due to the extremely small sizes and the use of adequate surfactants. Nanoemulsions can use hydrophobic and hydrophilic drugs because it is possible to make both w/o or o/w nanoemulsions (Sonneville-Aubrun, et al. 2004). They are non-toxic and non-irritant systems and they can be used for skin or mucous membranes, parenteral and non parenteral administration in general and they have been used in the cosmetic field. Nanoemulsions can be prepared by three methods mainly: high-pressure homogenization, microfluidization and phase inversion temperature. Transdermal delivery using nanoemulsions has been reduced due to the stability problems inherent to this dosage form. Some examples of drugs using nanoemulsions to transdermal drug delivery are gamma tocopherol, caffeine, plasmid DNA, aspirin, methyl salicylate, insulin and nimesulide (Shakeel & Ramadan, 2010).

8. Conclusions

Transdermal drug delivery has several potential advantages over other parenteral delivery methods. Apart from the convenience and noninvasiveness, the skin also provides a "reservoir" that sustains delivery over a period of days. Furthermore, it offers multiple sites to avoid local irritation and toxicity, yet it can also offer the option to concentrate drugs at local areas to avoid undesirable systemic effects. However, at present, the clinical use of transdermal delivery is limited by the fact that very few drugs can be delivered transdermally at a viable rate. This difficulty is because the skin forms an efficient barrier for most molecules, and few noninvasive methods are known to significantly enhance the penetration of this barrier.

In order to increase the range of drugs available for transdermal delivery the use of chemical and physical enhancement techniques have been developed in an attempt to compromise skin barrier function in a reversible manner without concomitant skin irritation. Recently, several alternative physical methods have emerged to transiently break the stratum corneum barrier and also the use of chemical enhancers continues expanding. The projectile methods use propelled microparticles and nanoparticles to penetrate the skin barrier. Microneedle arrays are inserted through the skin to create pores. "Microporation" creates arrays of pores in the skin by heat and radio frequency ablation. Also, ultrasound has been employed to disrupt the skin barrier. All these methods have their own advantages and drawbacks, but a reality is that new developments are expected in the future to make these methods even more versatile.

9. Acknowledgments

José Juan Escobar-Chávez wishes to acknowledge PAPIIT TA 200312 y PAPIIT IN 209709-3. The authors report no conflict of interests.

10. References

Aditya NP, Patankar S, Madhusudhan B, Murthy RSR & Souto EB. (2010). Arthemeter-loaded lipid nanoparticles produced by modified thin-film hydration: Pharmacokinetics, toxicological and *in vivo* anti-malarial activity. *European Journal of Pharmaceutical Sciences*, Vol. 40, pp.448-455, ISSN 0928-0987.

Agyralides, GG.; Dallas PP.; Rekkas, DM. (2004). Development and *in vitro* evaluation of furosemide transdermal formulations using experimental design techniques. *International Journal of Pharmaceutics*, Vol. 281, No.1-2, (August 2004), pp. 35-43, ISSN 0378-5173.

Akinbo, SR.; Aiyejusunle, CB.; Akinyemi, OA.; Adesegun, SA, & Danesi MA. (2007). Comparison of the therapeutic efficacy of phonophoresis and iontophoresis using dexamethasone sodium phosphate in the management of patients with knee ostheoarthritis. *Nigerian Postgraduate Medical Journal*; Vol. 14, No. 3, (September 2007), pp.190-94, ISSN 1117-1936.

Allan, G. Azone®. (1995). In: *Percutaneous Penetration Enhancers*, Smith EW, Maibach HI, Eds, pp. 129-3, Florida, Boca Raton.

Almeida AJ, Souto E. (2007). Solid lipid nanoparticles as a drug delivery system for peptides and proteins. *Advanced Drug Delivery Reviews,* vol. 59 pp.478-490, ISSN 0169-409X.

Al-Qallaf B, Das DB & Davidson A. (2009a). Transdermal drug delivery by coated microneedles: Geometry effects on drug concentration in blood. *Asia-Pacific Journal of Chemical Engineering*. Vol. 4, No. 6, (November/December 2009), pp. 845-857, ISSN 1932-2143.

Al-Qallaf B, Das DB. (2009b). Optimizing microneedle arrays to increase skin permeability for transdermal drug delivery. *Annals of the New York Academy of Sciences*. 1161: 83-94.

Alvarez-Roman R, Naik A, Kalia YN, Guy RH & Fessi H. (2004). Skin penetration and distribution of polymeric nanoparticles. *Journal of Controlled Release*, Vol. 99, pp.53-62, ISSN 0168-3659.

Alvarez-Román, R.; Merino, G.; Kalia, YN.; Naik, A, Guy & RH. (2003). Skin permeability enhancement by low frequency sonophoresis: Lipid extraction and transport pathways. *Journal of Pharmaceutical Sciences*, Vol. 92, No. 6, (June 2003), pp. 1138-46, ISSN 0022-3549.

Amnuaikit, C.; Ikeuchi, I.; Ogawara, K.; Higaki, K. & Kimura, T. (2005). Skin permeation of propranolol from polymeric film containing terpene enhancers for transdermal use. *International Journal of Pharmaceutics*, Vol. 289, No. 1-2, (January 2005), pp.167-78, ISSN 0378-5173.

Amrish, C. & Kumar SP. (2009). Transdermal delivery of ketorolac. *Yakugaku Zasshi*, Vol.129, No.3, (March 2009), pp. 373-9, ISSN 1347-5231.

Aoi, A.; Watanabe, Y, Mori S, et al. (2007). Herpes simplex virus thymidine kinase mediated suicide gene therapy using nano/microbubbles and ultrasound. *Ultrasound In Medicine & Biology*, Vol. 34, No. 39, (March 2008) pp. 425-434, ISSN *0301-5629*.

Arias JL, López-Viota M, López-Viota J & Delgado AV. (2009). Development of iron/ethylcellulose (core/shell) nanoparticles loaded with diclofenac sodium for arthritis treatment. *International Journal of Pharmaceutics*. Vol.382, pp.270-276, ISSN: 0378-5173.

Babu, RJ.; Dhanasekaran, M.; Vaithiyalingam, SR.; Singh, PN. & Pandit, JK. (2008). Cardiovascular effects of transdermally delivered bupranolol in rabbits: effect of chemical penetration enhancers. *Life Science*, Vol. 82, No. 5-6, (January 2008), pp. 273-8, ISSN 0024-3205.

Balaguer-Fernández, C.; Padula, C.; Femenía-Font, A.; Merino, V.; Santi, P. & López-Castellano A. (2010). Development and evaluation of occlusive systems employing polyvinyl alcohol for transdermal delivery of sumatriptan succinate. *Drug Delivery*, Vol. 17, No. 2, (February 2010), pp. 83-91, ISSN *1521-0464*.

Ball C, Thomson KR, Kavnoudias H. Irreversible Electroporation: A New Challenge in "Out of Operating Theater" Anesthesia. Anesthesia Analgesia, Vol. 110, No. 5, (May 2010), pp. 1305-9, ISSN 1526-7598.

Banga AK, Bose S & Ghosh TK. (1999). Iontophoresis and electroporation: comparisons and contrasts. *International Journal of Pharmaceutics*. Vol.179 pp. 1–19, ISSN: 0378-5173.

Bangham AD. (1993). Liposomes: the Babraham connection. *Chemistry and Physics of Lipids*. Vol. 64, pp.275-285, ISSN 0009-3084.

Barry, BW & Williams, AC. (1991). Terpenes and the lipid-protein-partititioning theory of skin penetration enhancement. *Pharmaceutical Research*, Vol. 8, No. 1, (January 1991), pp. 17–24, ISSN 1573-904X.

Barry, BW. (1983). *Dermatological Formulations: Percutaneous Absorption*, Marcel Dekker, ISBN 0824717295, New York.

Barry, BW. (2001). Novel mechanisms and devices to enable successful transdermal drug delivery. *European Journal of Pharmaceutical Sciences*, Vol. 14, No. 2, (September 2001), pp. 101–4, ISSN 0928-0987.

Becker SM, Kuznetsov AV. (2007). Numerical assessment of thermal response associated with *in vivo* skin electroporation: the importance of the composite skin model. Journal of Biomechanical Engineering, Vol. 129, No. 3, (June 2007), pp.330-40, ISSN 0148-0731.

Boucaud, A.; Machet, L.; Arbeille, B.; et al. (2001). In vitro study of low-frequency ultrasound-enhanced transdermal transport of fentanyl and caffeine across human and hairless rat skin. *International Journal of Pharmaceutics*, Vol. 228, No. 1-2, (October 2001), pp. 69-77, ISSN 0378-5173.

Bounoure, F.; Lahiani-Skiba, M.; Besnard, M.; Arnaud, P.; Mallet, E. & Skiba M. (2008). Effect of iontophoresis and penetration enhancers on transdermal absorption of metopimazine. *Journal of Dermatological Science*, Vol. 52, No. 3, (December 2008), pp. 170-7, ISSN *0923-1811*.

Byl, NN.; McKenzie, A.; Halliday, B.; Wong, T.& O'Connell J. (1993) The effects of phonophoresis with corticosteroids controlled pilots study. *Journal of Orthopaedic Sports Physical Therapy*, Vol. 18, No. 5, (November 1993), pp. 590-600, ISSN 0190-6011.

Cabak, A.; Maczewska, M.; Lyp, M.; Dobosz, J. & Gasiorowska U. (2005). The effectiveness of phonophoresis with ketoprofen in the treatment of epocondylopathy. *Ortopedia, Traumatologia, Rehabilitacja*; Vol. 37, No. 6, (December 2005), pp. 660-65. ISSN 1509-3492.

Cancel, LM.; Tarbell, JM. & Ben-Jebria A. (2004). Fluorescein permeability and electrical resistance of human skin during low frequency ultrasound application. *Journal of Pharmacuy and Pharmacology*, Vol. 56, No. 9, (September 2004), pp. 1109-18, ISSN 0022-3573.

Cázares-Delgadillo, J.; Naik, A.; Kalia, YN.; Quintanar-Guerrero, D. & Ganem-Quintanar A. (2005) Skin permeation enhancement by sucrose esters: A pH-dpendent phenomenon. *International Journal of Pharmaceutics*, Vol. 297, No. 1-2, (June 2005), pp. 204-212, ISSN 0378-5173.

Cevc G, Blume G. (1992). Lipid vesicles penetrate into intact skin owing to the transdermal osmotic gradients and hydration force. Biochimica et Biophysica Acta. *Vol.* 1104, pp. 226-232.

Chabri F, Bouris K, Jones T, Barrow D, Hann A, Allender C, Brain K & Birchall J. (2009). Microfabricated silicon microneedles for nonviral cutaneous gene delivery. *The British Journal of Dermatology*, Vol. 150, No. 5, pp. 869–77, ISSN: 0007-0963.

Chen B, Wei J, Tay FE, Wong YT & Iliescu C. (2008). Silicon microneedle array with biodegradable tips for transdermal drug delivery. *Microsystem Technologies*. Vol. 14, No. 7, pp. 1015-19, ISSN: 0946-7076.

Chen T, D'Addio SM, Kennedy MT, Swietlow A, Kevrekidis IG & Panagiotopoulos AZ. (2009). Protected Peptide Nanoparticles: Experiments and Brownian Dynamics Simulations of the Energetics of Assembly. Nano Letters, Vol. 9, pp. 2218-2222, ISSN: 1530-6984.

Cheng Y, Xu Z, Ma M & Xu T. (2008). Dendrimers as drug carriers: Applications in different routes of drug administration. *Journal of Pharmaceutical Sciences*, Vol. 97, pp.123-143, ISSN 0022-3549.

Clarke, L.; Edwards, A.; Graham, E. (2004) Acoustic streaming: an in vitro study. *Ultrasound In Medicine & Biology*, Vol. 30, No. 4, (April 2004), pp. 559–62, ISSN 0301-5629.

Cui Z, Han S, Padinjarae D & Huang L. (2005). Immunsotimulation mechanism of LPD nanoparticles as a vaccine carrier. Molecular Pharmacology, Vol. 2, pp. 22-28, ISSN: 0026-895X.

Dan Y, Liu H, Gao W & Chen S. (2010). Activities of essential oils from Asarum heterotropoides var. mandshuricum against five phytopathogens. *Crop Protection*. Vol. 29, No. 295-299. ISSN: 0261-2194.

Davis SP, Martanto W, Allen MG & Prausnitz MR. (2005). Hollow metal microneedles for insulin delivery to diabetic rats. IEEE T. *BioMedical Engineering*, Vol. 52, No 5, pp. 909-15, ISSN: 0018-9294.

Delgado-Charro MB, Guy RH. (1994). Characterization of convective solvent flow during iontophoresis. Pharmaceutical Research, Vol. 11, No. 7, (July 1994), pp. 29-35, ISSN 0724-8741.

Díaz-Torres, R. (2010). Transdermal nanocarriers. In: *Current Technologies to Increase the Transdermal Delivery of Drugs*, José Juan Escobar-Chávez/Virginia Merino (Eds.), pp., 120-40, Bentham Science Publishers, ISBN 978-1-60805-191-5, The Netherlands.

Dodla MC, Bellamkonda RV. (2008). Differences between the effect of anisotropic and isotropic laminin and nerve growth factor presenting scaffolds on nerve regeneration across long peripheral nerve gaps. *Biomaterials*. Vol. 29, pp.33-46, ISSN: 0142-9612.

Domínguez-Delgado C. L., Rodríguez-Cruz I. M. & López-Cervantes M. (2010). Chapter 1: The skin a valuable route for administration of drugs. In: José Juan Escobar-Chávez (Ed), *Current Technologies To Increase The Transdermal Delivery Of Drugs*. Bentham Science Publishers Ltd. ISBN: 978-1-60805-191-5, Bussum, The Netherlands.

Domínguez-Delgado C. L., Rodríguez-Cruz I. M., Escobar-Chávez J. J., Calderón-Lojero I. O., Quintanar-Guerrero David & Ganem-Quintanar Adriana. (2011). Triclosan nanoparticles as a novel option for acne treatment. *European Journal of Pharmaceutics and Biopharmaceutics*. IN PRESS, ISSN: 0928-0987.

Donnelly RF, Morrow DI, McCarron PA, Woolfson AD, Morrissey A, Juzenas P, Juzeniene A, Lani, V, McCarthy HO & Moan J. (2009). Microneedle arrays permit enhanced intradermal delivery of a preformed photosensitizer. *Photochemistry and Photobiology*. Vol. 85, pp. 195-204, ISSN 1751-1097.

Dubey V, Mishra D & Jain NK. (2007b). Melatonin loaded ethanolic liposomes: Physicochemical characterization and enhanced transdermal delivery. *European Journal of Pharmaceutics and Biopharmaceutics*. Vol. 67, pp. 398-405, ISSN: 0928-0987.

Dubey V, Mishra D, Dutta T, Nahar M, Saraf DK & Jain NK. (2007a). Dermal and transdermal delivery of an anti-psoriatic agent via ethanolic liposomes. *Journal of Controlled Release*, Vol. 123, pp.148-154, ISSN 0168-3659.

Dubey V, Mishra D, Nahar M, Jain V & Jain NK. (2010). Enhanced transdermal delivery of an anti-HIV agent via ethanolic liposomes. *Nanomedicine: Nanotechnology, Biology and Medicine*. Vol. 6. No. 4, (2010 August), pp. 590-6, ISSN: 1549-9634.

El Maghraby GM, Barry BW & Williams AC. (2008). Liposomes and skin: From drug delivery to model membranes. *European Journal of Pharmaceutical Sciences*, Vol. 34, pp.203-222, ISSN 0928-0987.

El-Kamel, AH.; Al-Fagih, IM. & Alsarra IA. (2008). Effect of sonophoresis and chemical enhancers on testosterone transdermal delivery from solid lipid microparticles:an in vitro study, *Current Drug Delivery*, Vol. 5, No. 1, (January 2008), pp. 20-26, ISSN 1567-2018.

Elnaggar YSR, El-Massik MA & Abdallah OY. (2009). Self-nanoemulsifying drug delivery systems of tamoxifen citrate: Design and optimization. *International Journal of Pharmaceutics*. Vol.380, pp.133-141, ISSN: 0378-5173.

Elsayed MMA, Abdallah OY, Naggar VF & Khalafallah NM. (2006). Deformable liposomes and ethosomes: Mechanism of enhanced skin delivery. *International Journal of Pharmaceutics*. Vol. 322, pp. 60-66, ISSN: 0378-5173.

Escobar-Chávez JJ, Bonilla-Martínez D, Villegas-González M.A. (2010b). Sonophoresis: A valuable physical enhancer to increase transdermal drug delivery. In: *Current Technologies to Increase the Transdermal Delivery of Drugs*, José Juan Escobar-Chávez/Virginia Merino (Eds.), pp. 53-76, Bentham Science Publishers, ISBN 978-1-60805-191-5, The Netherlands.

Escobar-Chávez JJ, Melgoza-Contreras LM, López-Cervantes M, et al. (2009c). The tape stripping technique as a valuable tool for evaluating topical applied compounds. In: *Frontiers in Drug Design & Discovery*, Gary W. Caldwell / Atta-ur-Rahman / Z.

Yan / M. Iqbal Choudhary (Eds.) Vol. 4, pp. 189-227, Bentham Science Publishers, eISBN 978-1-60805-202-8.

Escobar-Chávez JJ, Merino-Sanjuán V, López-Cervantes M, et al. (2009d). The use of iontophoresis in the administration of nicotine and new non nicotine drugs through the skin for smoking cessation. *Current Drug Discovery Technologies*, Vol. 6, No. 3, (September 2009), 171-185, ISSN 1570-1638.

Escobar-Chávez JJ, Quintanar-Guerrero D, and Ganem-Quintanar A. (2005). *In vivo* skin permeation of sodium naproxen formulated in PF-127 gels: Effect of Azone® and Transcutol®. *Drug Development and Industrial Pharmacy*; Vol. 31 No. 4-5, (May 2005), pp.447-54, ISSN 0363-9045.

Escobar-Chávez, JJ. & Merino, V. 2010a. *Current Technologies to increase the Transdermal Delivery of Drugs*, Bentham Science Publishers, ISBN: 978-1-60805-191-5, Bussum, The Netherlands.

Escobar-Chávez, JJ.; Bonilla-Martínez, D.; Villegas-González, A.; Rodríguez-Cruz, IM.; Domínguez-Delgado, CL. (2009a). The use of sonophoresis in the administration of drugs through the skin. *Journal of Pharmacy and Pharmaceutical Sciences*, Vol. 12, No. 1, (April 2009), pp. 88-115, ISSN: 1482-1826.

Escobar-Chávez, JJ.; Bonilla-Martínez, D.; Villegas-González, A.; Revilla-Vazquez, AL. (2009b). The electroporation as an efficient physical enhancer for transdermal drug delivery. *Journal of Clinical Pharmacology*, Vol. 49, No. 11, (August 2008), pp. 1262-83, ISSN: 0091-2700.

Escobar-Chávez, JJ.; López-Cervantes, M.; Naïk, A.; et al. (2006). Applications of the thermoreversible Pluronic F-127 gels in pharmaceutical formulations. *Journal of Pharmacy and Pharmceutical Sciences*; Vol. 9, No. 3, (November 2006), pp. 339-58, ISSN 1482-1826.

Escobar-Chávez, JJ.; Merino, V.; Díez-Sales, O.; Nácher-Alonso, A.; Ganem-Quintanar, A.; Herráez, M.; Merino-Sanjuán, M. (2008). The tape-stripping technique as a method for drug quntification in the skin. *Journal of Pharmacy and Pharmaceutical Sciences*, Vol. 11, No. 1, (March 2008):104-30, ISSN 1482-1826.

Escobar-Chávez, JJ.; Merino, V.; Díez-Sales, O.; Nácher-Alonso, A.; Ganem-Quintanar, A.; Herráez, M.; Merino-Sanjuán, M. (2011). Transdermal nortriptyline hydrocloride patch formulated within a chitosan matrix intended to be used for smoking cessation. *Pharmaceutical Development Technology*, Vol. 16, No. 2, (February 2010), pp. 162-9, ISSN *1083-7450*

Escribano, E.; Calpena, AC.; Queralt, J.; Obach, R.; Doménech J. (2003). Assessment of diclofenac permeation with different formulations: anti-inflammatory study of a selected formula, *European Journal of Pharmaceutical Sciences*, Vol. 19, No. 4, (July 2003), pp. 203-210, ISSN 0928-0987.

Essa EA, Bonner MC & Barry BW. (2004). Electrically assisted skin delivery of liposomal estradiol; phospholipid as damage retardant. *Journal of Controlled Release,* Vol. 95, pp.535-546, ISSN 0168-3659.

Fang J, Hung C, Liao M & Chien C. (2007). A study of the formulation design of acoustically active lipospheres as carriers for drug delivery. *European Journal of Pharmaceutics and Biopharmaceutics.* Vol. 67, pp. 67-75.

Fang JY, Lin HH, Chen HI, Tsai YH. (1998). Development and evaluation on transdermal delivery of enoxacin via chemical enhancers and physical iontophoresis. *Journal of Controlled Release*, Vol. 54, No. (August 1998), pp. 293-304, ISSN *0168-3659*.

Fang, JY.; Fang, CL.; Huang, YB.; Tsai, YH. (2002). Transdermal iontophoresis of sodium nonivamide acetate. V. Combined effect of pre-treatment by penetration enhancers. *International Journal of Pharm*aceutics, Vol. 235, No. 1-2, (March 2002), 95-105, ISSN 0378-5173.

Fang, JY.; Leu, YL.; Wang, YY.; Tsai, YH. (2002). *In vitro* topical application and *in vivo* pharmacodynamic evaluation of nonivamide hydrogels using Wistar rat as an animal model. *European Journal of Pharmaceutical Sciences*, Vol. 15, No. 5, (June 2002), pp. 417-23, ISSN 0928-0987.

García-González CA, Sampaio da Sousa AR, Argemí A, López Periago A, Saurina J, Duarte CM & Domingo C. (2009). Production of hybrid lipid-based particles loaded with inorganic nanoparticles and active compounds for prolonged topical release. *International Journal of Pharmaceutics*. Vol.382 No.1-2 (December 2009), pp.296-304. ISSN: 0378-5173.

Gardeniers HJ, Luttge R, Berenschot EJ, de Boer MJ, Yeshurun SY, Hefetz M, van't Oever R & van den Berg A. (2003). Silicon micromachined hollow microneedles for transdermal liquid transport. Journal of Medieval and Early Modern Studies. Vol. 12, pp 855-62.

Gill SH, Prausnitz RM. (2006). Coated microneedles for transdermal drug delivery. *Journal of Controlled Release*, Vol. 117, pp.227-37, ISSN 0168-3659.

Goswami S, Bajpai J & Bajpai AK. (2010). Designing Gelatin Nanocarriers as a Swellable System for Controlled Release of Insulin: An *In-Vitro* Kinetic Study. Journal of Macromolecular Science. Vol. 47, pp.119-130, ISSN 1060-1325.

Griffin, JE. & Touchstone, JC. (1972). Effects of ultrasound frequency on cortisone into swine tissue. *American Journal of Physcal Medicine*, Vol. 51, No. 2, (April 1972), pp. 62-78, ISSN 0002-9491.

Güngör, S.; Bektaş, A.; Alp, FI.; Uydeş-Doğan, BS.; Ozdemir, O.; Araman, A.; Ozsoy, Y. (2008). Matrix-type transdermal patches of verapamil hydrochloride: in vitro permeation studies through excised rat skin and pharmacodynamic evaluation in rats. *Pharmaceutical Development Technology*, Vol. 13, No. 4, pp. 283-9, ISSN *1083-7450*.

Guy RH, Kalia YN, Delgado-Charro MB, Merino V, Lopez A, Marro D. (2000). Iontophoresis: electrorepulsion and electroosmosis. Journal of Controlled Release, Vol. 64, No. 1-3, (February 2000), pp. 129-32, ISSN 0168-3659.

Hadgraft, J. & Lane, ME. (2005). Skin permeation: The years of enlightenment. *International Journal of Pharmaceutics*, Vol. 305, No. 1-2, (November 2005), pp. 2–12, ISSN 0378-5173.

Hadgraft, J.; Walters, KA. & Wotton, PK. (1985). Facilitated transport of sodium salicylate across an artificial lipid membrane by azone. *Journal of Pharmacy and Pharmacology*, Vol. 37, No. 10, (October 1985), pp. 725-727, ISSN 0022-3573.

Haq MI, Smith E, John DN, Kalavala M, Edwards C, Anstey A, Morrissey A & Birchall JC. (2009). Clinical administration of microneedles: skin puncture, pain and sensation. Biomedical Microdevices. Vol. 11, pp 35–47, ISSN: 1387-2176.

Hathout, RM.; Woodman, TJ.; Mansour, S.; Mortada, ND.; Geneidi, AS.; Guy, RH. (2010). Microemulsion formulations for the transdermal delivery of testosterone. *European Journal of Pharmaceutical Sciences*, Vol. 40, No. 3, (June 2010), pp. 188-96, ISSN 0928-0987.

Hehn, B. & Moll, F. (1996). Phonophoretic permeation of procaine hydrochloride through and MDCK cell monolayer. *Pharmazie*; Vol. 51, No. 5, (May 1996), pp. 341-5, ISSN 0031-7144.

Heller, R.; Jaroszeski, R.; Glass, LF.; et al. (1996). Phase I / II Trial for the treatment of cutaneous and subcutaneous tumor using electrochemotherapy, *Cancer*, Vol. 77, No. 5, (March 1996), pp. 964–971, ISNN 1097-0142.

Henry S, McAllister V D, Mark GA & Prausnitz RM. (1998). Microfabricated microneedles: A novel approach to transdermal drug delivery. *Journal of Pharmaceutical Sciences*, Vol. 87, pp.922-25, ISSN 0022-3549.

Herffernan M, Murthy N. (2005). Polyketal nanoparticles: A new pH-sensitive biodegradable drug delivery vehicle. *Bioconjugate Chemistry*. Vol. 16, pp.1340-1342,

Hippius, M.; Uhlemann, C.; Smolenski, U.; et al. (1998). In vitro investigations of drug release and penetration enhancing effect of ultrasound on transmembrane transport of flufenamic acid. *International Journal of Clinical Pharmacoloy & Therapeutics*, Vol. 36, No. 2, (September 1998), pp. 107 11, ISSN 0946-1965.

Hong M, Zhu S, Jiang Y, Tang G & Pei Y. (2009). Efficient tumor targeting of hydroxycamptothecin loaded PEGylated niosomes modified with transferrin. *Journal of Controlled Release*, Vol. 133, pp.96-102, ISSN 0168-3659.

Huang X, Du Y, Yuan H & Hu F. (2009). Preparation and pharmacodynamics of low-molecular-weight chitosan nanoparticles containing insulin. Carbohydrate Polymers. Vol. 76, pp. 368-373, ISSN: 0144-8617

Huang, JF.; Sung, KC.; Wang, JJ.; Lin, YH.; Fang, JY. (2005). The effects of electrically assisted methods on transdermal delivery of nalbuphine benzoate and sebacoyl dinalbuphine ester from solutions and hydrogels. *International Journal of Pharmaceutics*,Vol. 297, No. 1-2, (April 2005), pp. 162–171, ISSN 0378-5173.

Jin Y, Tong L, Ai P, Li M & Hou X. (2006). Self-assembled drug delivery systems: 1. Properties and *in vitro/in vivo* behavior of acyclovir self-assembled nanoparticles (SAN). *International Journal of Pharmaceutics*. Vol.309, pp.199-207, ISSN: 0378-5173.

Johnson S, Trejo J, Veisi M, Willhite GP, Liang JT & Berkland C. (2010). Effects of Divalent Cations, Seawater, and Formation Brine on Positively Charged Polyethylenimine/Dextran Sulfate/ Chromium(III) Polyelectrolyte Complexes and Partially Hydrolyzed Polyacrylamide/Chromium(III) Gelation. Journal of Applied Polymer Science. Vol. 115, pp.1008-1014, ISSN 1097-4628.

Joshi M, Patravale V. (2008). Nanostructured lipid carrier (NLC) based gel of celecoxib. *International Journal of Pharmaceutics*. Vol.346, pp.124-132, ISSN: 0378-5173.

Kabanov, V.A.; Zezin, A.B.; Rogacheva, V.B.; Gulyaeva, Z.G.; Zansochova, M.F.; Joosten, J.G.H. & Brackman, J. (1998). Polyelectrolyte behavior of astramol poly(propyleneimine) dendrimers. *Macromolecules*. Vol 31, pp.142-5144, ISSN 0024-9297.

Khaibullina, A.; Jang, BS.; Sun, H.; et al. (2008). Pulsed high intensity focused ultrasound enhances uptake of radiolabeled monoclonal antibody to human epidermoid tumor in nude mice. *Journal of Nuclear Medicine*, Vol. 49, No. 2, (February 2008), pp. 295-302, ISSN 0161-5505.

Kigasawa, K.; Kajimoto, K.; Watanabe, M.; Kanamura, K.; Saito, A.; Kogure, K. (2009). In vivo transdermal delivery of diclofenac by ion-exchange iontophoresis with geraniol. *Biological & Pharmaceutical Bullettin*, Vol. 32, No. 4, (April 2009), pp. 684-7, ISSN *0918-6158*.

Kim, TY.; Jung, DI.; Kim, YI.; Yang, JH.; Shin, SC. (2007). Anesthetic effects of lidocaine hydrochloride gel using low frequency ultrasound of 0.5MHz. *Journal of Pharmacy & Pharmaceutical Sciences*, Vol, 10, No. 1, (February 2007), pp. 1-8, ISSN 1482-1826.

Kushner IV, J.; Blankschtein, D. & Langer, R. (2008). Heterogeneity in skin treated with low-frequency ultrasound. *Journal of Pharmaceutical Sciences*, Vol. 97, No. 10, (October 2008), pp. 4119–28, ISSN 0022-3549.

Kwon S.-Y., (2006). Acne Treatment by a Dissolvable Microneedle Patch, *Proceedings of Controlled Release Society 33st Annual Meeting*; #115.

Larkin, JO.; Casey, GD.; Tangney, M.; et al. (2008). Effective tumor treatment using optimized ultrasound mediated delivery of bleomycin. *Ultrasound In Medicine & Biology*, Vol.34, No. 3, (March 2008), pp. 406-13, ISSN 0301-5629.

Lboutounne H, Chaulet J, Ploton C, Falson F & Pirot F. (2002). Sustained ex vivo skin antiseptic activity of chlorhexidine in poly(ε-caprolactone) nanocapsule encapsulated form and as a digluconate. *Journal of Controlled Release*, Vol. 82, pp.319-334, ISSN 0168-3659.

Leboulanger B, Aubry JM, Bondolfi G, Guy RH, Delgado-Charro MB. (2004). Lithium monitoring by reverse iontophoresis*invivo*. Clinical Chemistry, Vol. 50, No. 11, (November 2004), pp. 2091-100, ISSN 1530-8561.

Lee P, Peng S, Su C, Mi F, Chen H, Wei M, Lin, H & Sung H. (2008). The use of biodegradable polymeric nanoparticles in combination with a low-pressure gene gun for transdermal DNA delivery. *Biomaterials*. Vol.29, No. 6, (February 2008) pp. 742-751, ISSN: 0142-9612.

Lee WJ, Park J & Prausnitz RM. (2007). Dissolving microneedles for transdermal drug delivery. *Biomaterials*. Vol. 29, pp. 2113-24, ISSN: 0142-9612.

Lee, PJ.; Ahmad, N.; Langer, R.; Mitragotri, S.; Prasad Shastri, V. (2006). Evaluation of chemical enhancers in the transdermal delivery of lidocaine. *International Journal of Pharmaceutics*, Vol. 308, No. 1-2, (February 2006), pp. 33-9, ISSN *0378-5173*.

Lee, S.; Snyder, B.; Newnham, RE.; Smith, NB. (2004). Noninvasive ultrasonic transdermal insulin delivery in rabbits using the light weight cymbal array. *Diabetes Technology & Therapeutics*; Vol. 6, No. 6, (December 2004), pp. 808-15, ISSN 1520-9156.

Levenets, AA.; Shuvalov, SM.; Poliakov, AV. (1989). The effect of the disodium salt of ethylenediaminetetraacetate on the healing of experimental suppurative wounds. *Stomatologiia (Mosk)*; Vol. 68, No. 5, (September-October 1989), pp. 14-16, ISSN 0039-1735.

Li GP, Liu ZG, Liao B & Zhong NS. (2009). Induction of Th1-Type Immune Response by Chitosan Nanoparticles Containing Plasmid DNA Encoding House Dust Mite Allergen Der p 2 for Oral Vaccination in Mice. Cellular and Molecular Immunology. Vol. 6, pp.45-50, ISSN: 1672-7681.

Liu W, Hu M, Liu W, Xue C, Xu H & Yang X. (2008). Investigation of the carbopol gel of solid lipid nanoparticles for the transdermal iontophoretic delivery of triamcinolone acetonide acetate. *International Journal of Pharmaceutics.* Vol.364, pp.135-141, ISSN: 0378-5173.

Liu, H.; Li, S.; Pan, W.; et al. (2006). Investigation into the potential of low-frequency ultrasound facilitated topical delivery of Cyclosporin A. *International Journal of Pharmaceutics,* Vol. 326, No. 1-2, (December 2006), pp. 32-38, ISSN 0378-5173.

Lopez-Castellano, A & Merino V.(2010). Chapter 2: Chemical enhancers. In: José Juan Escobar-Chávez (Ed), *Current Technologies To Increase The Transdermal Delivery Of Drugs.* Bentham Science Publishers Ltd. ISBN: 978-1-60805-191-5, Bussum, The Netherlands.

Lu, MY.; Lee, D. & Rao, GS. (1992). Percutaneous absorption enhancement of leuprolide. *Pharmaceutical Research,* Vol. 9, No. 12, (December 1992), pp. 1575-9, ISSN 0724-8741.

Lubbers, J.; Hekkenberg, RT. & Bezemer, RA. (2003). Time to threshold (TT), a safety parameter for heating by diagnostic ultrasound. *Ultrasound In Medicine & Biology,* Vol. 29, No. 5, (May 2003), pp. 755-64, ISSN 0301-5629.

Luis, J.; Park, EJ.; Meyer, RJ.; Smith, NB. (2007). Rectangular cymbal arrays for improved ultrasonic transdermal insulin delivery. *Journal of the Acoustical Society of America,* Vol. 122, No. 4, (October 2007), pp. 2022-30, ISSN 0001-4966.

Ma, X.; Fang, L.; Guo, J.; Zhao, N.; He, Z. (2010). Effect of counter-ions and penetration enhancers on the skin permeation of flurbiprofen. *Journal of Pharmaceutical Sciences,* Vol. 99, No. 4, (April 2010), pp. 1826-37, ISSN 0022-3549.

Machet, L.; Pinton, J.; Patat, F.; Arbeille, B.; Pourcelot, L.; Vaillant, L. (1996). In vitro phonophoresis of digoxin across hairless mice and human skin: thermal effect of ultrasound. *International Journal of Pharmaceutics,* Vol. 133, No. 1-2, (May 1996), pp. 39-45, ISSN 0378-5173.

Maestrelli F, González-Rodríguez ML, Rabasco AM & Mura P. (2005). Preparation and characterisation of liposomes encapsulating ketoprofen–cyclodextrin complexes for transdermal drug delivery. *International Journal of Pharmaceutics.* Vol. 298, pp.55-67, ISSN: 0378-5173.

Maloney M, Bezzant JL, Stephen RL. (1992). Iontophoreric administration of lidocaine anesthesia in office practice. *Journal of Dermatologic Surgery & Oncology,* Vol. 18, No. , (November 1992), 937-40, ISSN 0148-0812.

Manosroi A, Kongkaneramit L & Manosroi J. (2004). Stability and transdermal absorption of topical amphotericin B liposome formulations. *International Journal of Pharmaceutics.* Vol. 270, pp.279-286, ISSN: 0378-5173.

Matinian, AL.; Nagapetian, KH.; Amirian, SS.; et al. (1990). Papain phonophoresis in the treatment of suppurative wounds and inflammatory processes. *Khirurgiia (Mosk),* Vol. 9, (September 1990), pp. 74-6, ISSN 0023-1207.

McCarron PA, Hall M. (2008). Incorporation of novel 1-alkylcarbonyloxymethyl prodrugs of 5-fluorouracil into poly(lactide-co-glycolide) nanoparticles. *International Journal of Pharmaceutics.* Vol. 348, pp. 115-124, ISSN: 0378-5173.

McElnay, JC.; Benson, HA.; Harland, R.; Hadgraft, J. (1993). Phonophoresis of methyl nicotinate. A preliminary study to elucidate the mechanism of action. *Pharmaceutical Research,* Vol. 10, No. 12, (December 1993), pp. 1726-31, ISSN 0724-8741.

Mei Z, Chen H, Weng T, Yang Y & Yang X. (2003). Solid lipid nanoparticle and microemulsion for topical delivery of triptolide. *European Journal of Pharmaceutics and Biopharmaceutics*. Vol. 56, No. 189-196, ISSN: 0928-0987.

Meidan, VM.; Walmsley, AD.; Docker, MF.; Irwin, WJ. (1999). Ultrasound enhanced diffusion into coupling gel during phonophoresis of 5-fluorouracil. *International Journal of Pharmaceutics*, Vol. 185, No. 2, (August 1999), pp. 205-13, ISSN 0378-5173.

Mélot, M.; Pudney, PD.; Williamson, AM.; Caspers, PJ.; Van Der Pol, A.; Puppels, GJ. (2009). Studying the effectiveness of penetration enhancers to deliver retinol through the stratum cornum by in vivo confocal Raman spectroscopy. *Journal of Controlled Release*, Vol. 138, No. 1, (August 2009), pp. 32-9, ISSN 0168-3659.

Menjoge AR, Kannan RM & Tomalia DA. (2010). Dendrimer-based drug and imaging conjugates: design considerations for nanomedical applications. *Drug Discovery Today*. Vol. 15, pp. 171-185, ISSN: 1359-6446.

Menon, GK.; Price, LF.; Bommannan, B.; et al. (1994). Selective obliteration of the epidermal calcium gradient leads to enhanced lamellar body secretion. *Journal of Investigative Dermatology*, Vol. 102, No. 5, (May 1994), pp. 789-95, ISSN 0022-202X.

Merino V, Kalia, YN, Guy RH. (1997). Transdermal therapy and diagnosis by iontophoresis. *Trends in Biotechnology*, Vol. 15, No. 8, (August 1997), pp. 288-90. ISSN 0167-7799.

Merino V, Lopez A, Kalia YN, Guy RH. (1999). Electrorepulsion versus electroosmosis: effect of pH on the iontophoretic flux of 5-fluorouracil. Pharmaceutical Research, Vol. 16, No. 5, (May 1999), pp. 758-61, ISSN 0724-8741.

Merino, G.; Kalia, YN. & Guy, RH. (2003). Ultrasound-Enhanced Transdermal Transport. *Journal of Pharmaceutical Sciences*, Vol. 92, No. 6, (June 2003), pp. 1125-37, ISSN 0022-3549.

Merino, V.; Micó-Albiñana, T.; Nácher, A.; Díez-Sales, O.; Herráez, M.; Merino-Sanjuán, M. (2008). Enhancement of nortriptyline penetration through human epidermis: influence of chemical enhancers and iontophoresis. *Journal of Pharmacy & Pharmacology*, Vol. 60, No. 4, (April 2008), pp. 415-20, ISSN 0022-3573.

Meshali, MM.; Abdel-Aleem, HM.; Sakr, FM.; et al. (2008). In vitro phonophoresis: effect of ultrasound intensity and mode at high frequency on NSAIDs transport across cellulose and rabbit skin membranes. *Pharmazie*; Vol. 63, No. 1, (January 2008), pp. 49-53, ISSN 0031-7144.

Mittal A, Sara UV, Ali A, Aqil M. (2008). The effect of penetration enhancers on permeation kinetics of nitrendipine in two different skin models. *Biology & Pharmaceutical Bulletin*, Vol. 31, No. 9, (September 2008), pp. 1766-72, ISSN 0918-6158.

Miyazaki, S.; Mizuoka, H.; Kohata, Y.; Takada, M. (1992). External control of drug release and penetration. Enhancing effect of ultrasound on the transdermal absorption of indomethacin from an oinment in rats. *Chemical & Pharmaceutical Bulletin (Tokyo)*; Vol. 40, No. 10, (October 1992), pp. 2826-2830, ISSN 0009-2363.

Montenegro, L.; Bucolo, C. & Puglisi, G. (2003). Enhancer effects on in vitro corneal permeation of timolol and acyclovir. *Pharmazie*, Vol. 58, No. 7, (July 2003), pp. 497-501, ISSN 0031-7144.

Monti, D.; Giannelli, R.; Chetoni, P.; Burgalassi, S. (2001). Comparison of the effect of ultrasound and of chemical enhancers on transdermal permeation of caffeine and morphine through hairless mouse skin in vitro. *International Journal of Pharmaceutics*, Vol. 229, No. 1-2, (October 2001), pp. 131-7, ISSN 0378-5173.

Morimoto, Y.; Mutoh, TM.; Ueda, H.; et al. (2005). Elucidation of the transport pathway in hairless rat skin enhanced by low-frequency sonophoresis based on the solute-water transport relationship and confocal microscopy. *Journal of Controlled Release*, Vol. 103, (April 2005), pp. 587–97, ISSN 0168-3659.

Mura, S.; Manconi, M.; Sinico, C.; Valenti, D.; Fadda, AM. (2009). Penetration enhancer-containing vesicles (PEVs) as carriers for cutaneous delivery of minoxidil. *International Journal of Pharmaceutics*, Vol. 380, No. 1-2, (October 2009), pp. 72-9, ISSN 0378-5173.

Murthy SN, Sen A, Zhao YL, Hui SW. (2004). Temperature influences the postelectroporation permeability state of the skin. Journal of Pharmaceutical Sciences, Vol. 93, No. 4, (April 2004), pp.908-15, ISSN 0928-0987.

Mutalik S, Parekh HS, Davies NM, Udupa N. (2009). A combined approach of chemical enhancers and sonophoresis for the transdermal delivery of tizanidine hydrochloride. *Drug Delivery*, Vol. 16, No. 2, (February 2009), pp. 82-91, ISSN 1071-7544.

Nair, V. & Panchagnula, R. (2003). Poloxamer gel as vehicle for transdermal iontophoretic delivery of arginine vasopressin: evaluation of in vivo performance in rats. *Pharmacology Research*, Vol. 47, No. 6, (June 2003), pp. 555-62, ISSN 1043-6618.

Ng, GY. & Wong, RY. (2008). Ultrasound phonophoresis of panax notoginseng improves the strength of repairing ligament: a rat model. *Ultrasound In Medicine & Biology*, Vol. 34, No. 12, (December 2008), pp. 1919-23, ISSN 0301-5629.

Niederhafner P, Šebestík J & Ježek J. (2005). Peptide dendrimers. *Journal of Peptide Science.* Vol. 11, pp. 757-788, ISSN: 1099-1387.

Novak, FJ. (1964). Experirnental wansmission of lidocalne through intact skin by ultrasound. *Archives of Physical Medicine & Rehabilitation*, Vol. 64, (May 1996), pp. 231-2, ISSN 0003-9993.

Ogiso T, Iwaki M & Paku T. (1995). Effect of various enhancers on transdermal penetration of indomethacin and urea, and relationship between penetration parameters and enhancement factors. *Journal of Pharmaceutical Sciences*, Vol. 84, pp.482–88, ISSN: 1520-6017.

Okino M, Mohri H. (1987). Effects of a high-voltage electrical impulse and an anticancer drug on *in vivo* growing tumors. Japanese Journal of Cancer Research, Vol. 78, (December 1987), pp. 1319-1321, ISSN 0910-5050.

Orlowskim S, Belehradek JJ, Paoletti C, Mir LM. (1988). Transient electropermeabilization of cells in culture. Increase of the cytotoxicity of anticancer drugs. Biochemical Pharmacology, Vol. 34, (December 1988), pp. 4727-4733, ISSN 0006- 2952.

Paliwal, S.; Menon, GK.; Mitragotri, S. (2006). Low-frequency sonophoresis: ultrastructural basis for stratum corneum permeability assessed using quantum dots. *Journal of Investigative Dermatology*, Vol. 126, No. 5, (May 2006), pp. 1095–1101, ISSN 0022-202X.

Parekh HS. (2007). The Advance of Dendrimers - A Versatile Targeting Platform for Gene/Drug Delivery. Current Pharmaceutical Design. Vol. 13, pp. 2837-2850, ISSN 1381-6128.

Park JH, Allen MG & Prausnitz MR. (2005). Biodegradable polymer microneedles: fabrication, mechanics and transdermal drug delivery. *Journal of Controlled Release*, Vol. 104, pp.51-66, ISSN 0168-3659.

Park JH. (2004). *Polymeric microneedles for transdermal drug delivery*. PhD Thesis. Georgia Institute of Technology.

Perennes F, Marmiroli B, Matteucci M, Tormen M, Vaccari L & Fabrizio ED. (2006). Sharp beveled tip hollow microneedle arrays fabricated by LIGA and 3D soft lithography with polyvinyl alcohol. Journal of Micromechanics and Microengineering. Vol. 16, pp. 473-79, ISSN 1361-6439.

Phillips, CA. & Michniak, BB. (1995). Transdermal delivery of drugs with differing lipophilicities using Azone analogs as dermal penetration enhancers. *Journal of Pharmaceutical Sciences*, Vol. 84, No. 12, (December 1995), pp. 1427-33, ISSN 0022-3549.

Pliquett U, Gallo S, Hui SW, GusbethCh, Neumann E. (2005). Local and transient structural changes in stratum corneum at high electric fields: contribution of Joule heating. Biolectrochemistry, Vol. 67, No.1, (September 2005), pp. 37-46, ISSN1567-5394.

Pliquett U, GusbethCh, Nuccitelli R. (2008). A propagating heat wave model of skin electroporation. Journal of Theoretical Biology, Vol. 251, No. 2, (March 2008), pp. 195-201, ISSN 0022-5193.

Prausnitz MR, Bose VG, Langer R, Weaver JC. (1993). Electroporation of mammalian skin: a mechanism to enhance transdermal drug delivery. Proceeding of the National Academy of Sciences of the united states of American, Vol. 90, No. 22, (November 1993), pp. 10504-8, ISSN 0027-8424.

Ragelis, Siu. (1981). Tetracycline penetration into tissue by modified electro and phonophoretic methods. *Antibiotiki*, Vol. 26, No. 9, (September 1981), pp. 699-703, ISSN 0003-5637.

Rizwan, M.; Aqil, M.; Talegaonkar, S.; Azeem, A.; Sultana, Y:, Ali, A. (2009). Enhanced transdermal drug delivery techniques: an extensive review of patents. Recent Patents on Drug Delivery & Formula*tions*, Vol. 3, No. 2, pp. 105-24, ISSN1872-2113.

Rodriguez-Justo O. & Moraes Â. M..(2011). Analysis of process parameters on the characteristics of liposomes prepared by ethanol injection with a view to process scale-up: Effect of temperature and batch volume. *Chemical Engineering Research and Design*. Vol. 89, No. 6, (June 2011), pp. 785-792, ISSN: 0263-8762.

Rojas-Oviedo I, Salazar-López RA, Reyes-Gasga J & Quirino-Barreda CT. (2007). Elaboration and structural analysis of aquasomes loaded with Indomethacin. *European Journal of Pharmaceutical Sciences*, Vol. 32, pp. 223-230, ISSN 0928-0987.

Rornanenko, IM. & Araviiskii, RA. (1991). Comparative levels of amphoteficin B in the skin and subcutaneous fatty tissue after cutaneous application of amphotericin ointment by phonophoresis and with preliminary treatment by dimethyl sulfoxide. *Antibiotiki i Khimioterapiia*; Vol. 36, No. 9, (September 1991), pp. 29-31, ISSN 0235-2990.

Rosim, GC.; Barbieri, CH.; Lanças, FM.; Mazzer, N. (2005). Diclofenac phonphoresis in human volunteers. *Ultrasound in Medicine & Biology*, Vol. 31, No. 3, (March 2005), pp. 337-43, ISSN 0301-5629.

Rossier-Miranda FJ, Schroën CGPH & Boom RM. (2009). Colloidosomes: Versatile microcapsules in perspective. Colloids and Surfaces A: Physicochemical and Engineering Aspects. Vol. 343, pp. 43-49, ISSN: 0927-7757.

Roxhed N, Samel B, Nordquist L, Griss P & Stemme G. (2008). Painless drug delivery through microneedle-based transdermal patches featuring active infusion. *IEEE Transactions in Biomedical Engineering*. Vol. 55 No.3, pp. 1063-71. ISSN: 0018-9294

Rzigalinski BA, Strobl JS. (2009). Cadmium-containing nanoparticles: Perspectives on pharmacology and toxicology of quantum dots. Toxicology and Applied Pharmacology. Vol. 238, pp. 280-288, ISSN: 0041-008X.

Saliba, S.; Mistry, DJ.; Perrin, DH.; Gieck, J.; Weltman, A. (2007). Phonophoresis and the absorption of dexamethasone in the presence of an occlusive dressing. Journal of Athletic Training, Vol. 42, No. 3, (July-September 2007), pp. 349-54, ISSN 1062-6050.

Sammoura F, Kang JJ, Heo YM, Jung TS & Lin L. (2007). Polymeric microneedle fabrication using a microinjection molding technique. Microsystem Technologies. Vol. 13, pp. 517-22, ISSN: 1432-1858.

Sanna V, Caria G & Mariani A. (2010). Effect of lipid nanoparticles containing fatty alcohols having different chain length on the ex vivo skin permeability of Econazole nitrate. Powder Technology. Vol. 201, pp. 32-36, ISSN: 0032-5910.

Santander-Ortega MJ, Stauner T, Loretz B, Ortega-Vinuesa JL, Bastos-González D, Wenz G, Schaefer UF, Lehr CM. (2010). Nanoparticles made from novel starch derivatives for transdermal drug delivery. Journal of Controlled Release, Vol. 141, pp.85-92, ISSN 0168-3659.

Santoianni, P.; Nino, M. & Calabro, G. (2004). Intradermal drug delivery by low frequency sonophoresis (25KHz). Dermatol Online Journal, Vol. 10, No. 2, (October 2004), pp. 24-33, ISSN 10872108.

Senyiğit, T.; Padula, C.; Ozer, O.; Santi, P. (2009). Different approaches for improving skin accumulation of topical corticosteroids. International Journal of Pharmaceutics, Vol. 380, No. 1-2, (October 2009), pp. 155-60, ISSN 0378-5173.

Serikov, NP. (2007). Efficacy of ibuprofen (nurofen gel) ultraphonophoresis for pain in ostheoarthritis. Terapevticheskii arkhiv, Vol. 79, No. 5, pp. 79-81, ISSN 0040-3660.

Shakeel F, Ramadan W. (2010). Transdermal delivery of anticancer drug caffeine from water-in-oil nanoemulsions. Colloids and Surfaces B: Biointerfaces. Vol. 75, pp. 356-362, ISSN: 0927-7765.

Sharma BB, Jain SK & Vyas SP. (1994). Topical liposome system bearing local anaesthetic lignocaine: preparation and evaluation. Journal of Microencapsulation. Vol. 11, pp. 279-286, ISSN 0265-2048.

Shelley WB, McConahy JC, Hesbacher EN. (1950). Effectiveness of antihistaminic compounds introduced into normal skin by iontophoresis. The Journal of Investigative Dermatology, Vol. 15, No. 5, (November 1950), pp. 343-4, ISSN 0022-202X.

Shen, Q.; Li, W. & Li, W. (2007). The effect of clove oil on the transdermal delivery of ibuprofen in the rabbit by in vitro and in vivo methods. Drug Development & Industrial Pharmacy; Vol. 33, No. 12, (December 2007), pp. 1369-74, ISSN 0363-9045.

Shim J, Seok Kang H, Park W, Han S, Kim J & Chang I. (2004). Transdermal delivery of mixnoxidil with block copolymer nanoparticles. Journal of Controlled Release, Vol. 97, pp.477-484, ISSN 0168-3659.

Skauen, DM. (1974). Heat production by ultrasonic equipment. Journal of Pharmaceutical Sciences, Vol. 163, No. 1, (January 1974), pp. 114-6, ISSN 0022-3549.

Smith, JC & Irwin, WJ. (2000). Ionisation and the effect of absorption enhancers on transport of salicylic acid through silastic rubber and human skin. International Journal of Pharmaceutics, Vol. 210, No. 1-2, (December 2000), pp. 69-82, ISSN 0378-5173.

Smith, NB.; Lee, S. & Shung, KK. (2003). Ultrasound-mediated transdermal in vivo transport of insulin with low profile cymbal arrays. *Ultrasound in Medicine & Biology*, Vol. 29, No. 8, (August 2003), pp. 1205-10, ISSN 0301-5629.

Sonneville-Aubrun O., Simonnet J. -T. & Alloret F. L. (2004). Nanoemulsions: a new vehicle for skincare products. Advances in Colloid and Interface Science. Vols. 108-109, (20 May 2004), pp. 145-149, ISSN 0001-8686.

Soppimath KS, Aminabhavi TM, Kulkarni AR & Rudzinski WE. (2001). Biodegradable polymeric nanoparticles as drug delivery devices. *Journal of Controlled Release*, Vol. 70, pp.1-20, ISSN 0168-3659.

Stoeber B, Liepmann D. (2005). Arrays of hollow out-of-plane microneedles for drug delivery. *Journal of* Microelectronic systems. Vol. 14, No. 3, pp. 472-79, ISSN 0026-2692.

Sung, KC.; Fang, J-Y.; Wang, JJ.; Hu O, Y-P.(2003).Transdermal delivery of nalbuphine and its prodrugs by electroporation. *European Journal of Pharmaceutical Sciences*, Vol. 18, No. 1, (January 2003), pp. 63–70, ISNN 0928-0987.

Svenson S, Tomalia DA. (2005). Dendrimers in biomedical applications – reflections on the field. *Advanced Drug Delivery Reviews*, vol. 57, pp. 2106-2129, ISSN 0169-409X.

Tachibana, K. & Tachibana, S. (1993). Use of ultrasound to enhance the local anesthetic effect of topically applied aqueous Lidocaine. *Anesthesiology*, Vol. 78, No. 6, (June 1993), pp. 1091-6, ISSN 0003-3022.

Tachibana, K. & Tachibana, S. (1999). Application of ultrasound energy as a new drug delivery system. *Nihon Yakurigaku Zasshi*; Vol. 114, No. 1, (October 1999), pp. 138P-141P, ISSN 1340-2544.

Tang, H.; Mitragotri, S.; Blankschtein, D.; Langer, R. (2001). Theoretical description of transdermal transport of hydrophilic permeants: application to low frequency sonophoresis. *Journal of Pharmaceutical Sciences*, Vol. 90, No. 5, (May 2001), pp. 543–66, ISSN 0022-3549.

Tartis MS, Kruse DE, Zheng H, Zhang H, Kheirolomoom A, Marik J & Ferrara KW. (2008). Dynamic microPET imaging of ultrasound contrast agents and lipid delivery. *Journal of Controlled Release*. Vol. 131: No. 3, (November, 2008) pp.160-166, ISSN 0168-3659.

Teeranachaideekul V, Souto EB, Junyaprasert VB & Müller RH. (2007). Cetyl palmitate-based NLC for topical delivery of Coenzyme Q10 – Development, physicochemical characterization and *in vitro* release studies. *European Journal of Pharmaceutical Sciences*, Vol. 67, pp. 141-148, ISSN 0928-0987.

Teo A L, Shearwood C, Kian C N, Jai L & Shabbiir M. (2005). Transdermal Microneedles for Drug Delivery Application. Materials Science and Engineering: B. Vol. 132, pp. 151-54. ISSN 0921-5093.

Tezel H, Dokka S, Kelly S, Hardee GE, Mitragotri S. (2004). Topical delivery of anti-sense oligonucleotides using low-frequency sonophoresis. *Pharmaceutical Research*, Vol. 21, No. 12, (December 2004), pp. 2219-25, ISSN 0724-8741.

Thote AJ, Gupta RB. (2005). Formation of nanoparticles of a hydrophilic drug using supercritical carbon dioxide and microencapsulation for sustained release. Nanomedicine: Nanotechnology, Biology and Medicine. Vol. 1, pp. 85-90, ISSN: 1549-9634.

Tiwari, SB.; Pai, RM.; Udupa, N. (2004). Influence of ultrasound on the percutaneous absorption of ketorolac tromethamine in vitro across rat skin. *Drug Delivery*, Vol. 11, No. 1, (January-February 2004), pp. 47-51, ISSN 1071-7544.

Ugazio E, Cavalli R & Gasco MR. (2002). Incorporation of cyclosporin A in solid lipid nanoparticles (SLN). *International Journal of Pharmaceutics.* Vol. 241, pp.341-344, ISSN: 0378-5173.

Vaddi, HK.; Wang, LZ.; Ho, PC.; Chan, SY. (2001) Effect of some enhancers on the permeation of haloperidol through rat skin in vitro. *International Journal of Pharmaceutics,* Vol. 212, No. 2, (January 2001), pp. 247-55, ISSN 0378-5173.

Walker, JJ. (1983). Ultrasound therapy for keloids. *South African Medical Journal,* Vol. 64, No. 8, (August 1983), pp. 270, ISSN 0256-9574.

Wang, YY.; Hong, CT.; Chiu, WT.; Fang, JY. (2001). In vitro and in vivo evaluations of topically applied capsaicin and nonivamide from hydrogels. *International Journal of Pharmaceutics,* Vol. 224, No. 1-2, (August 2001), pp. 89-104, ISSN 0378-5173.

Wells, PN. (1977). *Biomedical ultrasonics.* Academic Press, pp. 421-30, New York.

Wen Z, Fang L, He Z. (2009). Effect of chemical enhancers on percutaneous absorption of daphnetin in isopropyl myristate vehicle across rat skin in vitro. *Drug Delivery,* Vol. 16, No. 4, (May 2009), pp. 214-23, ISSN 1071-7544.

Williams, AC. & Barry, BW. (2004). Penetration enhancers. *Advance Drug Delivery Reviews,* Vol. 56, No. 5, (March 2004), 603–18, ISSN 0169-409X.

Williams, AR. (1990). Phonophoresis: an in vivo evaluation using three topical anaesthetic preparations. *Ultrasonics;* Vol. 28, No. 3, (May 1990), pp. 137-41, ISSN 0041-624X.

Xu DH, Zhang Q, Feng X, Xu X, Liang WQ. (2007). Synergistic effects of ethosomes and chemical enhancers on enhancement of naloxone permeation through human skin. *Pharmazie,* Vol. 62, No. 4, (April 2007), pp. 316-8, ISSN 0031-7144.

Yang, JH.; Kim, DK.; Yun, MY.; Kim, TY.; Shin, SC. (2006). Transdermal delivery system of triamcinolone acetonide from a gel using phonophoresis. *Archives of Pharmacal Research,* Vol. 29, No. 5, (May 2006), pp. 412-27, ISSN 0253-6269.

Yang, JH.; Kim, TY.; Lee, JH.; et al. (2008). Anti-hyperalgesic and anti-inflammatory effects of ketorolac tromethamine gel using pulsed ultrasound in inflamed rats. *Archives of Pharmacal Research,* Vol. 31, No. 4, (April 2008), pp. 511-17, ISSN 0253-6269.

Yoo HS, Lee JE, Chung H, Kwon IC & Jeong SY. (2005). Self-assembled nanoparticles containing hydrophobically modified glycol chitosan for gene delivery. *Journal of Controlled Release,* Vol. 103, pp.235-243, ISSN 0168-3659.

Zahn DJ, Trebotich D & Liepmann D. (2005). Microdialysis Microneedles for Continuous Medicla Monitoring. Biomedical Microdevices. Vol. 7, No. 1, pp. 59-69, ISSN 1387-2176.

Zhang, JY.; Fang, L.; Tan, Z.; Wu, J.; He, ZG. (2009). Influence of ion-pairing and chemical enhancers on the transdermal delivery of meloxicam. *Drug Development & Industrial Pharmacy,* Vol. 35, No. 6, (June 2009), pp. 663-70, ISSN 0363-9045.

Zheng J, Zhu R, He Z, Cheng G, Wang H & Yao K. (2010). Synthesis and Characterization of PMMA/SiO$_2$ Nanocomposites by In Situ Suspension Polymerization. Journal of Applied Polymer Science. Vol. 115, pp. 1975-1981, ISSN 0021-8995.

Zimmermann S, Fienbork D, Stoeber B, Flouriders WA & Liepmann D. A. (2003). Microneedle-Base Glucose Monitor: Fabricated on a Wafer-Level Using In-Devoce Enzyme Immobilization. *Proceedings of 12th International Conference on solid state sensors, actuators and Microsystems.* pp.99-102.

Part 2

Diagnostic

8

Closed-Loop Control of Anaesthetic Effect

Santiago Torres, Juan A. Méndez,
Héctor Reboso, José A. Reboso and Ana León
Universidad de La Laguna
Spain

1. Introduction

The interest in automation technologies applied to anaesthesia has been grown exponentially in last decade. The main difference with other fields of automation is that the presence of a human supervisor has been never questioned. In spite of this, the use of automation tools to monitor and control the main variables during surgery notably helps the anaesthetist during surgery. The basic functions of the automation systems in anaesthesia are monitoring and control of the main variables of the process. This leads to two expected benefits. First, the anaesthetist will be freed of some routinary tasks so that he can concentrate more on the state of the patient. On the other hand, using these tools contributes to improve the global performance of the process in terms of safety, costs reduction and patient comfort.

During the surgery operation three main variables have to be regulated: hypnosis, analgesia and muscle relaxation. To achieve this, drugs have to be properly administered to the patient. In recent years many efforts have been made in the development of new drug delivery technologies (Bressan et al., 2009). Most of the difficulties to calculate the proper drug rate to each patient were the inexistence of precise methods to monitor the anaesthetic state of the patient. In the past, patient monitoring was performed just by observing several patient signs (sweat, head lifting, movement, etc.). Nowadays the way that anaesthesia is monitored has changed considerably.

Concerning hypnosis regulation, many efforts have been made to provide the anaesthesiologist with reliable methods for monitoring. In particular, the introduction of the Bispectral Index (BIS) to measure the depth of anaesthesia was one of the key elements in the development of new ways of drug administration (Sigl and Chamoun, 94).

The other main problem in designing control algorithms to regulate hypnosis arises from the complexity of the patient response to drug infusion. This response can be divided in two subsystems. One is the Pharmacokinetics (PK) that refers to the adsorption, distribution, biotransformation and excretion of the drug. And the other is the Pharmacodynamics (PD) that describes the equilibrium relationship between concentration in the body and visible effect produced in the patient. In practice a linear model has been accepted to describe the PK and a nonlinear model for the PD part.

First works involved with anaesthesia control were focused in checking the performance of a fully automated controller compared with the results obtained in a process guided by an anaesthetist. In (Sakai et al., 2000) and (Morley et al., 2000) it is showed that proposed PID controller can assure intraoperative hemodynamic stability and a fast recover of the patient from the hypnosis effects of the drug using closed-loop techniques. In these works and in the works of Absalom (Absalom et al., 2002a, Absalom et al., 2002b, Absalom et al., 2003), it can be shown that the performance of the closed-loop system was as efficient as the observed in the process guided by the specialist, without demonstrating any clinical advantages over the manual techniques.

In the last decade, a lot of research related with automatic control of anaesthesia has been made. Most of them use the intravenous drug propofol as the hypnotic agent. It is important to mention the works that follow a signal-based control, as PID (Liu et al., 2006; Dumont et al., 2009) and fuzzy controllers (Gil, 2004), and the works that follow a model-based control. In this way, many different proposals have been made depending on the controller structure, the controlled variable and the prediction model used. In (Struys. et al., 2001; Sawaguchi et al., 2003; Furutani et al., 2005) the drug concentration in brain is used as controlled variable. In (Ionescu et al., 2008) and (Niño et al., 2009), were EPSAC tecniques are used as controller structure, in (Screenivas et al., 2008), were robust characteristics are added in the design of the controller, and in (S. Syafiie et al., 2009), were nonlinear techinques are used, the authors use predictive control techniques. In (Screenivas et al., 2009) a comparative study between predictive control and PID techniques applied to the control of anaesthetic is done.

The focus of this chapter will be in the regulation of depth of consciousness of patients under general anaesthesia with intravenous propofol.

2. Anaesthetic process: The control problem

The main variables that describe the anaesthetic process are depicted in figure 1. In this figure an input-output description of the system is shown. As can be observed, manipulated variables are anaesthetics, relaxants or serums. Perturbations in the system are signals that can occur at any time (surgical stimulation, blood loss, etc.). The output variables can be measurable and not measurable. The main interest in anaesthesia is focused in non-measurable variables: hypnosis, analgesia and muscular relaxation. Although these variables are not directly measurable, there are methods to estimate them that are used in clinical practice. These methods are based on the use of alternative variables whose behaviour allows the estimation of the non-measurable ones.

Hypnosis is a general term indicating loss of consciousness and absence of the memory of the intervention after awake. Currently, the techniques that have been considered more efficient for this are based in the processing of the patient electroencephalogram (EEG), (Kazama et al., 1999; Struys et al., 2000).

The description of the BIS dynamics has been done mainly with physiological based models. These models consist of a PK part to describe the drug distribution in the internal organs and a PD part to describe the drug effect on the physiological variables of interest.

The drug distribution in the body depends on transport and metabolic processes, which in many cases are not clearly understood. However, dynamical models based on conservation laws that capture the exchange of material between coupled macroscopic subsystems or compartments, are widely used to model these processes.

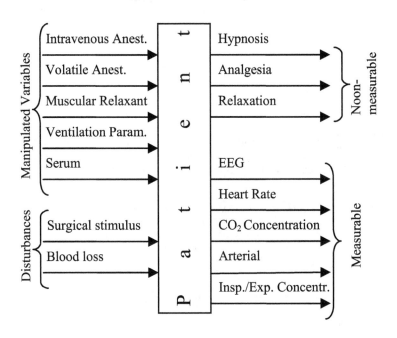

Fig. 1. Input-output description of the anaesthetic process.

2.1 The compartmental model

Figure 2 shows a model based in three compartments: central, fast and slow. The central compartment is the volume in which initial mixing of the drug occurs, and thus can be thought to include the vascular system (blood volume) and for some drugs the interstitial fluid. The fast peripheral compartment represents a compartment of the body that absorbs drug rapidly from the central compartment, and thus can be thought of as comprising tissues of the body that are well-perfused (such as muscles and vital organs). Finally the slow peripheral compartment is used to mathematically represent a compartment into which re-distribution occurs more slowly, and thus can be thought of as including tissues with a poor blood supply (such as adipose tissue).

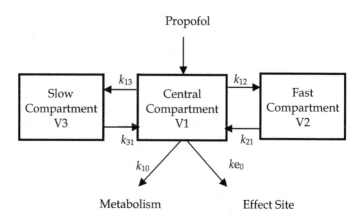

Fig. 2. Compartmental model.

The drug is infused in central compartment and then distributed to the slow and fast compartment and eliminated trough metabolism. Defining the drug concentration variable of the i-th compartment as C_i, the propofol distribution can be described as:

$$V_1 \frac{\partial C_1}{\partial t} = V_2 C_2(t) k_{21} + V_3 C_3(t) k_{31} - V_1 C_1(t)(k_{10} + k_{12} + k_{13}) + u(t) \qquad (1)$$

$$V_2 \frac{\partial C_2}{\partial t} = V_1 C_1(t) k_{12} - V_2 C_2(t) k_{21} \qquad (2)$$

$$V_3 \frac{\partial C_3}{\partial t} = V_1 C_1(t) k_{13} - V_3 C_3(t) k_{31} \qquad (3)$$

$$\frac{\partial C_e}{\partial t} = C_1(t) k_{e0} - C_e(t) k_{e0} \qquad (4)$$

where $u(t)$ represents the drug infusion rate in the central compartment and V_i is the volume of the i-th compartment. The dynamics of the compartmental model is defined by the following diffusion constants: k_{10} (rate constant for drug metabolism), k_{12} (rate constant for re-distribution of drug from central to fast peripheral compartment), k_{21} (rate constant for re-distribution of drug from fast to central compartment), k_{13} (rate constant for redistribution of drug from central to slow compartment) and k_{31} (rate constant for redistribution of drug from slow to central compartment). Common PK models for propofol are the Marsh model (Marsh et al., 1991) and the Schnider model (Schnider et al., 1998). Differences between both models can be seen in table 1.

From the point of view of hypnosis control, the variable of interest is not the blood concentration but the concentration in the place where the effect on the controlled variable is produced (effect site concentration). Thus, when there is a simultaneous measure of the drug concentration in blood and its effect on the brain, drug latency can be observed that produces a temporal displacement between the peak of blood concentration and the drug effect.

To include this dynamics in the model a fourth compartment is added. This compartment is known as effect site. It is assumed that this compartment is attached to the central compartment and has negligible volume. The diffusion constant of the effect site is k_{e0}.

	Marsh Model	**Schnider Model**
V_1	0.228 L/Kg	4.27L
k_{10}(min⁻¹)	0.119	0.0443+0.0107*(BW-77)-0.0159*(LBM-59)+0.0062*(HT-177)
k_{12}(min⁻¹)	0.112	0.302-0.0056*(Age-53)
k_{13}(min⁻¹)	0.0419	0.196
k_{21}(min⁻¹)	0.005	1.29-0.024*(Age-53)
k_{31}(min⁻¹)	0.0033	0.0035
ke_0(min⁻¹)	1.21	0.456

Table 1. Comparison of Marsh and Schnider models for PK of propofol. BW stands for Body Weight, LBM is Lean Body Mass and HT is Height.

On the other hand, the drug's pharmacodynamics, that represents the BIS in terms of the effect site concentration, is governed by:

$$BIS = f(C_e) \qquad (5)$$

The f function is usually taken as an EMAX model whose profile suits the described process:

$$\Delta BIS = \Delta BIS_{max} \frac{C_e^\gamma}{C_e^\gamma + EC_{50}^\gamma} \qquad (6)$$

$$\Delta BIS = BIS - BIS_0 \qquad (7)$$

$$\Delta BIS_{max} = BIS_{max} - BIS_0 \qquad (8)$$

BIS_0 corresponds to the awake state, BIS_{max} represents the minimum achievable BIS and EC_{50} represents the concentration in the effect site for which the effect is half the maximum value, γ represents the sensitivity of the patient to mall concentration variations in the effect site. This parameter can be seen as index that measures the degree of nonlinearity of the model.

2.2 The control problem

From the perspective of the control system three level of complexity can be distinguished. The basic procedure is the open-loop practice in which the anaesthetist, according to the parameters of the patient (age, weight, sex, ASA) directly uses predefined infusion rates of drugs. According to the response observed through his vital signs the drug rates can be modified (the anaesthetist is the controller).

In the next level, it appears the Target Controlled Infusion systems (TCI). In TCI the infusion rate is calculated from models of the pharmacokinetic of the patient, as can be seen in figure

3. Thus, the objective in TCI is to achieve a pre-set target plasma concentration. According to the model of the patient the TCI system (normally implemented in the infusion pump) delivers the adequate drug doses to achieve the objective.

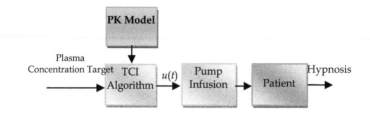

Fig. 3. Hypnosis control with TCI

There is a clear weakness in TCI related to the fact that the real plasma concentration cannot be online measured to compute the infusion rate. That is, TCI is also an open-loop control strategy. Closed-loop strategies appear to solve this problem. The main idea in closed-loop control is to use information of the state of the patient to automatically adjust the drug dosing. Many efforts have been made to provide the anaesthetist with more reliable methods for monitoring this state. In particular, the introduction of the Bispectral Index (BIS) to measure the depth of anaesthesia was one of the key elements in the development of new ways of drug administration (Sigl and Manchoun, 94). BIS has been demonstrated to correlate well with the depth of consciousness of the patient. Thus, it can be used as a feedback system to the controller in order to compute the adequate infusion rate, as can be seen in figure 4.

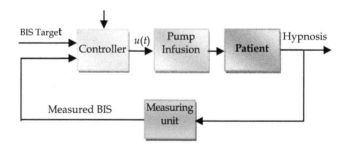

Fig. 4. Hypnosis control with closed-loop controller.

The controller algorithm used for anaesthesia control can be based on signals or in models. Signal based controllers are basically PID algorithms. The key feature of this algorithm is that no model is necessary to compute the infusion rate. Instead, the measured BIS is used to compute an error signal from which the drug dose is calculated. Model based controllers are an alternative to PID controller. The advantage of model-based controller is its ability to predict the behaviour of the patient and anticipate the changes in drug infusion to avoid undesirable responses.

In order to develop an adequate model-based control strategy, it is necessary to obtain a suitable model for the patient behaviour. One common practice is to simplify the model by means of linear approximations around a nominal state (corresponding to BIS target). On the other hand, models are also necessary for offline simulation of the controller structure. The most accepted models for patient representation are those based on compartments to represent the pharmacokinetic together with a nonlinear modelling that describes the PD.

3. Implementation of the closed-loop control of anaesthesia

The main elements that constitute the control system are depicted in figure 5. As can be observed there is a computer that centralizes the monitoring and control task in the system. The BIS monitor is a passive analyser of EEG, that allows monitor the deep of anaesthesia, and has the first objective of adjust in real time the dose of drugs administered to one patient to the actual need. The BIS correlated well with the level of responsiveness and provided an excellent prediction of the level of sedation and loss of consciousness for propofol and midazolam. In this work the Aspect® A-2000 monitor was used. The communication with the computer was implemented via a RS-232 serial interface. Concerning the actuator, the Graseby® infusion pump was used for drug infusion in the patient. The pump is also governed via a RS-232 serial interface.

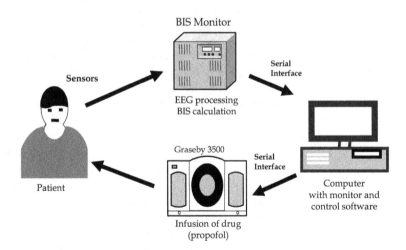

Fig. 5. Main elements of the closed-loop control system.

Apart from sending commands to the pump, the program in the PC reads continuously its state to detect eventual failures of any of the elements in the control loop, like missing BIS signal, excessive infusion rate in the pump syringe changes, etc. The program in the computer has all the routines to monitor and control the system.

The goal is to make a manual induction with propofol and remifentanil and maintain the BIS target during the maintenance of anaesthesia. Remifentanil infusion was adjusted manually and rocuronium was administered in bolus as needs. The operation conditions and the population in which the study was performed are explained in next section.

4. PI control

First control algorithm implemented was a PI controller. This algorithm has been extensively used in several automated closed loop systems. The administration of the drug is made based in the error between the BIS target and the current BIS, and the accumulated error during the operation. Both actions are regulated by gains, which are adjusted in an empirical way trying to get a smooth transitory and a stable response of the patient.

The goal is to make a manual induction with propofol and remifentanil and maintain a BIS target during the maintenance of anaesthesia. Reminfentanil infusion was adjusted manually and rocuronium was administered in bolus as needs. In the real proofs, a BIS target (BIS_r) of 50 is considered while the measurement and actuation period is 5 seconds. Before starting its operation, the software checks that all the security alarms are programmed.

This study was approved by the Ethical and Research Committee of the Hospital Universitario de Canarias and has written informed consent of the patients. The study was performed on a population of 15 patients of 30-60 years. In the real proofs with patients, a BIS target of 50 is considered while the measurement and actuation period is 5 seconds. Before starting its operation, the software checks that all the security alarms are programmed. In the operating room, the patient was connected to the BIS monitor, and the anaesthesia system was started in monitor mode. After the patient had breathed 100% oxygen for 3 min, the system was switched to manual mode, and anaesthesia was induced by means of nearly 2mg/Kg propofol manual bolus. Once the patient achieves a BIS closed to 50, the system is switched to automatic and the interest control algorithm is responsible to regulate the BIS around the objective.

The adjustment of the controller gains was made in an empirical way trying to get a smooth transitory and a stable response. This task was done following standard procedures in online process control engineering. For this, it was necessary the presence of a control expert together with the anaesthesiologist in the operating theatre. Thus, after several trials adequate values for PI controller where found to be $Kp=0.67$, $Ki=0.055$. This set of values was tested in the whole population of the study with satisfactory results. Figures 6 and 7 present the evolution of the anaesthesia for two different patients: patient 1 and patient 2. As can be observed, in both cases the system remains stabilised around the reference value with an oscillation of near ±10 units in the worst case (patient 2).

The results obtained with the population submitted to proofs show the patient remains stabilised around the reference value with an oscillation of near ±10 units in the worst case.

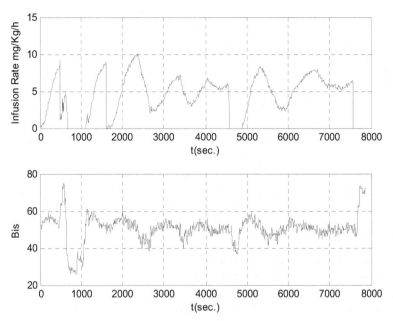

Fig. 6. Results of anaesthesia automatic control on patient 1.

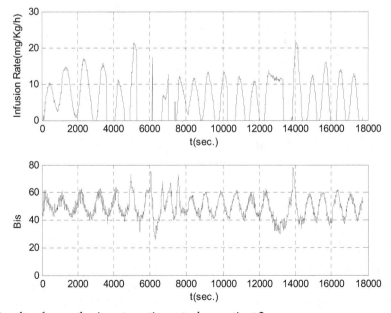

Fig. 7. Results of anaesthesia automatic control on patient 2.

The study revealed that although results are satisfactory, eventually the performance of the controller could decrease. There are two main factors that contribute to this. First of all, the variability between patients implies that the nominal PI parameters chosen are not the best choice for all the patients. Together with this, the dead time present in the system also contributes to reduce the phase margin of the closed loop system. The origin of this time-delay is the period of time since the drug is infused until it causes the adequate effect in the patient. The main effect observed is that the evolution of the BIS is quite oscillatory (see figure 7) around the reference value.

5. Dead-time compensation

In previous section it can be viewed that PI controller usually gives a response with oscillations around the BIS reference value. In this section, the control algorithm is modified in order to compensate these oscillations and get a better transitory. The results shown in this paper are in simulation after having adjusted the patient dynamical model.

The first method implemented to improve the results obtained with the fixed PI controller is to compensate the dead-time present in the system. To do this, a dead-time compensator based on the Smith Predictor theory (Smith, 72) is proposed to act with the PI controller. The basis of the Smith Predictor is to consider the feedback of the controlled variable BIS without delay. As this is variable is not available, the predictor estimates this value and uses this estimation as the feedback signal. To correct the deviations between this estimation and the real value, a correction term, resulting from the error between the estimation and the measured BIS, is added to the feedback signal, as can be seen in the figure 8.

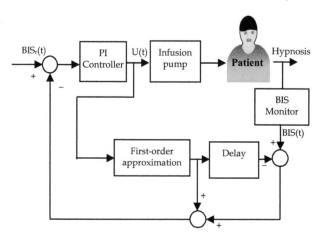

Fig. 8. PI Controller with Smith Predictor for patient hypnosis control.

The basics of this compensation algorithm consider the formulation of the Smith Predictor for linear systems. To apply the Smith Predictor to the nonlinear model of the patient, a first-order plus a time-delay approximation of the patient model is considered. A delay between 90 and 120 seconds is considered.

5.1 Model adjustment

In order to make the simulations proofs of the proposed algorithm, a physiology model of the patient dynamics was designed. As it was told, the model has two parts: pharmacokinetics and pharmacodynamics. The parameters adjustment was made in simulation using the real results obtained from a female, 56 years old patient, 84 Kg. weight, 160 cm. height.

After obtaining a satisfactory manual adjustment, the values for the pharmacokinetics model are k10=0.006, k12=11.0; k21=14.04, k13=10.02, k31=283.50 and ke0=0.0063. The values for the pharmacodynamics model are EC50=610.0, γ=1.5, BIS_0 =100 and BIS_{max}=0.

To validate the model the simulated response is compared with the real one. The obtained results, shown in figure 9a), prove the goodness of the model.

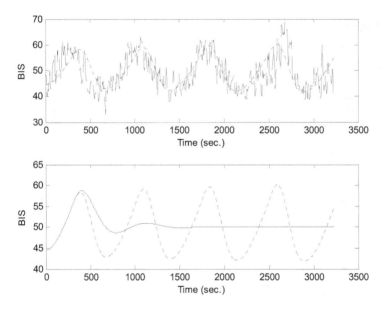

Fig. 9. a) Simulated BIS output (dotted) and real patient BIS output (solid) obtained under the action of a PI controller. b) PI controlled output (dotted) and PI with delay-time compensation output (solid).

5.2 Smith predictor (dead-time compensation)

The proposal here is to improve the performance of the closed-loop system by means of a compensation of the system time-delay. The origin of this time-delay is the period of time between from the infusion pump starts until the drug is distributed along the central compartment. The majority of the works in the literature do not explicitly consider the presence of this time-delay in the proposed models. In fact, in model equations (1)-(4), time-delay is not considered. But in real proofs, some delays between 1 and 2 minutes have to be considered to have a realistic model of the dynamics. Under this hypothesis, a time-delay compensator based on the Smith Predictor theory has been proposed to be added to the PI controller.

5.3 Results with PI controller with dead-time compensation

As it is well known, the basics of this compensation algorithm consider the formulation of the Smith Predictor for linear systems. To apply the Smith Predictor to the nonlinear model of the patient, a first-order plus a time-delay approximation of the patient model is considered. Thus, the configuration employed can be seen in figure 8. A delay between 90 and 120 seconds is considered in the simulations. In figure 9b the results obtained with the patient are shown. The evolution of the BIS signal with the Smith Predictor (in solid line) is much better than with the PI controller (in dotted line), and does not show oscillations around the reference BIS value.

5.4 Self-adaptive dead-time compensation

The main advantage of the time-delay compensation for the PI controller is a better performance in the transitory of the BIS signal. This advantage is conditioned to obtain a good fist-order approximation of the system. However, this model has to be changed in at least two situations. First, when the operation point changes due to a change in the BIS reference for the same patient. Second, when the controller is applied in a different patient, whose physiologic model has to be estimated.

In order to improve the efficiency of that controller, an adaptation of the first-order model patient is added. The aim of this algorithm is to make the time-delay compensator independent of the model assumed for the patient. In order to obtain a simple adaptive algorithm that guarantees the closed-loop stability, model reference adaptive controller – MRAC- (Aström and Wittenmark, 94) is used, as can be seen in figure 10.

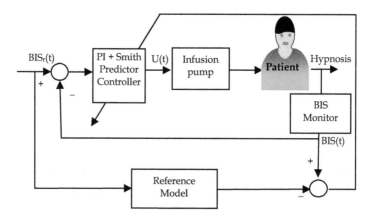

Fig. 10. PI with Smith Predictor controller inserted in the adaptive control scheme MRAC. The error between the system output and the model reference output is used to update the parameters of the PI with Smith Predictor controller.

Following this control scheme, the controller parameters are adjusted by an adaptation law that depends on the error between the system output (BIS) and the model reference output defined for this closed-loop. Minimising a certain cost-function involving this error, an adaptation law of the adjustable controller parameters is obtained. In this case, the adjustable parameters are the static gain and the time constant of the approximated first-order model used in the Smith Predictor.

5.5 Results with the PI controller with self-adaptive dead-time compensation

Several simulation experiments has been made for the patient simulated in previous sections, choosing as the reference model a second-order model with poles, expressed in the z-plane discrete formulation, in z=0.98 and z=-0.75.

The results are shown in figure 11a), where the evolution of the BIS under the self-adaptive compensator algorithm is drawn in solid line and compared with the results obtained in figure 9b) –PI and PI+compensator controllers-. In figure 11b) the evolution of the static gain under this self-adaptive scheme is shown. As it can be observed, some extra oscillations are produced with respect to the previous algorithm, which corresponds to the period of time in that the parameter is adapting.

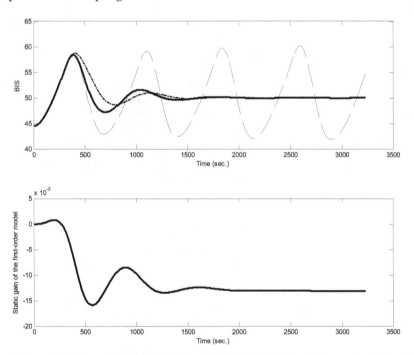

Fig. 11. a) PI controlled system output (dotted), PI with Smith Predictor controlled output (dashed), and self-adaptive time-delay compensation controlled output (solid) compared for the same patient. b) Evolution of the static gain of the first-order approximation model of the time-delay compensation.

Once the optimal values for the parameters are reached, the performance of the system is very similar to the previous controller. In that case, the static gain took a value of -0.037. In this case, the stabilising value for this parameter is near the half. However, the performance is also satisfactory. Moreover, no assumptions over the system had to been made, which is the main advantage of this new algorithm.

Comparing the results obtained with the previous algorithm, some extra oscillations are produced, which corresponds to the period of time in that the parameter is adapting. Once the optimal values for the parameters are reached, the performance of the system is very similar to the previous controller. Moreover, no assumptions over the system had to been made, which is the main advantage of this control algorithm.

6. PI control with self-adaptive gains

Another method to avoid the problem of the oscillations around the BIS reference value occurred with the PI controller is using an adaptive scheme to obtain the gains of the PI controller. The method is based on assuring a desired performance of the closed loop, by emplacing its poles as required, in order to obtain a smooth transition to the BIS reference value.

This method is part of a kind of adaptive controllers, known as self-tuning regulators –STR– (Aström and Wittenmark, 94). They are based on two steps. First, an identification of the system is made in order to get the dynamics in each instant of time. This assures that the controller takes into account the variations in the dynamics of the system. Second step is to compute the control law assuming that the identification results are true. The variety of STR schemes differs in the method used to compute the control law. In this work, an adjustable PI controller is used, which gains are tuned by trying that the closed loop performance of the system be as similar as possible to a desired reference model. This is obtained by emplacing the poles of the reference model into the desired values to get a satisfactory response of the system.

STR controllers have two different parts. The most important part is that they provide an observer in order to identify the dynamics of the system to control. This is an essential point due to the results of the system identification are taken into account to compute the adaptive control law. In this case, a recursive least-squares method based is used to provide the parameters of the dynamics of the observed system.

The second part of the controller is to compute the control law to apply to the system. The results of the identification part are taken to obtain the control action. In this way, the controller takes into account the variations of the dynamics of the system, if they occur. Another advantage of this scheme is its flexibility to be applied to different systems, with the same dynamics but with different parameters, because the identification process adapts the controller to the new situation.

In this case, a pole placement controller is used. Considering the dynamics of the patient as a first order system, and using a PI controller with adaptive gains, the closed loop performance results in a second order system, which dynamics are set by emplacing its poles to the desired values for the closed loop system. Next subsections describe these two parts of the proposed controller.

6.1 Patient dynamics identification

To obtain the dynamics of the patient, a stochastic recursive least-squares method is employed. It consists of an observer of the discrete system that tries to minimize the following cost function:

$$J = \frac{1}{2}\varepsilon^2(k) \tag{9}$$

where $\varepsilon(k)$ is the residual error between the output of the system, $BIS(k)$, and the observed model, being k the instant of time.

Consider the following first order model as an approximation of the patient dynamics, with $u(k)$ being the drug infusion rate of applied to the patient, and $BIS(k)$ the BIS value obtained:

$$BIS(k) + a_1 BIS(k-1) = b_1 u(k-1) \tag{10}$$

It can be expressed by:

$$y(k) = \phi^T(k)\theta \tag{11}$$

$$\varphi(k) = \begin{bmatrix} -BIS(k-1) & u(k-1) \end{bmatrix}^T \tag{12}$$

$$\theta = \begin{bmatrix} a_1 & b_1 \end{bmatrix}^T \tag{13}$$

In each instant of time, the values of output and input of the system are measured. The iterative process to obtain the best parameters θ that reproduce the performance of the patient is given by the equations:

$$e(k) = y(k) - \phi^T(k)\theta(k-1) \tag{14}$$

$$\theta(k) = \theta(k-1) + W(k)\phi(k)e(k) \tag{15}$$

where:

$$W(k) = \frac{c}{k} \tag{16}$$

being c a constant.

6.2 Pole placement controller

The control law considered for the system is obtained by applying a PI controller. This controller has two gains to adjust: the proportional gain, Kp, and the integer gain, Ki. The discrete version of this controller is given by:

$$G_c(k) = \frac{\alpha + \beta z^{-1}}{1 - z^{-1}} \tag{17}$$

where the relation with the gains is given by:

$$\alpha = K_p + K_i \frac{T}{2} \tag{18}$$

$$\beta = -K_p + K_i \frac{T}{2} \tag{19}$$

being T the sampling time of the system. Considering for the patient the model (10) and for the controller the expression (17), the poles of the closed loop are given by the roots of the following polynomial:

$$D(z^{-1}) = (1 + a_1 z^{-1})(1 - z^{-1}) + b_1 z^{-1}\left(\alpha + \beta z^{-1}\right) \tag{20}$$

Consider the following specification for the closed-loop:

$$Q(z^{-1}) = (1 - q_1 z^{-1})(1 - q_2 z^{-1}) \tag{21}$$

where q_1 and q_2 are the location of the desired poles for the system. It is easy to obtain from (20) and (21) the resulted gains of the PI controller:

$$\alpha = \frac{-1}{b_1}\left(1 + q_1 + q_2 + a_1\right) \tag{22}$$

$$\beta = \frac{1}{b_1}\left(q_1 q_2 + a_1\right) \tag{23}$$

The parameters of the system are obtained in each instant of time form the identification process (15). With the values (22) and (23), the gains of the PI controller are obtained, using (18) and (19), by:

$$K_p = \frac{\alpha - \beta}{2} \tag{24}$$

$$K_i = \frac{\alpha + \beta}{T} \tag{25}$$

6.3 Results with the PI self-adaptive controller

The results shown here correspond to a female of 40 years old, 70 Kg. weight and 170 cm height. The Schnider model presented in section 2 gives an accurate response with the real values obtained for the patient, where the following parameters for (6)-(8) equations are chosen: $BIS_0=95$, $BIS_{max}=8.9$, $EC_{50}=4.94$ µg/ml and $\gamma=2.69$. Initially, the patient is infused with a bolus of 1.45 mg/Kg during 2 minutes in order to carry the patient near the desired value for the degree of hypnosis. The reference value is $BIS_r=50$. After that, the compensated adaptive controller starts controlling the system.

To define the controller, the following assumptions are considered. First, the model for the patient is chosen as:

$$BIS(k) - 0.812BIS(k-1) = -25.389u(k-1) \qquad (26)$$

For the second-order reference model, the poles are located in $0.997 \pm 0.0027j$ that correspond to a system with natural frequency 0.05 rad/sec and delta coefficient 0.75. For initiating the identification algorithm (15), the parameters used in (26) are chosen. c constant in (16) is set to 0.005.

Figure 12 shows the evolution of the BIS and the parameters of the PI controller in this case. As it can be seen, after the application of the initial bolus, the PI controller varies its gains and the patient remains its degree of freedom around the desired value of 50, but with oscillations.

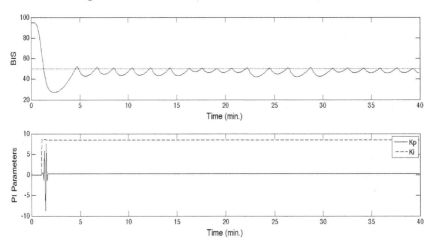

Fig. 12. Results of the PI self-adaptive controller. First graph shows the BIS evolution with respect to BIS_r and second graph are the gains evolution of the PI controller.

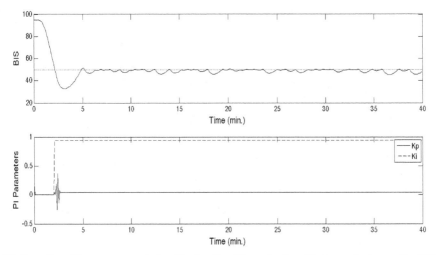

Fig. 13. Results of the compensated self-adaptive PI controller. First graph shows the BIS evolution with respect to BIS_r and second graph are the gains evolution of the PI controller.

To avoid these oscillations in the stationary, the compensation of the time delay by means of a Smith predictor is done in this case. To do that, the time delay considered is 1 minute. Figure 13 shows the results obtained in this case. The oscillations around the objective value are considerably reduced and the performance of the closed loop systems results better than in previous case.

7. Model Predictive Control (MPC)

As an alternative to signal based controllers proposed before, it is shown an algorithm that uses explicitly the model of the patient to compute the drug infusion rate. The objective is to improve the performance of other techniques as those based in PI controllers. Figure 14 shows the structure of the proposed controller. As can be observed, the drug infusion rate is computed as a sum of two terms:

$$u(t) = u_n + \delta u \tag{27}$$

The first term (u_n) is obtained by inverting the model of the patient and is computed to take the BIS variable to the nominal value (BIS$_r$=50, x_n). That is, from the target BIS (BIS$_r$) and using the model of the patient (PK+PD) it can be obtained the infusion rate that leads the BIS signal to the desired value. To do this, the inverse dynamics of the system model is evaluated, assuming that the system is approximated by (1)-(5). Taking matrix notation for this model, it can be expressed by:

$$\dot{x} = Ax + Bu \tag{28}$$

where $x = \begin{bmatrix} C_1 & C_2 & C_3 & C_e \end{bmatrix}^T$.

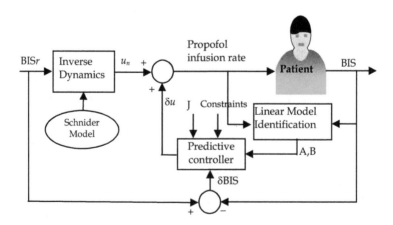

Fig. 14. Structure of the proposed model-based predictive controller.

Assuming that the target state is an equilibrium state $x_n = \begin{bmatrix} C_{1n} & C_{2n} & C_{3n} & C_{en} \end{bmatrix}^T$, the nominal input can be obtained by solving:

$$Ax_n + Bu_n = 0 \tag{29}$$

C_{en} is computed by using the EMAX model (6), (7) and (8):

$$C_{en} = \exp\left(\frac{1}{\gamma} \ln\left(EC_{50}^\gamma \frac{\alpha}{1-\alpha} \right) \right) \tag{30}$$

with:

$$\alpha = \frac{BIS_r - BIS_0}{BIS_{max} - BIS_0} \tag{31}$$

Finally, to compute the nominal input u_n and the nominal state x_n equation (29) is solved to obtain the following solution:

$$x'_n = M^{-1}N \tag{32}$$

where $x'_n = \begin{bmatrix} C_{1n} & C_{2n} & C_{3n} & u_n \end{bmatrix}^T$ and:

$$M = \begin{bmatrix} A_{11} & A_{12} & A_{13} & B_1 \\ A_{21} & A_{12} & A_{23} & B_2 \\ A_{31} & A_{32} & A_{33} & B_3 \\ A_{41} & A_{42} & A_{43} & B_4 \end{bmatrix} \tag{33}$$

$$N = -\begin{bmatrix} A_{14}C_{en} \\ A_{24}C_{en} \\ A_{34}C_{en} \\ A_{44}C_{en} \end{bmatrix} \tag{34}$$

In Fig. 15, a simulation of the BIS in a patient with only this nominal input (u_n) is presented.

As can be observed, the BIS tends to the nominal value (BIS_r=50) if only this input is applied. In practice, several considerations have to be taken into account. The first one is related to the modeling errors in the patient dynamics. In the simulation presented here no modeling errors were considered. In the real implementation, a deviation of the response of the system with respect to this ideal trajectory will be observed. On the other hand, as can be observed, the response exhibits a sluggish behavior that in real practice is undesirable. That is why this action is complemented with an additional term that tries to correct the deviations of the system from the nominal trajectory and also improves the transient response of the BIS curve.

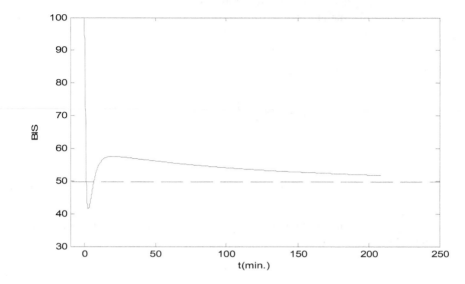

Fig. 15. Simulation of the BIS in a patient applying only the nominal input u_n.

This action is computed considering that the deviations of the BIS from the nominal value can be described by a linear approximation:

$$\delta\dot{x} = A\delta x + B\delta u \tag{35}$$

$$\delta BIS = C\delta x + D\delta u \tag{36}$$

where $\delta x = x - x_n$ and $\delta BIS = BIS - BIS_r$.

Then the control law δu_k can be obtained from an optimization problem (model based predictive controller). The problem can be formulated as obtaining the control law δu_k so that a specified cost function is minimized under a receding horizon strategy. Consider for example the following index:

$$J_k = \sum_{j=1_1}^{N} \gamma(j)\left[w(k+j) - \hat{y}(k+j\,|\,t)\right]^2 + \sum_{j=1}^{NU} \lambda(j)\left[\delta u(k+j-1)\right]^2 \tag{37}$$

where N is the prediction horizon and NU is the control horizon. The problem is to find the sequence δu_{k+j} so that J_k is minimized. Assuming a receding horizon strategy, only the first value of the sequence is applied and the procedure is repeated at $k+1$. In this optimization, constraints can also be included, although the computational complexity is greatly increased.

Figure 16 shows a simulation of this strategy. Initial condition was BIS=39. As can be observed, the response of the system is now much faster than that observed in figure 14 and achieves a very acceptable error quite soon.

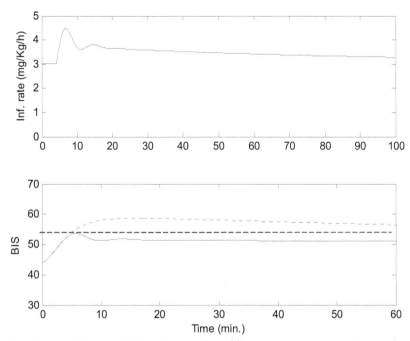

Fig. 16. Simulation of the model-based controller of figure 14 on a patient. Nominal input (dashed line) and nominal+predictive controller (solid line).

8. Conclusion

In this chapter both results on modelling and control of patients under general anaesthesia with propofol is presented. First results presented refer to the synthesis of linear models for use in model-based controllers. The anaesthetic process was segmented into several phases, according to the state of the surgery (consciousness, hypnosis, intubation, incision, etc.). The propofol infusion rate in ml/h was used as the input variable $u(t)$, while the BIS represented the output. Validation of the proposed model was done with real data patients.

For simulation purposes a PK/PD model based on compartmental approaches as obtained. The model was adjusted using information of real data from patients. The obtained model was used to simulate the response of the patients with the different controllers.

Concerning hypnosis control, this chapter presents a review of the state of the art of the closed-loop control of anaesthesia. Then, a description of approaches based on signal feedback and model based controllers are presented.

The chapter proposed an advanced PI controller with several important features. First, an adaptive module is included that adapts the controller to the specific patient behaviour. On the other hand, the controller incorporates a dead-time compensation system that improves notably the performance of the controller. The performance of this compensation is improved by self-adapting the approximation of the patient model used in the Smith Predictor scheme.

The last part of the chapter is devoted to the design of model-based controllers. In particular, a model-based predictive controller is presented that corrects efficiently the transient evolution of the BIS, offering a smooth evolution of this signal to the reference value.

9. Acknowledgment

This work is under the auspicious of the Research Project DPI2010-18278 supported by "Ministerio de Educación y Ciencia" of the Spanish Government.

10. References

Absalom, A.R., Sutcliffe, Kenny, G.N.C., (2002a). *Closed-loop Control of Anesthesia Using Bispectral Index. Performance Assessment in Patients Undergoing Major Orthopedic Surgery under Combined General and Regional Anesthesia.* Anesthesiology; 96. pp.67–73.

Absalom, A.R.; Leslie, K.; Kenny, G.N.C. (2002b). *Closed loop control of sedation for colonoscopy using the Bispectral Index.* Anaesthesia, 57. pp. 690–709.

Absalom, A.R.; Kenny, G.N.C. (2003). *Closed-loop control of propofol anaesthesia using bispectral indexTM: performance assessment in patients receiving computer controlled propofol and manually controlled remifentanil infusions for minor surgery.* British Journal of Anaesthesia 90, No. 6. pp. 737-741.

Åström, K.J.; Wittenmark, B. (1994). *Adaptive Control (2nd ed.).* Addison-Wesley Publishing Company, Inc.

Bressan, N.; Moreira, A.P.; Amorim, P.; Nunes, C.S. (2009). *Target controlled infusion algorithms for anesthesia: Theory vs practical implementation.* Engineering in Medicine and Biology Society, EMBC 2009. Annual International Conference of the IEEE, pp. 6234-6237.

Dumont, G.A.; Martinez, A.; Ansermino, J.M. (2009). *Robust control of depth of anesthesia.* International Journal of Adaptive Control and Signal Processing, No. 23. pp. 435-454.

Furutani, E.; Sawaguchi, Y.; Shirakami, G.; Araki, M.; Fukuda, K. (2005). *A hypnosis control system using a model predictive controller with online identification of individual parameters.* Proceedings of the 2005 IEEE Conference on Control Applications. Toronto, Canada, August, pp. 28-31.

Gil, F.G. (2004). *Sistema de ayuda a la toma de decisiones mediante logica fuzzy en anestesia intravenosa: modelo farmacocinetico/farmacodinamico del propofol.* PhD. Thesis, Universidad de Murcia, España.

Ionescu, C.M.; De Keyser, R.; Torrico, B.C.; De Smet, T.; Struys, M.M.; Normey-Rico, J.E. (2008). *Robust Predictive Control Strategy Applied for Propofol Dosing Using BIS as a Controlled Variable During Anesthesia.* IEEE Transactions On Biomedical Engineering, Vol. 55, No. 9, pp. 2161-2170.

Kazama, T.; Ikeda, K.; Morita, K.; Kikura, M.; Doi, M.; Ikeda, T.; Kurita, T.; Nakajima, Y. (1999). *Comparison of the Effect-site keO s of Propofol for Blood Pressure and EEG Bispectral Index in Elderly and Younger Patients*. Anesthesiology, Vol. 90, No. 6, June, pp. 1517-1527.

Liu, N.; Chazot, T.; Genty, A.; Landais, A.; Restoux, A.; McGee, K.; Laloë, P.A.; Trillat, B.; Barvais, L.; Fischler, M. (2006). *Titration of Propofol for Anesthetic Induction and Maintenance Guided by the Bispectral Index: Closed-loop versus Manual Control. A Prospective, Randomized, Multicenter Study*. Anesthesiology, No. 104. pp. 686–695.

Marsh, B. ; White, M. ; Morton N. ; Kenny, G.N.C. (1991). *Pharmacokinetic model driven infusion of propofol in children*. Br J Anaesth., Vol. 67, pp. 41-48.

Morley, A., Derrick, J., Mainland, P., Lee, B. B. and Short, T. G. (2000). *Closed loop control of anaesthesia: an assessment of the bispectral index as the target of control*. Anaesthesia, 55. pp. 953-959.

Niño J.; De Keyser, R.; Syafiie, S.; Ionescu, C.; Struys, M.M. (2009). *EPSAC-controlled anesthesia with online gain adaptation*. International Journal of Adaptive Control and Signal Processing, No. 23, pp. 455–471.

Sawaguchi, Y.; Purutani, E.; Shirakami, G.; Araki, M.; Fukuda, K. (2003). *A model predictive sedation control system under total intravenous anesthesia*. Proceedings of the IEEE EMBS Asian-Pacific Conference on Biomedical Engineering, pp. 358- 359.

Sakai, T.; Matsuki A.; White P.F.; Giesecke A.H. (2000). *Use of an EEG-bispectral closed-loop delivery system for administering propofol*. Anaesthesiologica Scandinavica, 44. pp. 1007-1010.

Schnider, T.W.; Minto, C.F.; Gambus, P.L.; Anderson, C.; Goodale, D.B.; Shafer S.L.; Youngs, E.J. (1998). *The Influence of method of administration and covariates on the pharmacokinetics of propofol in adult volunteer*. Anesthesiology, Vol. 88, pp. 1170–1182.

Sigl, J.C.; Chamoun, N.G. (1994). *An introduction to bispectral analysis for the electroencephalogram*. Journal of Clinical Monitoring, Vol. 10, No.6, pp. 392-404.

Smith, C. (1972). *Digital Computer Process Control*. Intext Education Publishers. Scranton PA.

Sreenivas, Y.; Samavedham, L.; Rangaiah, G. P. (2008). *Advanced Regulatory Controller for Automatic Control of Anesthesia*. Proceedings of the 17th World Congress of The International Federation of Automatic Control, Seoul, Korea, July, pp. 6-11.

Sreenivas, Y.; Samavedham, L. Rangaiah, G. P. (2009). *Advanced Control Strategies for the Regulation of Hypnosis with Propofol*. Ind. Eng. Chem. Res., No. 48, pp. 3880–3897.

Struys, M.M.; De Smet, T.; Depoorter, B.; Versichelen, L.F.; Mortier, E.P.; Dumortier, F.J.; Shafer, S.L.; Rolly, G. (2000). *Comparison of plasma compartment versus two methods for effect compartment-controlled target controlled infusion for propofol*. Anesthesiology, Vol. 92, No. 2, pp. 399–406.

Struys, M.M.; De Smet, T.; Versichelen, L.F.; Van De Velde, S.; Van den Broecke, R.; Mortier, E.P. (2001). *A Comparison of Closed-loop Controlled Administration of Propofol Using Bispectral Index as the Controlled Variable versus "Standard Practice" Controlled Administration*. Anesthesiology, No. 95. pp. 6–17.

Syafiie, S.; Niño, J.; Ionescu, C.; De Keyser, R. (2009). *NMPC for Propofol Drug Dosing during Anesthesia Induction*. L. Magni et al. (Eds.): Nonlinear Model Predictive Control, LNCIS, No. 384, pp. 501–509.

9

Application of Matrix-Assisted Laser Desorption/Ionization Imaging Mass Spectrometry

Nobuhiro Zaima

Department of Applied Biological Chemistry,
Graduate School of Agriculture, Kinki University
Japan

1. Introduction

The clarification of metabolic dynamics in lesion areas is important. Many approaches, such as high performance liquid chromatography mass spectrometry, gas chromatography mass spectrometry, immunohistochemistry, are used to define disease-related abnormalities. Matrix-assisted laser desorption/ionization imaging mass spectrometry (MALDI-IMS) is attracting attention as a new valuable tool. MALDI-IMS is a two-dimensional MALDI mass spectrometric technique used to visualize the spatial distribution of molecules without extraction, purification, separation, or labeling of biological samples (Cornett et al., 2007; Zaima et al., 2010b). MALDI-IMS has revealed the characteristic distribution of several biomolecules, including proteins (Caprioli et al., 1997; Groseclose et al., 2007; Morita et al., 2010), peptides (Chansela et al., 2011; Stoeckli et al., 2002), amino acids (Goto-Inoue et al., 2010b; Zaima et al., 2010a), lipids (Hayasaka et al., 2009; Murphy et al., 2009; Zaima et al., 2011a), and carbohydrates (Goto-Inoue et al., 2010b), in various tissues. The versatility of MALDI-IMS has opened a new frontier in several fields, such as pharmacology, medicine, agriculture, biology, and pathology. In this review, we describe the methodology and applications of MALDI-IMS for biological samples.

2. MALDI-MS

MALDI-MS was developed from laser desorption/ionization mass spectrometry (LDI-MS). The first LDI-MS experiment for high-mass molecules was reported in 1987 (Tanaka et al., 1987). In this experiment, a powder of cobalt metal in glycerol was used for the observation of ions with a mass to charge (m/z) ratio of 34,000. Soon afterward, MALDI-MS results of serum albumin (67,000 Da) were reported using nicotinic acid as the matrix (Karas & Hillenkamp, 1988). It was reported that MALDI-MS can detect a wide range of molecules ranging from small (m/z <1000) to large molecules (m/z >1,000,000) (Yates, 1998). The schema of MALDI-MS is shown in Figure 1.

In routine MALDI-MS analysis (i.e., non-imaging analysis), the analyte can be mixed with an excess of matrix. On the other hand, molecular imaging of tissue sections using MALDI-IMS requires the tissue surface to be homogeneously covered by a matrix. On-tissue application of matrix results in the *in situ* extraction of molecules from biological tissues. The cocrystal of matrix and analyte molecules in tissue is irradiated with a pulsed laser of appropriate energy, leading to desorption and ionization of the matrix and analyte molecules. The fragmentation of analyte molecules is prevented by the incorporation of the analyte molecules into matrix crystals. The role of the optical absorption of the matrix in the transfer of energy from the laser beam to the analyte molecules is governed by Beer's law, as described previously (Karas et al., 1985). However, the mechanisms underlying the formation of charged matrix and analyte molecules in the MALDI process are not fully understood.

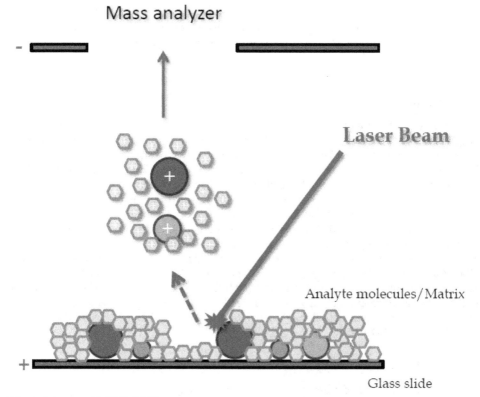

Fig. 1. Schema of MALDI-MS.

The matrix molecules absorb the laser energy and facilitate desorption and ionization of analyte molecules in the tissue. The homogeneous matrix cover is important for MALDI-IMS, because a heterogeneous distribution of matrix results in different ionization efficiencies of analyte molecules based on their location.

3. Methodology of MALDI-IMS

The important experimental steps for visualizing endogenous molecules or administered pharmaceutical agents in tissue using MALDI-IMS are sample preparation (such as fixation, sectioning, and washing), choice of matrix and matrix application, measurement, and data analysis. To obtain meaningful biological images, all steps need to be carefully controlled. In this section, the basic experimental MALDI-IMS procedures are described. The schema of MALDI-IMS is presented in Figure 2.

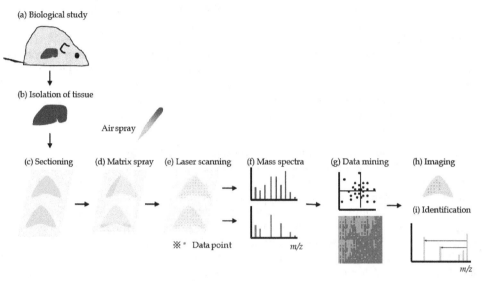

Fig. 2. Schema of MALDI-IMS.

After biological study (a), the tissue of interest should be appropriately isolated (b). A thin section of isolated tissue is mounted on a glass slide (c), coated with matrix (d), and measured by a mass spectrometer (e). The resultant mass spectra (f) can be used for a data mining approach (g). Molecules of interest can be visualized (f) and identified by MS/MS on tissue (f).

3.1 Biological sample preparation

The samples for MALDI-IMS come from a variety of biological sources, including organs, whole animal body dosed with a pharmaceutical compound, or pathological tissues. Optimization of the sample preparation procedure according to the chemical and physical properties of analytes is important. Here, the basic sample preparation steps for MALDI-IMS are described.

3.1.1 Sample condition for MALDI-IMS

Collection and treatment procedures need to be sufficiently fast to prevent rapid tissue degradation, because the sample degradation process starts immediately after the cessation of blood flow. The most preferred sample for MALDI-IMS is a chemically unmodified fresh-frozen one. Fresh-frozen samples can be prepared using dry ice, liquid nitrogen, or liquid nitrogen-chilled isopentane, and can be preserved in a deep freezer until required. The samples should be well sealed to prevent drying during storage, and it is important to ensure that the tissue section morphology is well preserved before MALDI-IMS.

3.1.2 Fixation and embedding

Fixation of samples, such as formalin fixation, is preferably avoided because the protein crosslinking introduced by formalin fixation makes MALDI-IMS analysis difficult. However, many medical samples are routinely formaldehyde-fixed and paraffin-embedded (FFPE) just after dissection. To address this problem, the on-tissue proteolytic digestion method, in which proteins are denatured and digested by enzymes, has been developed (Djidja et al., 2009; Groseclose et al., 2007; Lemaire et al., 2007; Morita et al., 2010). The on-tissue proteolytic digestion method includes a paraffin removal step using xylene and ethanol. In the paraffin removal step, lipophilic molecules are lost; therefore, FFPE samples cannot be used for lipid imaging. When the samples are formaldehyde-fixed without paraffin-embedding, lipid imaging can be performed (Zaima et al., 2011c). However, the detected ion intensities of lipids in formaldehyde-fixed samples are lower than those in fresh-frozen ones are.

Embedding of the tissue samples in supporting material, such as an optimal cutting temperature (OCT) compound, allows the maintenance of tissue morphology and precise sample sectioning. However, supporting materials are often ionized during MALDI-MS analysis and sometimes act as ion suppressors of molecules of interest (Schwartz et al., 2003). Therefore, samples should not be embedded if precise sample sections can be prepared without embedding. When it is difficult to prepare a sample section, the use of carboxymethylcellulose (CMC) or gelatin as embedding material is recommended. Sodium CMC (2%) is reported to be used as an alternative embedding compound that does not interfere with the detection sensitivity of biomolecules in MALDI-IMS analysis (Stoeckli et al., 2006; Zaima et al., 2010a). Chen et al. reported that gelatin provides a cleaner signal background than OCT (Chen et al., 2009). Researchers should ensure compatibility between the supporting material and the biomolecules of interest.

3.1.3 Sectioning

The basic sectioning procedure for MALDI-IMS samples is same as that for pathological examination. Sections for MALDI-IMS can be prepared using a cryostat. The sample stage temperature is typically maintained between -5 and -20°C. To obtain high quality sections from tissues with high fat content (e.g., brain), or atherosclerotic lesions, breast tissue, or lipid storage disease samples lower temperatures are required. In general, 5–20-μm-thick sections are prepared for the analysis of low-molecular-weight molecules. The use of thinner tissue sections (2–5 μm thick) has been recommended for the analysis of high-molecular-weight molecules (range, 3–21 kDa) (Goodwin et al., 2008). Sections are usually thaw-mounted on a stainless steel conductive stage or on commercially available indium-tin oxide (ITO)-coated glass slides. We recommend the use of ITO-coated glass slides because these transparent slides enable microscopic observation of the section after MALDI-IMS. Use of adhesive film is suitable for samples for which thaw-mounted preparation of sections is challenging (e.g., bone or whole-body sections) (Stoeckli et al., 2006; Zaima et al., 2010a). The procedure for sectioning using adhesive film is shown in Figure 3. The prepared section should be immediately dried in a vacuum desiccator to avoid moisture condensation that could cause delocalization of analyte molecules in the tissue. Moisture condensation can be avoided by placing the prepared section in a dry and cold container until return to room temperature.

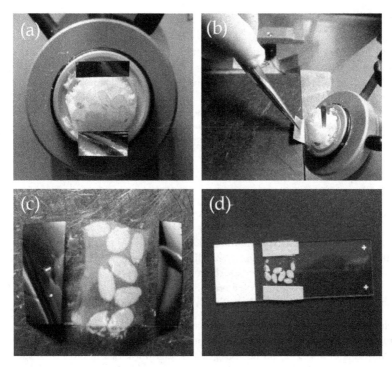

Fig. 3. Procedure for sectioning using adhesive film.

Attachment of adhesive film to the sample block (a). The end of the adhesive film must be anchored with tweezers to prevent adhesion of the film to the sample stage (b). After the sample section is obtained (c), the sample section on the adhesive film is attached to a glass slide (d).

3.1.4 Washing

Washing is required for peptide or protein analysis because their detection is often prevented by large amounts of easily ionized lipid species. Lipid removal simplifies mass spectra in the range of m/z 400–1000; thus, lipid removal enables the detection of low-mass peptides that are usually masked by lipid peaks. The washing method should be optimized for the target imaging molecules. Several washing protocols using organic solvents have been reported (Aerni et al., 2006; Andersson et al., 2008; Groseclose et al., 2007; Lemaire et al., 2006; Schwartz et al., 2003).

Washing is also used for removing the matrix from the tissue section after MALDI-IMS analysis. The matrix can be removed using the solvent that is used for preparing the matrix solution. For example, 2,5-dihydroxybenzoic acid (DHB) can be rapidly removed by methanol. Matrix removal enables the microscopic observation of a tissue section followed by pathological staining, such as hematoxylin and eosin (HE) staining, toluidine blue staining etc.

3.2 Matrix application

The matrix plays a central role in MALDI-MS soft ionization (Karas & Hillenkamp, 1988; Karas & Kruger, 2003). Biomolecules are softly ionized in the cocrystal with the matrix, which absorbs the laser beam energy and protects biomolecules from the disruptive energy. Protonated ion ([M + H]+) or deprotonated ion ([M − H]−) molecules are generally detected. Sodium adduct ion ([M + Na]+) and potassium adduct ion ([M + K]+) are often observed by biological sample analysis. It is very important to choose appropriate matrices for obtaining meaningful biomolecular images. An overview of the matrices used for IMS can also be found in other reviews (Chughtai & Heeren, 2010; Kaletas et al., 2009).

3.2.1 Choice of matrix

The choice of matrix used for MALDI-IMS depends on the mass range and chemical properties of the analytes. Among the many kinds of matrices, sinapinic acid (3,5-dimethoxy-4-hydroxycinnamic acid [SA]) is generally used for high-molecular-weight molecules, such as proteins, while α-cyano-4-hydroxycinnamic acid (CHCA) is often used for medium-molecular-weight molecules, such as peptides. 2,6-dihydroxyacetophenone (DHA), DHB, or 9-aminoacridine (9-AA) is generally used for low-molecular-weight molecules, such as pharmaceutical compounds, lipids, or metabolites (Hattori et al., 2010; Hayasaka et al., 2009; Khatib-Shahidi et al., 2006; Sugiura et al., 2009; Woods & Jackson, 2006).

The development of new matrices is still being reported. We and other research groups recently reported the use of nanoparticles as new matrices (Hayasaka et al., 2010; McLean et al., 2005; Moritake et al., 2009; Su & Tseng, 2007; Sugiura & Setou, 2010). For example, iron oxide nanoparticles enable the visualization of sulfatide and phospholipid distribution (Ageta et al., 2009; Taira et al., 2008), silver nanoparticles can be used for the analysis of fatty acids (Hayasaka et al., 2010), and gold nanoparticles are appropriate for the sensitive detection of glycosphingolipids, such as sulfatides and gangliosides (Goto-Inoue et al., 2010a).

3.2.2 Matrix application

There are various methods for applying the matrix onto the section, such as deposition, spraying, and sublimation. The matrix application method also influences analyte extraction efficiency. Compared to other methods, the deposition of matrix solution using automatic depositing robotic devices, such as a chemical inkjet printer (ChIP-1000; Shimadzu Corporation, Kyoto, Japan), increases signal sensitivity, but decreases spatial resolution (Aerni et al., 2006; Chansela et al., 2011; Morita et al., 2010). The other limitation of the inkjet printer is capillary clogging, which occurs when highly concentrated matrix solutions are used. Spraying is the most frequently used method in MALDI-IMS. Using this method, an entire tissue section can be homogeneously coated with relatively small crystals in a short time without special equipment. For its operation, several instruments, including Thin layer chromatography (TLC) sprayers and artistic airbrushes, are available; we use a metal airbrush with a 0.2-mm nozzle because of its simple and easy-to-handle design. This method requires skillful operation because some airbrush parameters are hand-operated. If there is an excess of matrix solution on the tissue, an inhomogeneous crystal can be formed with analytes that have migrated from their original location; on the other hand, if not enough matrix solution is sprayed and it evaporates without sufficiently moisturizing the tissue section, analytes cannot be adequately extracted from the tissue section. The operation should be performed at a constant room temperature and humidity. Beginners are recommended to practice spraying until homogeneous matrix spraying can be reproducibly achieved. Sublimation is a new method for applying matrix to tissue sections (Hankin et al., 2007). Using this technique, a matrix can be applied uniformly over a large sample plate in a few minutes without solvents. Additionally, previous reports demonstrated that this method increases analyte signal and that the fine microcrystals formed from the condensed vapor reduce the image resolution limitation caused by crystal size (Dekker et al., 2009; Vrkoslav et al., 2010).

3.3 Measurement and data analysis

3.3.1 Measurement

MALDI-IMS should be performed as soon as possible after matrix application, regardless of the coating method. The procedure to obtain a good spectrum in MALDI-IMS is almost the same as that for traditional MALDI-MS; mass range, detector gain, and laser power must be optimized. From the mechanical setting perspective, there are 3 differences between MALDI-MS and MALDI-IMS. The first difference is the above-mentioned matrix application. The second difference is the need for focusing of the laser beam. To obtain meaningful biological images by MALDI-IMS, the laser spot size should be reduced to 10–50 μm. The third difference is that a two-dimensional region must be set for analyses. The scan pitch, which signifies the distance between laser irradiation spots, must be fixed. The limitation of the scan pitch, which decides the spatial resolution of the image, depends on the laser spot size and mechanical movement control of the mass spectrometer sample stage. We have developed a new instrument (Mass Microscope) that can move the sample stage by 1 μm, and in which the finest size of the laser diameter is approximately 10 μm (Harada et al., 2009). The measurement time depends on the number of data spots, the frequency of the laser, the number of shots per spot, and the time required to move the sample stage. For example, when researchers select the region of interest as a 1×1 mm^2 area with a 10-μm scan pitch (10,000 data points), it takes about 1 h to complete the measurement using a mass microscope equipped with a 1000-Hz laser (100 shots/data point).

MALDI-IMS ionizes numerous compounds in a tissue at the same time. Sometimes, we detect multiple molecules with the same m/z value. In such cases, a new imaging technique, "MS/MS imaging," is effective. Using this technique, we can separate each ion derived from their specific fragment ions. Some reports have described the use of MS/MS imaging for IMS of endogenous metabolites and an exogenous drug (Khatib-Shahidi et al., 2006; Porta et al., 2011). Additionally, the combination of ion-mobility separation with MALDI-IMS provides a unique separation dimension to further enhance the capabilities of IMS (Jackson et al., 2007; McLean et al., 2007; Stauber et al., 2010). It can be used to produce images without interference from background ions of similar mass, and this can remove ambiguity from imaging experiments and lead to a more precise localization of the compound of interest.

3.3.2 Data analysis

A large amount of data (a few gigabytes) is obtained from MALDI-IMS; therefore, visualization software packages that can rapidly and efficiently analyze enormous spectra have been developed. BioMap (a free software; Novartis, Basel, Switzerland), FlexImaging

(Bruker Daltonics, Bremen, Germany), and ImageQuest (Thermo Fisher Scientific, CA, USA) are generally used for visualization. For biomarker analysis of the MALDI-IMS dataset, data mining should be used (Hayasaka et al., 2011; Zaima et al., 2011b; Zhang et al., 2004). Data mining software effectively reduce the number of biomarker candidates (Hayasaka et al., 2011; Zhang et al., 2004). We previously reported the use of principal component analysis (PCA) to discover different biomolecules in starvation-induced fatty livers and normal livers (Zaima et al., 2009). Hierarchical clustering was also used to analyze the data obtained from gastric cancer and non-neoplastic mucosa tissue sections (Deininger et al., 2008). Several studies have reported the discovery of biomarkers using MALDI-IMS (Bakry et al., 2011; Ducret et al., 2006; Hong & Zhang, 2011; Solassol et al., 2009; Zaima et al., 2011b).

4. Instruments

The requirement for performing IMS is the availability of an *x-axis-y-axis* moving stage with electronic controls. Most modern MS instruments produced by major MS hardware companies (*i.e.*, Shimadzu, ThermoFisher Scientific, Bruker Daltonics, Applied Biosystems, Waters) can be adapted for MALDI-IMS. Time of flight (TOF) is the most widely used technology. TOF analyzers allow the separation of ionized accelerated molecules according to their m/z ratio. TOF-MS offers suitable performance for MALDI-IMS, namely, good transmission ratio (50–100%), sensitivity, mass range, and repetition rate. However, TOF-MS lacks the capability to perform effective tandem MS experiments. This disadvantage of TOF-MS was overcome with the introduction of hybrid analyzers, such as a combination of quadrupole mass analyzer and TOF (so-called qTOF), combination of quadrupole ion trap (QIT) and TOF (so-called QIT-TOF), combination of ion mobility spectrometry (IMS) and TOF (so-called IMS-TOF), or a combination of two TOF mass spectrometers (so-called TOF-TOF). These combination systems revolutionized the application of TOF-MS systems for structural analysis with tandem MS. In general, the first system is used to select a precursor ion for fragmentation, while the second TOF system is employed for fragment analysis. Other mass analyzers (and their combinations), such as linear ion trap (LIT) (Landgraf et al., 2009; Wiseman et al., 2006; Zaima et al., 2010a), triple quadrupole (QqQ) (Hopfgartner et al., 2009; Porta et al., 2011), and Fourier transform ion cyclotron resonance (FTICR) (Taban et al., 2007), are used for MALDI-IMS. The advantages of commercially available LIT instruments are miniaturization, capability of sample analysis on nonconductive glass slides, MALDI performance at intermediate pressure, and superior performance on multistage MS. The QqQ system allows quantitative analysis and single or multiple reaction monitoring (SRM/MRM). The FTICR system offers very high mass resolving power and high mass measurement accuracy.

5. Applications of MALDI-IMS

5.1 Imaging mass spectrometry-based histopathologic examination

Recently, we applied MALDI-IMS for pathologic examination of atherosclerotic aorta (Fig. 4). We named it imaging mass spectrometry-based histopathologic examination (IbHE) (Zaima et al., 2011c). IbHE revealed the characteristic distribution of biomolecules in smooth muscle cells, lipid-rich regions, and calcified regions of an atherosclerotic lesion obtained from aortic roots of apolipoprotein E (ApoE)-deficient mice. We found that phosphatidylcholine (PC), which contains arachidonic acid (20:4) (m/z 804.5), was distributed in the smooth muscle cells of the atherosclerotic lesion. Cholesterol linoleate (CE

18:2) (*m/z* 671.6) and cholesterol oleate (CE 18:1) were characteristically distributed in lipid-rich regions, and the ion at *m/z* 566.9 was localized in the calcified region. These biomolecules were hardly detected in the normal aortic roots of ApoE-deficient mice. We applied this method to other vascular diseases, such as varicose veins, arteriovenous fistulae, abdominal aortic aneurysm, and triglyceride deposit cardiomyovasculopathy, and observed the characteristic distribution of biomolecules (Tanaka et al., 2010; Tanaka et al., 2011). In the analysis of several vascular diseases with atherosclerotic lesions, we often observed ectopic TG distribution. Although the role of TG in the evolution of atherosclerosis remains unknown, there is a possibility that TG plays an important role in the evolution of some kinds of atherosclerosis, as we previously found that characteristic atherosclerosis accumulated TG in aortic lesions, while the accumulated cholesterol was normal (Hirano et al., 2008). The reexamination of vascular diseases by IbHE may result in new findings, because IbHE can visualize the localization of low-molecular-weight molecules, which are rarely visualized by other techniques. We believe IbHE is of considerable value as a new histopathological examination because IbHE can visualize metabolic abnormalities in disease.

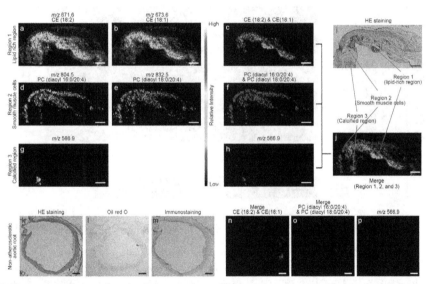

Fig. 4. Representative molecular images of specific ions in a mouse atherosclerotic lesion.

Visualization of biomolecules in atherosclerotic roots (a-j). Scale bar, 100 μm. Specific ion images of region 1 (a and b) and the combined image of *m/z* 671.6 and 673.6 (c). Specific ion images of region 2 (d and e) and the combined image of *m/z* 804.5 and 832.5 (f). Specific ion images of region 3 (g) and the monochrome image of *m/z* 566.9 (h). Comparison of HE staining (i) and the merge images of regions 1, 2, and 3 (j). An image of non-atherosclerotic aortic roots of mice at 12 weeks of age (k-m). Scale bar, 200 μm. HE staining after IMS (k). Oil red O staining (l). Immunostaining of α-actin, which is a marker for smooth muscle cells (m). Merge image of CE (18:2) and CE (18:1) (n). Merge image of PC (diacyl 16:0/20:4) and PC (diacyl 18:0/20:4) (o). Ion image of *m/z* 566.9 (p). "Reprinted from Atherosclerosis, 217. 2, Zaima et al., Imaging mass spectrometry-based histopathologic examination of atherosclerotic lesions, 430., Copyright (2011), with permission from Elsevier."

5.2 IMS for exogenous drugs

MALDI-IMS is a powerful tool for visualizing the distribution of exogenous drugs and their metabolites. Porta et al. reported the visualization of the distribution of cocaine and its metabolites down to a concentration of 5 ng/mg in intact single hair samples from chronic users (Porta et al., 2011) (Fig. 5).

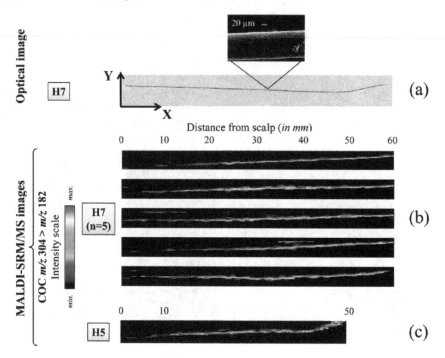

Fig. 5. Imaging of cocaine in hair samples H7 and H5. (H7 and H5 are sample names used in this article)

Optical image of hair sample H7 (a). MALDI-SRM/MS image based on the SRM trace of COC (m/z 305 > m/z 182) for five replicates of single hair samples from individual H7 (b) and single hair analysis from individual H5 (c). The quantitative results from LC-SRM/MS routine analysis were as follows: 130 ng/mg (H7, whole sample); 4.9 ng/mg (H5, segment 0–10 mm), and 8.5 ng/mg (H5, segment 10–50 mm). SRM; selected reaction monitoring. "Reprinted with permission from Porta et al., 2011. Copyright 2011 American Chemical Society."

MALDI-IMS is also applicable to pharmacokinetic analysis. As a Food and Drug Administration (FDA)-mandated pharmacokinetic test, whole-body autoradiography (WBA) is widely performed to determine spatial and quantitative information about a drug compound. Although much information can be acquired by WBA, it has several limitations. First, WBA requires the compound of interest to be radioactively labeled. Furthermore, the detected signal does not distinguish between the original radiolabeled compound and its metabolites that have retained the radiolabel. To complement the disadvantage of WBA, MALDI-IMS and WBA have recently been used together. The combination of MALDI-IMS and

WBA makes it possible to obtain more reliable data for absorption, distribution, metabolism, and excretion of drugs (Atkinson et al., 2007; Caprioli et al., 2008; Clench et al., 2008; Stoeckli et al., 2006). The application of MALDI-IMS to pharmacokinetics in a whole-body mouse section was first reported by Rohner et al. in 2005 (Rohner et al., 2005). In this study, they showed a good correlation between WBA and MALDI-IMS data. Figure 5 shows the simultaneous visualization of drug and metabolites in a whole-rat sagittal tissue section (Khatib-Shahidi et al., 2006). Khatib-Shahidi et al. visualized the temporal distribution of dosed olanzapine (brand name Zyprexa) (8 mg/kg) and its metabolites. In this study, MALDI-IMS was further extended to detect proteins from organs present in a whole-body section.

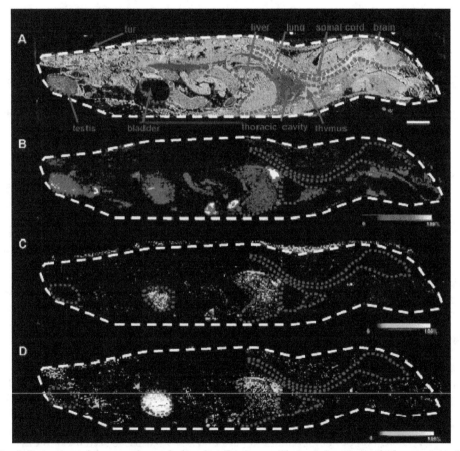

Fig. 6. Detection of drug and metabolite distribution at 6 h post-dose in a whole-rat sagittal tissue section by a single IMS analysis.

Optical images of a 6 h post-olanzapine (OLZ)-dosed rat tissue section across 4 gold MALDI target plates (A). Organs are outlined in red. MS/MS ion image of OLZ (m/z 256) (B). MS/MS ion image of N-desmethyl metabolite (m/z 256) (C). MS/MS ion image of 2-hydroxymethyl metabolite (m/z 272) (D). Scale bar, 1 cm. "Reprinted with permission from Khatib-Shahidi et al., 2006. Copyright 2006 American Chemical Society."

6. Conclusions

MALDI-IMS can be applied to pathological examinations leading to the discovery of potential targets for new drugs, and for the distributional analysis of exogenous drugs in animal and human tissues. We recently used MALDI-IMS in the discovery of metabolites that have pharmacological effects on natural resources. MALDI-IMS will become an essential tool for molecular imaging in pharmacology in the near future.

7. Acknowledgement

This work was supported by the Program for Promotion of Basic and Applied Research for Innovations in Bio-oriented Industry (BRAIN).

8. References

Aerni, H. R., Cornett, D. S., & Caprioli, R. M. (2006). Automated acoustic matrix deposition for MALDI sample preparation. *Anal Chem* 78.3, pp.827-34

Ageta, H., Asai, S., Sugiura, Y., Goto-Inoue, N., Zaima, N., & Setou, M. (2009). Layer-specific sulfatide localization in rat hippocampus middle molecular layer is revealed by nanoparticle-assisted laser desorption/ionization imaging mass spectrometry. *Med Mol Morphol* 42.1, pp.16-23

Andersson, M., Groseclose, M. R., Deutch, A. Y., & Caprioli, R. M. (2008). Imaging mass spectrometry of proteins and peptides: 3D volume reconstruction. *Nat Methods* 5.1, pp.101-108

Atkinson, S. J., Loadman, P. M., Sutton, C., Patterson, L. H., & Clench, M. R. (2007). Examination of the distribution of the bioreductive drug AQ4N and its active metabolite AQ4 in solid tumours by imaging matrix-assisted laser desorption/ionisation mass spectrometry. *Rapid Commun Mass Spectrom* 21.7, pp.1271-6

Bakry, R., Rainer, M., Huck, C. W., & Bonn, G. K. (2011). Protein profiling for cancer biomarker discovery using matrix-assisted laser desorption/ionization time-of-flight mass spectrometry and infrared imaging: A review. *Analytica Chimica Acta* 690.1, pp.26-34

Caprioli, R. M., Cornett, D. S., & Frappier, S. L. (2008). MALDI-FTICR imaging mass spectrometry of drugs and metabolites in tissue. *Analytical Chemistry* 80.14, pp.5648-5653

Caprioli, R. M., Farmer, T. B., & Gile, J. (1997). Molecular imaging of biological samples: localization of peptides and proteins using MALDI-TOF MS. *Anal Chem* 69.23, pp.4751-60

Chansela, P., Goto-Inoue, N., Zaima, N., Sroyraya, M., Sobhon, P., & Setou, M. (2011). Visualization of neuropeptides in paraffin-embedded tissue sections of the central nervous system in the decapod crustacean, Penaeus monodon, by imaging mass spectrometry. *Peptides*

Chen, R., Hui, L., Sturm, R. M., & Li, L. (2009). Three dimensional mapping of neuropeptides and lipids in crustacean brain by mass spectral imaging. *J Am Soc Mass Spectrom* 20.6, pp.1068-77

Chughtai, K., & Heeren, R. M. (2010). Mass spectrometric imaging for biomedical tissue analysis. *Chem Rev* 110.5, pp.3237-77

Clench, M. R., Trim, P. J., Henson, C. M., Avery, J. L., McEwen, A., Snel, M. F., Claude, E., Marshall, P. S., West, A., & Princivalle, A. P. (2008). Matrix-Assisted Laser Desorption/Ionization-Ion Mobility Separation-Mass Spectrometry Imaging of Vinblastine in Whole Body Tissue Sections. *Analytical Chemistry* 80.22, pp.8628-8634

Cornett, D. S., Reyzer, M. L., Chaurand, P., & Caprioli, R. M. (2007). MALDI imaging mass spectrometry: molecular snapshots of biochemical systems. *Nat Methods* 4.10, pp.828-833

Deininger, S. O., Ebert, M. P., Futterer, A., Gerhard, M., & Rocken, C. (2008). MALDI Imaging Combined with Hierarchical Clustering as a New Tool for the Interpretation of Complex Human Cancers. *J Proteome Res* 7.12, pp.5230-5236

Dekker, L. J., van Kampen, J. J., Reedijk, M. L., Burgers, P. C., Gruters, R. A., Osterhaus, A. D., & Luider, T. M. (2009). A mass spectrometry based imaging method developed for the intracellular detection of HIV protease inhibitors. *Rapid Commun Mass Spectrom* 23.8, pp.1183-8

Djidja, M. C., Francese, S., Loadman, P. M., Sutton, C. W., Scriven, P., Claude, E., Snel, M. F., Franck, J., Salzet, M., & Clench, M. R. (2009). Detergent addition to tryptic digests and ion mobility separation prior to MS/MS improves peptide yield and protein identification for in situ proteomic investigation of frozen and formalin-fixed paraffin-embedded adenocarcinoma tissue sections. *Proteomics* 9.10, pp.2750-63

Ducret, A., Meistermann, H., Norris, J. L., Aerni, H. R., Cornett, D. S., Friedlein, A., Erskine, A. R., Augustin, A., Mudry, M. C. D., Ruepp, S., Suter, L., Langen, H., & Caprioli, R. M. (2006). Biomarker discovery by imaging mass spectrometry - Transthyretin is a biomarker for gentamicin-induced nephrotoxicity in rat. *Molecular & Cellular Proteomics* 5.10, pp.1876-1886

Goodwin, R. J., Pennington, S. R., & Pitt, A. R. (2008). Protein and peptides in pictures: imaging with MALDI mass spectrometry. *Proteomics* 8.18, pp.3785-800

Goto-Inoue, N., Hayasaka, T., Zaima, N., Kashiwagi, Y., Yamamoto, M., Nakamoto, M., & Setou, M. (2010a). The detection of glycosphingolipids in brain tissue sections by imaging mass spectrometry using gold nanoparticles. *J Am Soc Mass Spectrom* 21.11, pp.1940-3

Goto-Inoue, N., Setou, M., & Zaima, N. (2010b). Visualization of spatial distribution of gamma-aminobutyric acid in eggplant (Solanum melongena) by matrix-assisted laser desorption/ionization imaging mass spectrometry. *Anal Sci* 26.7, pp.821-5

Groseclose, M. R., Andersson, M., Hardesty, W. M., & Caprioli, R. M. (2007). Identification of proteins directly from tissue: in situ tryptic digestions coupled with imaging mass spectrometry. *J Mass Spectrom* 42.2, pp.254-62

Hankin, J. A., Barkley, R. M., & Murphy, R. C. (2007). Sublimation as a method of matrix application for mass spectrometric imaging. *J Am Soc Mass Spectrom* 18.9, pp.1646-52

Harada, T., Yuba-Kubo, A., Sugiura, Y., Zaima, N., Hayasaka, T., Goto-Inoue, N., Wakui, M., Suematsu, M., Takeshita, K., Ogawa, K., Yoshida, Y., & Setou, M. (2009). Visualization of volatile substances in different organelles with an atmospheric-pressure mass microscope. *Anal Chem* 81.21, pp.9153-7

Hattori, K., Kajimura, M., Hishiki, T., Nakanishi, T., Kubo, A., Nagahata, Y., Ohmura, M., Yachie-Kinoshita, A., Matsuura, T., Morikawa, T., Nakamura, T., Setou, M., & Suematsu, M. (2010). Paradoxical ATP Elevation in Ischemic Penumbra Revealed by Quantitative Imaging Mass Spectrometry. *Antioxid Redox Signal*

Hayasaka, T., Goto-Inoue, N., Ushijima, M., Yao, I., Yuba-Kubo, A., Wakui, M., Kajihara, S., Matsuura, M., & Setou, M. (2011). Development of imaging mass spectrometry (IMS) dataset extractor software, IMS convolution. *Anal Bioanal Chem* 401.1, pp.183-93

Hayasaka, T., Goto-Inoue, N., Zaima, N., Kimura, Y., & Setou, M. (2009). Organ-specific distributions of lysophosphatidylcholine and triacylglycerol in mouse embryo. *Lipids* 44.9, pp.837-48

Hayasaka, T., Goto-Inoue, N., Zaima, N., Shrivas, K., Kashiwagi, Y., Yamamoto, M., Nakamoto, M., & Setou, M. (2010). Imaging mass spectrometry with silver nanoparticles reveals the distribution of fatty acids in mouse retinal sections. *J Am Soc Mass Spectrom* 21.8, pp.1446-54

Hirano, K., Ikeda, Y., Zaima, N., Sakata, Y., & Matsumiya, G. (2008). Triglyceride deposit cardiomyovasculopathy. *N Engl J Med* 359.22, pp.2396-8

Hong, D., & Zhang, F. Q. (2011). Elastic net-based framework for imaging mass spectrometry data biomarker selection and classification. *Statistics in Medicine* 30.7, pp.753-768

Hopfgartner, G., Varesio, E., & Stoeckli, M. (2009). Matrix-assisted laser desorption/ionization mass spectrometric imaging of complete rat sections using a triple quadrupole linear ion trap. *Rapid Commun Mass Spectrom* 23.6, pp.733-6

Jackson, S. N., Ugarov, M., Egan, T., Post, J. D., Langlais, D., Albert Schultz, J., & Woods, A. S. (2007). MALDI-ion mobility-TOFMS imaging of lipids in rat brain tissue. *J Mass Spectrom* 42.8, pp.1093-8

Kaletas, B. K., van der Wiel, I. M., Stauber, J., Guzel, C., Kros, J. M., Luider, T. M., & Heeren, R. M. (2009). Sample preparation issues for tissue imaging by imaging MS. *Proteomics* 9.10, pp.2622-33

Karas, M., Bachmann, D., & Hillenkamp, F. (1985). Influence of the Wavelength in High-Irradiance Ultraviolet-Laser Desorption Mass-Spectrometry of Organic-Molecules. *Analytical Chemistry* 57.14, pp.2935-2939

Karas, M., & Hillenkamp, F. (1988). Laser desorption ionization of proteins with molecular masses exceeding 10,000 daltons. *Anal Chem* 60.20, pp.2299-301

Karas, M., & Kruger, R. (2003). Ion formation in MALDI: the cluster ionization mechanism. *Chem Rev* 103.2, pp.427-40

Khatib-Shahidi, S., Andersson, M., Herman, J. L., Gillespie, T. A., & Caprioli, R. M. (2006). Direct molecular analysis of whole-body animal tissue sections by imaging MALDI mass spectrometry. *Anal Chem* 78.18, pp.6448-56

Landgraf, R. R., Conaway, M. C. P., Garrett, T. J., Stacpoole, P. W., & Yost, R. A. (2009). Imaging of Lipids in Spinal Cord Using Intermediate Pressure Matrix-Assisted Laser Desorption-Linear Ion Trap/Orbitrap MS. *Anal Chem* 81.20, pp.8488-8495

Lemaire, R., Menguellet, S. A., Stauber, J., Marchaudon, V., Lucot, J. P., Collinet, P., Farine, M. O., Vinatier, D., Day, R., Ducoroy, P., Salzet, M., & Fournier, I. (2007). Specific MALDI imaging and profiling for biomarker hunting and validation: fragment of the 11S proteasome activator complex, Reg alpha fragment, is a new potential ovary cancer biomarker. *J Proteome Res* 6.11, pp.4127-34

Lemaire, R., Wisztorski, M., Desmons, A., Tabet, J. C., Day, R., Salzet, M., & Fournier, I. (2006). MALDI-MS direct tissue analysis of proteins: Improving signal sensitivity using organic treatments. *Anal Chem* 78.20, pp.7145-53

McLean, J. A., Ridenour, W. B., & Caprioli, R. M. (2007). Profiling and imaging of tissues by imaging ion mobility-mass spectrometry. *J Mass Spectrom* 42.8, pp.1099-105

McLean, J. A., Stumpo, K. A., & Russell, D. H. (2005). Size-selected (2-10 nm) gold nanoparticles for matrix assisted laser desorption ionization of peptides. *J Am Chem Soc* 127.15, pp.5304-5

Morita, Y., Ikegami, K., Goto-Inoue, N., Hayasaka, T., Zaima, N., Tanaka, H., Uehara, T., Setoguchi, T., Sakaguchi, T., Igarashi, H., Sugimura, H., Setou, M., & Konno, H. (2010). Imaging mass spectrometry of gastric carcinoma in formalin-fixed paraffin-embedded tissue microarray. *Cancer Sci* 101.1, pp.267-73

Moritake, S., Taira, S., Sugiura, Y., Setou, M., & Ichiyanagi, Y. (2009). Magnetic nanoparticle-based mass spectrometry for the detection of biomolecules in cultured cells. *J Nanosci Nanotechnol* 9.1, pp.169-76

Murphy, R. C., Hankin, J. A., & Barkley, R. M. (2009). Imaging of lipid species by MALDI mass spectrometry. *J Lipid Res* 50 Suppl. pp.S317-22

Porta, T., Grivet, C., Kraemer, T., Varesio, E., & Hopfgartner, G. (2011). Single hair cocaine consumption monitoring by mass spectrometric imaging. *Anal Chem* 83.11, pp.4266-72

Rohner, T. C., Staab, D., & Stoeckli, M. (2005). MALDI mass spectrometric imaging of biological tissue sections. *Mech Ageing Dev* 126.1, pp.177-85

Schwartz, S. A., Reyzer, M. L., & Caprioli, R. M. (2003). Direct tissue analysis using matrix-assisted laser desorption/ionization mass spectrometry: practical aspects of sample preparation. *J Mass Spectrom* 38.7, pp.699-708

Solassol, J., Mange, A., Chaurand, P., Perrochia, H., Roger, P., & Caprioli, R. M. (2009). Liquid Chromatography-Tandem and MALDI Imaging Mass Spectrometry Analyses of RCL2/CS100-Fixed, Paraffin-Embedded Tissues: Proteomics Evaluation of an Alternate Fixative for Biomarker Discovery. *Journal of Proteome Research* 8.12, pp.5619-5628

Stauber, J., MacAleese, L., Franck, J., Claude, E., Snel, M., Kaletas, B. K., Wiel, I. M., Wisztorski, M., Fournier, I., & Heeren, R. M. (2010). On-tissue protein identification and imaging by MALDI-ion mobility mass spectrometry. *J Am Soc Mass Spectrom* 21.3, pp.338-47

Stoeckli, M., Staab, D., & Schweitzer, A. (2006). Compound and metabolite distribution measured by MALDI mass spectrometric imaging in whole-body tissue sections. *Int J Mass Spectrom* 260.2-3, pp.195-202

Stoeckli, M., Staab, D., Staufenbiel, M., Wiederhold, K. H., & Signor, L. (2002). Molecular imaging of amyloid beta peptides in mouse brain sections using mass spectrometry. *Anal Biochem* 311.1, pp.33-9

Su, C. L., & Tseng, W. L. (2007). Gold nanoparticles as assisted matrix for determining neutral small carbohydrates through laser desorption/ionization time-of-flight mass spectrometry. *Anal Chem* 79.4, pp.1626-33

Sugiura, Y., Konishi, Y., Zaima, N., Kajihara, S., Nakanishi, H., Taguchi, R., & Setou, M. (2009). Visualization of the cell-selective distribution of PUFA-containing phosphatidylcholines in mouse brain by imaging mass spectrometry. *J Lipid Res* 50.9, pp.1776-88

Sugiura, Y., & Setou, M. (2010). Matrix-assisted laser desorption/ionization and nanoparticle-based imaging mass spectrometry for small metabolites: a practical protocol. *Methods Mol Biol* 656. pp.173-95

Taban, I. M., Altelaar, A. F. M., Van der Burgt, Y. E. M., McDonnell, L. A., Heeren, R. M. A., Fuchser, J., & Baykut, G. (2007). Imaging of peptides in the rat brain using MALDI-FTICR mass spectrometry. *J Am Soc Mass Spectrom* 18.1, pp.145-151

Taira, S., Sugiura, Y., Moritake, S., Shimma, S., Ichiyanagi, Y., & Setou, M. (2008). Nanoparticle-assisted laser desorption/ionization based mass imaging with cellular resolution. *Anal Chem* 80.12, pp.4761-6

Tanaka, H., Zaima, N., Yamamoto, N., Sagara, D., Suzuki, M., Nishiyama, M., Mano, Y., Sano, M., Hayasaka, T., Goto-Inoue, N., Sasaki, T., Konno, H., Unno, N., & Setou, M. (2010). Imaging mass spectrometry reveals unique lipid distribution in primary varicose veins. *Eur J Vasc Endovasc Surg* 40.5, pp.657-63

Tanaka, H., Zaima, N., Yamamoto, N., Suzuki, M., Mano, Y., Konno, H., Unno, N., & Setou, M. (2011). Distribution of phospholipid molecular species in autogenous access grafts for hemodialysis analyzed using imaging mass spectrometry. *Anal Bioanal Chem* 400.7, pp.1873-80

Tanaka, K., Ido, Y., Akita, S., Yoshida, Y., & Yoshida, T. (1987). Detection of High Mass Molecules by Laser Desorption Time-Of-Flight Mass Spectrometry. *Proc. Japan-China Joint Symp. Mass Spectrom.*, pp.185

Vrkoslav, V., Muck, A., Cvacka, J., & Svatos, A. (2010). MALDI imaging of neutral cuticular lipids in insects and plants. *J Am Soc Mass Spectrom* 21.2, pp.220-31

Wiseman, J. M., Ifa, D. R., Song, Q., & Cooks, R. G. (2006). Tissue imaging at atmospheric pressure using desorption electrospray ionization (DESI) mass spectrometry. *Angew Chem Int Ed Engl* 45.43, pp.7188-92

Woods, A. S., & Jackson, S. N. (2006). Brain tissue lipidomics: direct probing using matrix-assisted laser desorption/ionization mass spectrometry. *AAPS J* 8.2, pp.E391-5

Yates, J. R., 3rd (1998). Mass spectrometry and the age of the proteome. *J Mass Spectrom* 33.1, pp.1-19

Zaima, N., Goto-Inoue, N., Adachi, K., & Setou, M. (2011a). Selective analysis of lipids by thin-layer chromatography blot matrix-assisted laser desorption/ionization imaging mass spectrometry. *J Oleo Sci* 60.2, pp.93-8

Zaima, N., Goto-Inoue, N., Hayasaka, T., Enomoto, H., & Setou, M. (2011b). Authenticity assessment of beef origin by principal component analysis of matrix-assisted laser desorption/ionization mass spectrometric data. *Anal Bioanal Chem* 400.7, pp.1865-71

Zaima, N., Goto-Inoue, N., Hayasaka, T., & Setou, M. (2010a). Application of imaging mass spectrometry for the analysis of Oryza sativa rice. *Rapid Commun Mass Spectrom* 24.18, pp.2723-9

Zaima, N., Hayasaka, T., Goto-Inoue, N., & Setou, M. (2010b). Matrix-assisted laser desorption/ionization imaging mass spectrometry. *Int J Mol Sci* 11.12, pp.5040-55

Zaima, N., Matsuyama, Y., & Setou, M. (2009). Principal component analysis of direct matrix-assisted laser desorption/ionization mass spectrometric data related to metabolites of fatty liver. *J Oleo Sci* 58.5, pp.267-73

Zaima, N., Sasaki, T., Tanaka, H., Cheng, X. W., Onoue, K., Hayasaka, T., Goto-Inoue, N., Enomoto, H., Unno, N., Kuzuya, M., & Setou, M. (2011c). Imaging mass spectrometry-based histopathologic examination of atherosclerotic lesions. *Atherosclerosis* 217.2, pp.427-32

Zhang, X., Leung, S. M., Morris, C. R., & Shigenaga, M. K. (2004). Evaluation of a novel, integrated approach using functionalized magnetic beads, bench-top MALDI-TOF-MS with prestructured sample supports, and pattern recognition software for profiling potential biomarkers in human plasma. *J Biomol Tech* 15.3, pp.167-75

Permissions

The contributors of this book come from diverse backgrounds, making this book a truly international effort. This book will bring forth new frontiers with its revolutionizing research information and detailed analysis of the nascent developments around the world.

We would like to thank Luca Gallelli, for lending his expertise to make the book truly unique. He has played a crucial role in the development of this book. Without his invaluable contribution this book wouldn't have been possible. He has made vital efforts to compile up to date information on the varied aspects of this subject to make this book a valuable addition to the collection of many professionals and students.

This book was conceptualized with the vision of imparting up-to-date information and advanced data in this field. To ensure the same, a matchless editorial board was set up. Every individual on the board went through rigorous rounds of assessment to prove their worth. After which they invested a large part of their time researching and compiling the most relevant data for our readers. Conferences and sessions were held from time to time between the editorial board and the contributing authors to present the data in the most comprehensible form. The editorial team has worked tirelessly to provide valuable and valid information to help people across the globe.

Every chapter published in this book has been scrutinized by our experts. Their significance has been extensively debated. The topics covered herein carry significant findings which will fuel the growth of the discipline. They may even be implemented as practical applications or may be referred to as a beginning point for another development. Chapters in this book were first published by InTech; hereby published with permission under the Creative Commons Attribution License or equivalent.

The editorial board has been involved in producing this book since its inception. They have spent rigorous hours researching and exploring the diverse topics which have resulted in the successful publishing of this book. They have passed on their knowledge of decades through this book. To expedite this challenging task, the publisher supported the team at every step. A small team of assistant editors was also appointed to further simplify the editing procedure and attain best results for the readers.

Our editorial team has been hand-picked from every corner of the world. Their multi-ethnicity adds dynamic inputs to the discussions which result in innovative outcomes. These outcomes are then further discussed with the researchers and contributors who give their valuable feedback and opinion regarding the same. The feedback is then collaborated with the researches and they are edited in a comprehensive manner to aid the understanding of the subject.

Apart from the editorial board, the designing team has also invested a significant amount of their time in understanding the subject and creating the most relevant covers. They scrutinized every image to scout for the most suitable representation of the subject and create an appropriate cover for the book.

The publishing team has been involved in this book since its early stages. They were actively engaged in every process, be it collecting the data, connecting with the contributors or procuring relevant information. The team has been an ardent support to the editorial, designing and production team. Their endless efforts to recruit the best for this project, has resulted in the accomplishment of this book. They are a veteran in the field of academics and their pool of knowledge is as vast as their experience in printing. Their expertise and guidance has proved useful at every step. Their uncompromising quality standards have made this book an exceptional effort. Their encouragement from time to time has been an inspiration for everyone.

The publisher and the editorial board hope that this book will prove to be a valuable piece of knowledge for researchers, students, practitioners and scholars across the globe.

List of Contributors

Pedro J. Camello, Cristina Camello-Almaraz and Maria J. Pozo
Department of Physiology, University of Extremadura, Cáceres, Spain

Adela Voican
Universitatea de Medicina din Craiova (AV, LN), Romania Univ Paris-Sud, Faculté de Médecine Paris-Sud UMR-S693, Le Kremlin Bicêtre, France

Bruno Francou, Liliana Novac, Nathalie Chabbert-Buffet, Marianne Canonico, Geri Meduri, Marc Lombes, Pierre-Yves Scarabin, Jacques Young, Anne Guiochon-Mantel and Jérôme Bouligand
Univ Paris-Sud, France

Bill J. Duke
Child Psychopharmacology Institute, USA

Carlos Olmeda-Gómez, Ma-Antonia Ovalle-Perandones and Antonio Perianes-Rodríguez
Carlos III University of Madrid, Spain

Alberto Lázaro, Sonia Camaño, Blanca Humanes and Alberto Tejedor
Renal Physiopathology Laboratory, Department of Nephrology, Hospital General Universitario Gregorio Marañón, Madrid, Spain

John M. Corkery, Fabrizio Schifano and A. Hamid Ghodse
University of Hertfordshire & St George's, University of London, United Kingdom

José Juan Escobar-Chávez
Unidad de Investigación Multidisciplinaria, Laboratorio 12: Materiales Nanoestructurados y Sistemas Transdérmicos, México Facultad de Estudios Superiores Cuautitlán-Universidad, Nacional Autónoma de México, Carretera Cuautitlán–Teoloyucan, San Sebastián Xhala, Cuautitlán Izcalli, Estado de México, México

Isabel Marlen Rodríguez-Cruz and Clara Luisa Domínguez-Delgado
Departamento de Ingeniería y Tecnología, Sección de Tecnología Farmacéutica, Facultad de Estudios Superiores Cuautitlán-Universidad Nacional Autónoma de México, Cuautitlán Izcalli, Estado de México, México

Santiago Torres, Juan A. Méndez, Héctor Reboso, José A. Reboso and Ana León
Universidad de La Laguna, Spain

Nobuhiro Zaima
Department of Applied Biological Chemistry, Graduate School of Agriculture, Kinki University, Japan

Printed in the USA
CPSIA information can be obtained
at www.ICGtesting.com
JSHW011420221024
72173JS00004B/611